Year Book of
MEDICINE
2020

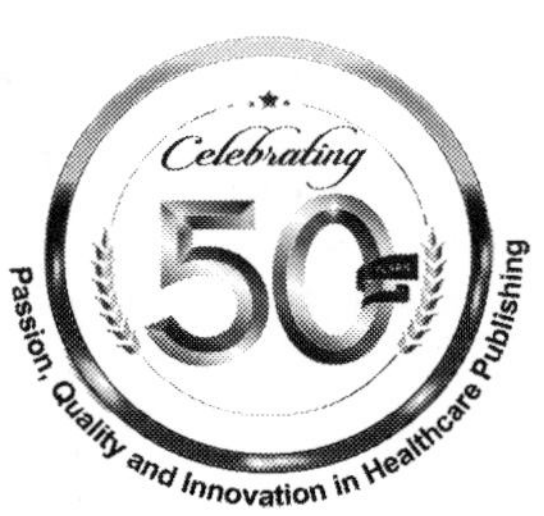

Year Book of
MEDICINE
2020

Chief Editor

Gurpreet S Wander MD DM

Professor and Head
Department of Cardiology
Hero DMC Heart Institute
Dayanand Medical College and Hospital
Ludhiana, Punjab, India

Section Editors

Siddharth N Shah

Surinder K Jindal

VK Bahl

Ajay Kumar

Vivekanand Jha

R Rajasekar

Rohini Handa

Jyotirmoy Pal

Gagandeep Singh

Foreword

Siddharth N Shah

YP Munjal

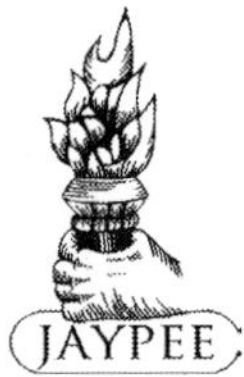

JAYPEE BROTHERS MEDICAL PUBLISHERS
The Health Sciences Publisher
New Delhi | London

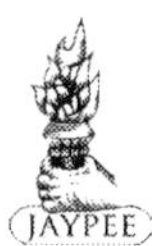 **Jaypee Brothers Medical Publishers (P) Ltd**

Headquarter

Jaypee Brothers Medical Publishers (P) Ltd
4838/24, Ansari Road, Daryaganj
New Delhi 110 002, India
Phone: +91-11-43574357
Fax: +91-11-43574314
Email: jaypee@jaypeebrothers.com

Overseas Office

J.P. Medical Ltd
83 Victoria Street, London
SW1H 0HW (UK)
Phone: +44 20 3170 8910
Fax: +44 (0)20 3008 6180
Email: info@jpmedpub.com

Website: www.jaypeebrothers.com
Website: www.jaypeedigital.com

Year Book of Medicine 2020

First Edition: **2020**

ISBN: 978-93-90020-68-3

Printed at Replika Press Pvt. Ltd.

Dedication

This book is dedicated to

Our parents; who taught us how to read

Our teachers; who taught us how to understand what we read

Our patients; who taught us how to use the knowledge we
acquire by reading, for the benefit of humanity.

CONTRIBUTORS

Chief Editor

Gurpreet S Wander MD DM
Professor and Head
Department of Cardiology
Hero DMC Heart Institute
Dayanand Medical College and Hospital
Ludhiana, Punjab, India

Section Editors

Siddharth N Shah MD FACP (Hon)
FRCP (Edin)
PG Teacher, University of Mumbai
Consultant, Bhatia, SL Raheja
Saifee, and Sir HN Reliance Hospitals
Mumbai, Maharashtra, India

Surinder K Jindal MD
Medical Director
Jindal Clinics
Emeritus-Professor
Postgraduate Institute of Medical
Education and Research
Chandigarh, India

VK Bahl MD DM
Principal Director
Max Health Care
Ex-Dean and Ex-Head
Department of Cardiology
All India Institute of Medical
Sciences
New Delhi, India

Ajay Kumar MD DM
Chairman
BLK Liver and Digestive Diseases
Institute
New Delhi, India

Vivekanand Jha MD DM
Executive Director
George Institute for Global Health
India, New Delhi, India
Chair of Global Kidney Health
Imperial College
London, United Kingdom

R Rajasekar MD
Senior Consultant Physician and
Diabetologist
Heart and
Diabetes Therapy Centre
Kumbakonam, Tamil Nadu, India

Rohini Handa MD DNB
Senior Consultant
Department of Rheumatology
Apollo Indraprastha Hospitals
New Delhi, India

Jyotirmoy Pal MD
Professor
Department of Medicine
RG Kar Medical College
Kolkata, West Bengal, India

Gagandeep Singh MD DM
Professor and Head
Department of Neurology
Dayanand Medical College
and Hospital
Ludhiana, Punjab, India

Associate Editors

Ragini Maheshwari MBBS
Consulting Diabetologist
Rohit Diabetes Centre and
Seven Hills Hospital
Mumbai, Maharashtra, India

Naveen Mittal MD DM
Professor
Department of Endocrinology
Dayanand Medical College and
Hospital
Ludhiana, Punjab, India

Aditya Jindal DNB DM
Senior Consultant and
Interventionalist
Jindal Clinics
Chandigarh, India

Uma M Krishnaswamy MD DM
Professor and Head
Department of Pulmonary
Medicine
St. John's National Academy of
Health Sciences
Bengaluru, Karnataka, India

Uma Devaraj MBBS DNB
Professor
Department of Pulmonary
Medicine
St. John's National Academy of
Health Sciences
Bengaluru, Karnataka, India

Kavitha V MD DM
Assistant Professor
Department of Pulmonary
Medicine
St. John's National Academy of
Health Sciences
Bengaluru, Karnataka, India

Gurpreet S Wander MD DM
Professor and Head
Department of Cardiology
Hero DMC Heart Institute
Dayanand Medical College and
Hospital
Ludhiana, Punjab, India

Tiny Nair MD DM
Professor and Head
Department of Cardiology
PRS Hospital
Thiruvananthapuram, Kerala, India

Dinkar Bhasin MD DM
Assistant Professor
Department of Cardiology
Vardhman Mahavir Medical
College and Safdarjung Hospital
New Delhi, India

Sandeep Lakhtakia MD DM
Director - Endoscopy & EUS
Asian Institute of
Gastroenterology
Hyderabad, Telangana, India

Manav Wadhawan MD DM
Director
BLK Institute of Digestive and Liver
Diseases
New Delhi, India

Vineet Ahuja MD DM
Professor
Department of Gastroenterology
and Human Nutrition
All India Institute of Medical
Sciences
New Delhi, India

Gopesh K Modi MD DM
Consultant
Department of Nephrology
Noble Samarpan Kidney Centre
Bhopal, Madhya Pradesh, India

Joyita Bharati MD DM
Assistant Professor
Department of Nephrology
Postgraduate Institute of Medical
Education and Research
Chandigarh, India

Packiamary Jerome MD
Deputy General Superintendent
Head of Department of Medicine
In charge ICU and RCU
Neyveli Lignite Corporation
Neyveli, Tamil Nadu, India

M Ananthi MD
Consultant Physician
Neyveli Lignite Corporation
Hospital
Neyveli, Tamil Nadu, India

Aman Sharma MD
Professor
Clinical Immunology and
Rheumatology Wing
Department of Internal Medicine
Postgraduate Institute of Medical
Education and Research
Chandigarh, India

Durga Prasanna Misra MD DM
Assistant Professor
Department of Clinical
Immunology
Sanjay Gandhi Postgraduate
Institute of Medical Sciences
Lucknow, Uttar Pradesh, India

Atanu Chandra MD
Assistant Professor
Department of General Medicine
RG Kar Medical College and
Hospital
Kolkata, West Bengal, India

Subhra Sankar Sen MBBS
Post Graduate Trainee
Department of General Medicine
Midnapore Medical College and
Hospital
Midnapore, West Bengal, India

Uddalak Chakraborty MD
Senior Resident
Department of General Medicine
College of Medicine and Sagore
Dutta Hospital
Kolkata, West Bengal, India

Gurleen Wander MD
Specialist Registrar
Chelsea and Westminster Hospital
London, United Kingdom

U Meenakshisundaram
MD DM
Director of Neurology
SRM Institutes for Medical Science
Chennai, Tamil Nadu, India

Jeyaraj Durai Pandian MD DM
Principal and Professor of
Neurology
Christian Medical College
Ludhiana, Punjab, India

FOREWORD

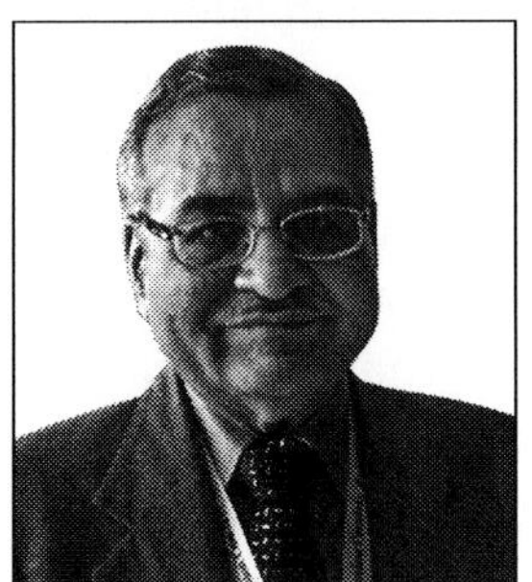

Siddharth N Shah MD FACP (Hon) FRCP (Edin)
PG Teacher, University of Mumbai
Consultant, Bhatia, SL Raheja
Saifee, and Sir HN Reliance Hospitals
Mumbai, Maharashtra, India

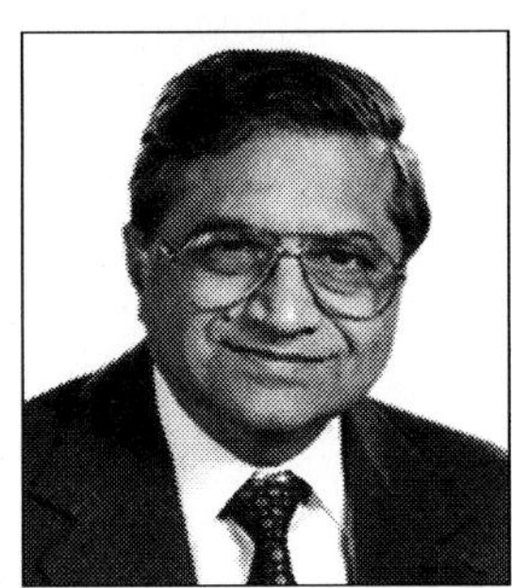

YP Munjal MD MAMS FRCP (Edin)
Medical Director and Honorary Senior Consultant
Diabetes and Life Style Disease Center
Banarsidas Chandiwala Institute of Medical Sciences
New Delhi, India

We are happy to note that the *"Year Book of Medicine, 2020"* is being published by the same group of experts of various subspecialties. It is nice to see it for third year in succession. As in previous years, the authors have picked up landmark articles with good clinical relevance from high-impact medical journals. This comprehensive collection of articles will enable any postgraduate student or practicing physician to get an overview of the new developments in various subspecialties of medicine. The uniformity in the pattern of commentaries, simple expressive language, and associated clinical message are distinguished features of this book. The abstracts of the article tell you the science and evidence on the topic. The commentaries give you an expert's opinion on the interpretation of these trials published in 2019.

In today's era of super specialization, an internist needs to be aware of the latest developments in various fields. This helps us to know what all situations can be handled by a physician and in what situation do we need to refer patients to a superspecialist. Knowledge is power for any physician. It has to be used effectively so that it translates into better clinical practices and patient care. Any activity by a physician is of benefit only if it ends up with better patient management. We urge upon the readers to translate the knowledge acquired from this book into routine clinical use. Physician inertia to adopt newer developments has to be shunned. Interpretation of clinical trials and use of this knowledge for patient care needs discussion among each other. The commentaries by the distinguished editors will be of use in that respect. We live in an era of evidence-based medicine. Medicine is under evaluation and scrutiny more than ever before. Scientifically based patient care with compassion is the best combination. Artificial intelligence, machine learning, and various omics including genomics, metabolomics, and proteomics are all entering into the arena of research and clinical practice. Many studies based on these modern methods have been included in the book. Role of genetics in patient management will increase in the coming years. Diagnostics through wearables and other sensors are now available for better patient- and disease-related information. Electronic medical records (EMRs) will soon be a reality and will become available to us with greater information about the patient's profile and past illnesses. The effort of every student of medicine has to be to acquire the latest knowledge and then use it watchfully for the benefit of the patient. Usually, a single trial will not influence our practices although some large randomized multicentric trials are so highly powered that these change the guidelines for management of some disorders. This book is a comprehensive compilation of all the significant trials of 2019. If one goes through all three "Year Books of 2018, 2019, and 2020", one will get to know most of the recent developments in medicine and its subspecialties. We hope this exercise will continue in the coming years and we wish good luck to the editors for this scientific activity.

"To study the phenomenon of disease without books is to sail uncharted sea, while to study books without patients is not going to the sea at all."

–Sir William Osler

We are happy to bring the "*Year Book of Medicine, 2020*" for the postgraduate students and practicing physicians. This is the third year in succession. You already have the "Year Books of Medicine, 2018 and 2019". Like the previous years, we have the same 9 sections with an expert in the field as the editor. We are happy that largely it is the same team which started 3 years back. Each section has approx 21 articles from high-impact factor journals and some important Indian journals. Idea is to include those studies which will have a long-term effect on our practice of medicine. A title is given to each commentary, which gives the main message of the trial. The commentary discusses the article and relevant issues. In the end, there are 2–3 key messages, which convey the current evidence-based thinking on the subject.

We have tried to include variety of research articles, which cover the range of each section. The articles chosen have been the choice of the section editor and the sub-editors of that particular section. The chief editor did not make a choice for the other sections. A few review articles have also been included. Only articles, which were published in 2019, have been included in this book. In the previous Year Books 2018 and 2019, we had articles published in 2017 and 2018, respectively. So, in case any library or individual has all three successive Year Books, one can go through a catalog or articles in the last 3 years. This is the only book of its kind in the world. The previous two books were widely read and we had excellent reviews. We have made some improvements based on the suggestions. One major change is that in the editors' choice, we have summarized 15 articles of 2019, which the section editors did not choose but I still felt that we needed to share that information.

We have all learned a lot in the process of compilation of this book about our and even, the other subspecialties. We hope you will also enjoy reading this book. The abstracts provide the original data and its interpretation is given by the experts in the commentaries. Most abstracts have been published as such after due permission. Wherever we could not get the permissions, we have rewritten them in our own language retaining the main message of the trial.

I have no words to express my gratitude to the editors and the sub-editors who put in so many hours to first choose the articles and then write the commentaries. Mr Jitendar Pal Vij, Group Chairman of Jaypee Brothers Medical Publishers (P) Ltd., has taken personal interest in this book. In fact, it started on his idea only and the format took shape later. It is an honor and a privilege for us to work with him. Dr Richa Saxena, Associate Director (Professional Publishing), is a very capable person, she is also very pleasant to work with. She absorbs a lot of stresses in the process. Her associate Prerna Bajaj (Development Editor) is a very useful member of our team. In my team, Muskan Sharma is the one who coordinates all the activities and without her, this book would not have been possible. We are lucky to have Mr Iqbal with us now who has gelled very well and the trio of us made an enjoyable and productive group.

Since coronavirus disease (COVID-19) came in 2020 only, no article on that is there in this book since all publications started from January 2020. The next Year Book will surely have a lot of articles on COVID-19. Meanwhile, stay safe and enjoy reading the latest information in Medicine.

Gurpreet S Wander

CONTENTS

Section 2: Chest and Critical Care
Section Editor: Surinder K Jindal

Associate Editors: Aditya Jindal, Uma M Krishnaswamy, Uma Devaraj, Kavitha V

Section 3: Diabetes and Metabolic Disorders
Section Editor: Siddharth N Shah

Associate Editors: Ragini Maheshwari, Naveen Mittal

Section 4: Gastroenterology/Hepatology
Section Editor: Ajay Kumar

Associate Editors: Sandeep Lakhtakia, Manav Wadhawan, Vineet Ahuja

Section 5: Infectious Diseases, HIV and TB
Section Editor: R Rajasekar

Associate Editors: Packiamary Jerome, M Ananthi

Section 6: Miscellaneous (Geriatrics, Genetics, and Pregnancy Related)
Section Editor: Jyotirmoy Pal

Associate Editors: Atanu Chandra, Subhra Sankar Sen, Uddalak Chakraborty, Gurleen Wander

Section 7: Nephrology and Hypertension
Section Editor: Vivekanand Jha

Associate Editors: Gopesh K Modi, Joyita Bharati

Section 8: Neurology
Section Editor: Gagandeep Singh

Associate Editors: U Meenakshisundaram, Jeyaraj Durai Pandian

Section 9: Rheumatology and Immunology
Section Editor: Rohini Handa

Associate Editors: Aman Sharma, Durga Prasanna Misra

Editors Choice

There have been some other significant publications and developments, which need to be covered as short communications since these will have significant impact on clinical medicine in future. These are some studies, which have not been included in the various sections but are important developments of 2019.

"Every great advance in science has issued from a new audacity of imagination."
—John Dewey

E-cigarette use (vaping) associated lung injury (EVALI)[1,2]

E-cigarettes became available 10 years back. They are being abused by youngsters and this is a matter of concern since they contain nicotine, flavoring agents, and other addictive substances. They are being sold with the hope that they aid in smoking cessation, but they are themselves habit forming and harmful. In 2019, two important observational studies were published in New England Journal of Medicine (NEJM) and the Lancet from Illinois and Utah in USA. In fact, besides these studies, a total of 2,400 patients with EVALI have been admitted in USA. There have been 52 deaths. The Centers for Disease Control and Prevention (CDC) identified tetrahydrocannabinol-containing products as the chemical, which damages the lungs. Patients are admitted with pulmonary infiltrates, shortness of breaths, gastrointestinal (GI) symptoms such as nausea, vomiting, and constitutional symptoms of fever and weight loss. The CDC and FDA are being asked by many experts to ban E-cigarettes in USA. In fact, E-cigarettes have been banned in India. This new disease entity is a matter of concern, since it can leave permanent functional and structural pulmonary effects.

Gene therapy[3]

Gene therapy has opened avenues for diseases, which were beyond cure earlier. It is a recent development. Since 2016, the FDA has given approval to six gene therapy products. Two for B-cell cancers and four for monogenic diseases including primary immunodeficiency syndrome, spinal muscular atrophy, a rare vision loss, and most importantly β-thalassemia. The therapeutic gene, which is inserted in diseased individual, is called "transgene". This can be done in two ways. Ex vivo with the use of stem cells so that gene reaches every cell. In the second in vivo method, gene is delivered to a slowly dividing post-mitotic cell directly like any pharmaceutical agents. The ex vivo system is used in hematopoietic stem cells implantation. This has been used for β-thalassemia, sickle cell anemia, and immunodeficiency syndrome. Presently, phase 3 trial for beta thalassemia and four gene therapy trials are ongoing for sickle cell anemia. In vivo gene therapy is being tried for hemophilia A and for spinal muscular atrophy. FDA has given approval for gene therapy for melanoma, non-Hodgkin's lymphoma, and some head and neck squamous cell carcinoma. Gene therapy is very expensive and these trials are being heavily funded since it opens vistas for a new form of therapy for genetic diseases especially monogenic diseases. At present, there are more than 800 gene therapy programs being developed at various institutions.

Two negative trials on use of vitamin D3[4,5]

Vitamin D deficiency is common and has been correlated with various diseases. Risk of type 2 diabetes mellitus has been linked to vitamin D deficiency (25-hydroxyvitamin D). In this large trial, called the D2d trial (Vitamin D and Type 2 Diabetes Trial) published in July 2019 issue of NEJM, 2,400 patients of prediabetes who were at increased risk of diabetes were randomly assigned to 4,000 IU of vitamin D3 or placebo. The incidence of diabetes over 2.5 years was looked at. There was no difference in new-onset diabetes with vitamin D3 supplementation. Although there was significant increase in vitamin D levels in the treated group. In previous studies from Norway and Japan, mild nonsignificant benefits were seen and hence this large trial was done, which is a negative trial for any benefit.

In a second large trial published in 2019 in December in the NEJM, high-dose vitamin D3 was given in critically ill vitamin D-deficient patients; this is a NHLBI funded trial, which is part of the PETAL network of studies. In this study, called the VIOLET trial (Vitamin D Improve Outcomes by Leveraging Early Treatment), enteral vitamin D was given in a dose of 540,000 IU. About 1,360 patients with vitamin D levels of <20 ng/mL were taken. This high dose of vitamin D resulted in significant increase in vitamin D levels. However, there was no decrease in 90-day mortality in these acutely sick patients in intensive care unit (ICU), who were on ventilator. This is also a negative trial, which does not show any benefit of vitamin D supplementation in acutely sick ICU patients.

Two reports in Lancet on *Plasmodium vivax* malaria[6,7]

The June 19, 2019 issue of Lancet carries an article from the global burden of disease study (GBD study). It looks at the prevalence of *Plasmodium vivax* (PV) malaria over 17 years from year 2000 to 2017. Globally, there were 25 million cases of PV malaria in 2000, which have decreased to 15 million in 2017. Thus, globally, there has been a decrease of 42% in PV malaria. Malaria peaked in 2005 in the world and has been decreasing since then. We all know *Plasmodium falciparum* malaria is the most common and most virulent type of malaria. It is still common in sub-Saharan Africa. PV is the second most common and is most widespread world over. It is not so benign as was thought earlier, because it has relapses since there is a dormant liver stage (Hypnozoites), which can cause relapses. The PV malaria has been eliminated from Europe, Sri Lanka, and Paraguay. It is nearly eliminated from China.

The 8-aminoquinoline drugs are effective in the liver stage and can prevent recurrences in PV malaria. However, they cause hemolytic anemia in glucose-6-phosphate-dehydrogenase (G6PD)-deficient individuals. Primaquine is the only available hypnozoites. It has to be given for 14 days for elimination of PV from liver. In another study published in Lancet, July 18, 2019, a short 7-day course of primaquine for PV in a dose of 1 mg/kg/day was compared with 14-day course of 0.5 mg/kg/day and placebo. It was found that 7-day double-dose course was as effective as the 14-day tended course. Thus, after doing G6PD and ruling out its deficiency, we can give a 7-day course according to this study. This will improve the compliance. In USA and Australia, 62,018 and thus primaquine analog called Tafenoquine is available. It can be given as single dose. However, it can only be used when G6PD activity is >70%.

Precision medicine and big data can overdiagnose abnormalities[8]

In an article published in September, 2019 in British Medical Journal (BMJ), the authors discussed some issues with big data. The human genome project was completed in 1990. This paved the way for precision medicine (personalized medicine) since we can judge the genetic makeup of an individual. Our ability to diagnose this and other processes in the body as resulted in a term called "omics". This includes genomics (DNA), proteomics (proteins), metabolomics (metabolites), and transcriptomics (RNA). Since we can derive information on these parameters of the body, we feel that we now can judge an individual's makeup better than what we could do earlier. Also, we have access to multiple images from imaging technologies, electronic medical records (EMRs), and biosensors. The biosensors can give us information on blood, sweat, and environment. Since we have all this information on an individual, we feel we can provide more precise treatment to an individual based on the genetic and metabolic makeup. This is the basis for precision medicine.

Big data implies that we can collate hundreds of these parameters in a given individual and by applying machine learning technologies, we can derive at information, which tells us risk profile of an individual and livelihood of disease occurrence. Big data gives us more information that it can cause overdiagnosis and over medicalization. Three early big data prestudies are a proof of this. One such study PIONEER 100 wellness project (P100) looked at 108 healthy people. In detailed genome study of 219 clinical tests, 643 metabolics, 262 proteins, and 4,616 microbes were evaluated. They found 95 had vitamin D deficiency, 81 had high mercury levels, 52 had prediabetes, and 73 had dyslipidemia of some variety. It shows virtually everyone had something wrong. Same findings were observed in the precision medicine creaming study and in longitudinal big data approach for precision medicine. The more parameter you evaluate more is the likelihood of something wrong be detected in an individual. The culture of more data, earlier data, and cellular information can cause problem of overdiagnosis. We will identify conditions that are not likely to cause harm. This will be exploited by modern technology companies such as Facebook and Amazon. Self-monitoring will result in balanced decisions and unnecessary overdiagnosis. Important challenge to precision medicine is to evaluate the likelihood that these abnormalities will cause disease. Precision medicine is useful because more information about an individual allows us to be more precise in our approach. However, we need to use this extensive new data pertinently for patient benefit.

Management of MDR (multidrug resistance) tuberculosis[9]

In a series of article published in September 14th, 2019 in Lancet, treatment of MDR is discussed in detail. World over, its prevalence is 4.5%. In some countries such as Ukraine and Kazakhstan, it is as high as 25% when resistance to rifampicin and isoniazid both is there and it is called MDR. Isoniazid resistance alone is more common and is 7%. Regimens of rifampicin, levofloxacin, pyrazinamide, and ethambutol all four are given for 6 months. Treatment of MDR is more difficult; it requires long duration regimen of 18–20 months. Recently, in March 28, 2019, issue of NEJM, the STREAM study collaborators compared the 2011 WHO guidelines 20-month regimen with a 9–11-month regimen used in Bangladesh. The shorter regimen had excess of 78% and longer one of 79%. 30% patients have HIV. Study was done in four countries. However, more recently with the availability of oral drugs, the injectable regimens are being avoided. At present, 15 regimens are being tested for MDR. WHO has divided drugs for MDR into three groups. Group A consists of drugs, which are highly effective and strongly recommended. It includes bedaquiline, levofloxacin and moxifloxacin, and linezolid. Group B drugs are agents of second choice. This includes clofazimine and cycloserine. Group C drugs are used when regimen cannot be completed with group A and B drugs. This includes amikacin, streptomycin, delamanid, ethambutol, ethionamide, prothionamide, imipenem, meropenem, and nPAS. Whole drugs have to be used for a period of 20 months.

Rapid drug susceptibility test (DST) has recently become available with the automatic cartridge-based molecular testing with GeneXpert platform. This has revolutionized treatment of MDR tuberculosis. Alternative semiautomatic method is line probe assay; it enables diagnosis in 1–5 days. The third method, next-generation whole genome sequencing, is the best but is more expensive. Treatment of MDR has been discussed in detail. It has become systematic and more successful after the publication of the STREAM trial according to this article.

Phase-3 positive trial of tetravalent dengue vaccine[10]

The November 6, 2019 issue of NEJM has results of a phase-3 study with tetravalent dengue vaccine by Takeda vaccines. The study is published by TIDES study group. WHO has ranked dengue as one of the top 10 threats to global health. It is a mosquito-borne viral disease caused by virus of genus *Flavivirus*. Half of the world population lives in endemic area for dengue. It has four serotypes DENV-1 through 4. Earlier in 2014, a trial on tetravalent dengue vaccine was published in NEJM by Sanofi. Subsequently, their vaccine Dengvaxia has been licensed in several countries. However, that vaccine is not effective in seronegative individuals.

The present study is a phase-3 study done in 20,000 subjects. Two injections are given 3 months apart. Study shows efficacy of 80%. Efficacy against hospitalization was 95%. There were no side effects compared to placebo. Thus, we will now have effective vaccine against dengue in the coming years. The study is ongoing with further recruitment and this is the primary finding of the trial.

Role of nutrition in health: What is a good diet for adults! [11-13]

In a series of above-mentioned articles published in the Lancet, the issue of nutrition and health is addressed in great detail. In a 46-page article titled Food in the Anthropocene: EAT–Lancet commission report is published in February, 2019. A healthy reference diet should be high in vegetables, fruits, whole grains, legumes, nuts, and unsaturated oils. All these are helpful in reducing noncommunicable diseases (NCD). There can be low-to-moderate amount of seafood and poultry as sources of protein. The following diets should be avoided as far as possible since they increase the risk of NCD. Red meat, processed meat, preserved food, salt, added sugar, refined grains, and starchy vegetables all should be avoided.

At present, the world population is 8 billion and is expected to increase to 10 billion by 2050. Presently, 2 billion people are overweight or obese. This number will go up unless diet issues are addressed. Unsaturated oil is much better than ghee and butter from animal sources. In fact, ghee and butter are very high in saturated fats. As healthy diet, the proportion of unsaturated oil can be 20% of each olive, soybean, rapeseed, sunflower, and peanut oil. The Mediterranean diet, which was used by Greek who had longest life expectancy, was typically low in red meat and high in plant-based olive oil.

Energy intake of an adult is 2,500 kcal/day. Proteins provide 10% of energy intake. This should increase to 12–15%. Red meat (beef, pork, and lamb) should be avoided and white meat (poultry and fish) is to be preferred. Plant proteins (legumes, soy foods, and nuts) are the best. Carbohydrates should be reduced to <60% of calories. Higher use causes high triglyceride (TG), low high-density lipoprotein (HDL), high BP, insulin resistance, and increase in mortality. Whole grain is the best carbohydrate. Fiber intake is presently <20 g/day. It should increase to 25–30 g/day. Recent review from ARIC study (atherosclerosis risk in communities) published in JAHA-2019 showed diet rich in wholegrain, apple, pear, citrus, green vegetables, and salad causes 19% decrease in cardiovascular (CV) mortality and 11% decrease in all-cause mortality. Refined carbohydrates should be avoided. Diet high in fiber and whole grain has been shown to reduce diabetes mellitus (DM), coronary artery disease (CAD), stroke, and breast, colon, and esophageal cancer. The third component of diet is fat. These should be <30% of the total calories, with saturated fat being <10%. The saturated fat from ghee butter and lard can be substituted by unsaturated vegetable oils, especially those high in polyunsaturated fats and omega-3 fatty acids. Avoid palm oil, since it is the only vegetable oil high in saturated fat. Rapeseed oil is also called canola oil. It is high in monounsaturated fats and omega-3 fatty acids. It was used in Finland where significant reduction of CAD was achieved. In the carbohydrates, sugar and sweeteners should be avoided.

In Lancet May 11, 2019, data from global burden of disease (GBD) is published over 2000–2017. It also shows that increased sodium, low whole grain, fruits, vegetables, nuts, and omega-3 fatty acids each accounts for 2% of global deaths. In south Asia, 19% of deaths can be attributable to unhealthy diets. Role of healthy diet has thus been discussed and defined in multiple papers published in 2019 as mentioned above.

Ustekinumab, a monoclonal antibody, an interleukin-12 and -23 antagonist, can be useful in ulcerative colitis[14]

Ustekinumab is an antagonist of p40 component of interleukin-12 and -23. It is a monoclonal antibody. It is already approved for use in patients with psoriasis, psoriatic arthritis, and Crohn's disease. There is a previous phase-3 trial in patients with Crohn's disease in whom it was found to be beneficial. In the present study, which is a UNIFI phase-3 study, ustekinumab has been evaluated in patients with moderate-to-severe ulcerative colitis. About 960 patients were randomly assigned to this drug, initially in an 8-week induction therapy phase and 44-

week maintenance phase. Patients who were assigned to the drug had greater remission induction and maintenance than the placebo group. This was seen by improvement in partial Mayo scores and in histological and endoscopic mucosal healing. More patients were, in corticosteroid-free remission, on this drug. There were seven patients who developed cancer on the drug and one patient in the placebo group. This increase in cancer needs further evaluation. This study is a positive study and shows benefit in induction and maintenance of remission in patients with moderate-to-severe ulcerative colitis

Menopausal hormonal therapy (MHT) and increased risk of breast cancer[15]

In a meta-analysis, the collaborative group on hormonal factors in breast cancer looked at prospective follow-up data on 1 lakh postmenopausal women who developed breast cancer and had used menopausal hormone therapy (MHT). The incidence of breast cancer was increased significantly among users of MHT. 5 years of MHT with estrogens plus daily progestogen preparation increased risk of breast cancer by 1 in 50, use of estrogens plus intermittent progestogen increased by 1 in 70, and estrogens alone preparation increased by 1 in 200 users with 5 year of MHT use. The risk increased to double of this with 10 years of MHT use. Breast cancer risk decreases after menopause. Use of MHT keeps the women in premenopausal state and so the menopausal reduction of cancer risk does not happen. Obesity and MHT both are risk factors for breast cancer. MHT was used more commonly before 2000. Publication of women's health initiative trial in 2002 and 2004 showed increased risk of breast cancer with combination MHT. MHT is also called as hormone replacement therapy (HRT). Since 2004, its use declined, since awareness of increased breast cancer risk had increased. MHT is used for relief of perimenopausal symptoms. Now, it is recommended that MHT should be used for minimum possible time since its use increases risk of breast cancer.

For left main CAD, CABG and PCI have similar 5-year outcomes[16]

Five-year results of this trial are presented here. 1,900 patients with left main disease were randomly assigned to angioplasty [percutaneous coronary intervention (PCI)] or coronary artery bypass graft (CABG). At 5 years, there was no significant difference in primary outcome of death, stroke, or myocardial infarction (MI). Left main PCI is now commonly done in most centers. Unlike triple vessel disease (TVD) where CABG has been shown to be better than PCI, left main coronary artery disease (CAD) patients have similar outcomes. After publication of this trial, there has been some criticism that the definition of MI used was not appropriate. However, the study shows PCI is a viable alternative to CABG when the lesion anatomy is favorable.

Efficacy and safety of low-dose colchicine after myocardial infarction[17]

Inflammation is known to play a role in the pathogenesis of atherosclerosis and in acute coronary events. In this trial, called the COLCOT trial, anti-inflammatory agent colchicine has been used in a dose of 0.5 mg daily. About 4,500 patients were enrolled within 1 month after myocardial infarction (MI). Over 2-year follow-up primary endpoint of death, MI or stroke was observed in 5.5% of colchicine group and 7.1% of placebo group. Colchicine significantly reduced the risk of ischemic cardiovascular (CV) events.

In 2017, a large trial, the CANTOS trial, looked at a monoclonal antibody canakinumab, which inhibits interleukin-1β. This anti-inflammatory agent also caused modest reduction in CV events and lowering of high-sensitivity C-reactive protein (hs-CRP) level, which is a marker of inflammation. The COLCOT study again indicates role of inflammation in progression of atherosclerosis and causation of acute coronary syndrome.

The evolution of the use of fecal microbiota transplantation (FMT) for treating various disorders[18]

The gut microbiota comprises bacteria, viruses, fungi, and archaea. The role of gut microbiota in health and disease is being recognized increasingly now. This has happened after microbial genome sequencing. Alteration in gut microbiota is called as "dysbiosis". Changes in gut microbiota are seen in gastrointestinal (GI) and non-GI disorders such as metabolic syndrome and obesity. The cause and effect relationship is not clear.

Fecal microbiota transplant (FMT) is being evaluated for various diseases. Presently, it is the treatment of choice for recurrent *Clostridioides difficile* previously called as *Clostridium difficile* (*C. difficile*). *C. difficile* infection occurs in individuals who are given prolonged antibiotics especially fluoroquinolones, clindamycin, and cephalosporins. It has a recurrence of 20–30%. The standard treatment presently is vancomycin and fidaxomicin. Previously, metronidazole was also used for this. FMT is now emerging as preferred treatment for recurrence of *C. difficile*, which is seen in one-third patients. FMT can be done from above through Ryle's tube or UGI endoscopy. It can be given from below by colonoscopy, sigmoidoscopy, or enema. Although it is being used world over for last 15 years, it has not yet been approved by FDA for this indication.

Besides *C. difficile* infection, FMT is also being evaluated for inflammatory bowel disease especially ulcerative colitis, hepatic encephalopathy, primary sclerosing cholangitis, irritable bowel syndrome and functional bowel disorders, hematopoietic stem cell transplant recipients, autistic spectrum disorders, and metabolic syndromes. Generally, stool is taken from stool bank and frozen samples are equally effective. Healthy stool donors are used for stool donation. This field is emerging and evolving. Randomized trials are being conducted for the above-mentioned potential indications. Presently, recurrent *C. difficile* infection is the only standard accepted indication.

Preeclampsia and hypertension in pregnancy are markers of subsequent ASCVD[19]

This study shows that hypertension in pregnancy (HIP) and preeclampsia are markers of subsequent increased risk of stroke by a hazard ratio (HR) of 1.9, cardiovascular events by 1.8, heart failure by 1.7, and atrial fibrillation by HR of 2.1. The risk with preeclampsia is more than that with HIP.

This is a large study using electronic health records of 1.3 million women from UK over a period of 20 years from 1997 to 2016. The American Heart Association and European Society of Cardiology already consider it as a screening tool for CAD and stroke. This UK study shows that HIP and preeclampsia are natural screening tools for premature cardiovascular events and these women should be closely observed and counseled for CV preventive practices.

Preeclampsia affects 2–8% of all pregnancies worldwide. Preeclampsia is responsible for 40% of maternal deaths. In this study, incidence of pre-eclampsia was 2.4% of all pregnancies. The study shows that these women should be kept on follow-up after pregnancy and preventive strategies for CVD need to be pursued aggressively.

Lipoprotein(a) [Lp(a)] now recognized as independent genetic risk factor for ASCVD[20]

Lipoprotein(a) [Lp(a)] is now being increasingly recognized as a risk factor for cardiovascular disease (CVD), calcific aortic valve disease, chronic kidney disease, and heart failure. It was discovered in 1963 as a new antigen associated with low-density lipoprotein (LDL) cholesterol. Geneticist Berg discovered it and named it Lp(a). It affects the endothelial function, plaque stability, and inflammation. Recently, the National Heart, Lung, and Blood Institute (NHLBI) has estimated that in 2018, around 1.4 billion people in the world have Lp(a) levels of >50 mg. This gives a prevalence of 10–30% in different ethnicities. Lp(a) is a genetic risk factor. It is determined by *Lp(a)* gene located on chromosome 6q26. It is not affected by age, activity, or diet. It has been shown to be higher in south Asians. Lp(a) levels are not affected by statins. The use of PCSK9 inhibitors in two trials, of evolocumab in the FOURIER trial and alirocumab in ODYSSEY OUTCOMES trial, shows that these agents can reduce LDL by 60% and Lp(a) by 30%. Lp(a) should now be considered as major risk factor for ASCVD. The 2018 AHA cholesterol guidelines recognize it as an independent risk factor. Lp(a) levels of <20 are considered optimal, 20–50 borderline, and >50 increase the risk of CAD by 2–3 times. When Lp(a) levels are high, treatment of LDL has to be more aggressive. The INTER-HEART study has shown that Lp(a) levels are especially important in South Asians. Africans have the highest Lp(a) levels and Chinese have the lowest Lp(a) levels. Lp(a) lowering will have greater value in South Asians. We should proactively screen young MI and young stroke patients for Lp(a) levels.

In March 19, 2019 issue of Circulation, two studies are published which underline the value of Lp(a) for screening. It should be done in all subjects with premature CVD and in those with statin resistant or familial hypercholesterolemia. In an editorial in same issue of Circulation, the authors feel that trials with targeted therapy for Lp(a) are now required and will make a difference in our approach, if they are found to be positive.

These are some of the clinical trials and review articles published in 2019, which have not been covered in respective sections and are hence summarized here conveying the basic message from these trials and articles.

REFERENCES

1. Layden JE, Ghinai I, Pray I, Kimball A, Layer M, Tenforde MW, et al. Pulmonary Illness Related to E-Cigarette Use in Illinois and Wisconsin—Final Report. N Engl J Med. 2020;382:903-16.

2. Blagev DP, Harris D, Dunn AC, Guidry DW, Grissom CK, Lanspa MJ. Clinical presentation, treatment, and short-term outcomes of lung injury associated with e-cigarettes or vaping: A prospective observational cohort study. Lancet. 2019;394:2073-83.

3. High KA, Roncarolo MG. Gene Therapy. N Engl J Med. 2019;381:455-64.

4. Pittas AG, Dawson-Hughes B, Sheehan P, Ware JH, Knowler WC, Aroda VR, et al. Vitamin D Supplementation and Prevention of Type 2 Diabetes. N Engl J Med. 2019;381:520-30.

5. The National Heart, Lung, and Blood Institute PETAL Clinical Trials Network. Early High-Dose Vitamin D3 for Critically Ill, Vitamin D–Deficient Patients. N Engl J Med. 2019;381:2529-40.

6. Battle KE, Lucas TCD, Nguyen M, Howes RE, Nandi AK, Twohig KA, et al. Mapping the global endemicity and clinical burden of *Plasmodium vivax*, 2000–17: A spatial and temporal modelling study. Lancet. 2019;394:332-43.

7. Taylor WRJ, Thriemer K, von Seidlein L, Yuentrakul P, Assawariyathipat Y, Assefa A, et al. Short-course primaquine for the radical cure of *Plasmodium vivax* malaria: A multicentre, randomised, placebo-controlled non-inferiority trial. Lancet. 2019;394:929-38.

8. Vogt H, Green S, Ekstrøm CT, Brodersen J. How precision medicine and screening with big data could increase overdiagnosis. BMJ. 2019;366:l5270.

9. Lange C, Dheda K, Chesov D, Mandalakas AM, Udwadia Z, Horsburgh CR Jr. Management of drug-resistant tuberculosis. Lancet. 2019;394:953-66.

10. Biswal S, Reynales H, Saez-Llorens X, Lopez P, Borja-Tabora C, Kosalaraksa P, et al. Efficacy of a Tetravalent Dengue Vaccine in Healthy Children and Adolescents. N Engl J Med. 2019;381:2009-19.

11. GBD 2017 Diet Collaborators. Health effects of dietary risks in 195 countries, 1990–2017: A systematic analysis for the Global Burden of Disease Study. Lancet. 2019;393:1958-72.

12. Willett W, Rockström J, Loken B, Springmann M, Lang T, Vermeulen S, et al. Food in the Anthropocene: The EAT–Lancet Commission on healthy diets from sustainable food systems. Lancet. 2019;393:447-92.

13. Kim H, Caulfield LE, Garcia-Larsen V, Steffen LM, Coresh J, Rebholz CM. Plant-based diets are associated with a lower risk of incident cardiovascular disease, cardiovascular disease mortality, and All-Cause mortality in a general population of Middle-Aged adults. J Am Heart Assoc. 2019;8:e012865.

14. Sands BE, Sandborn WJ, Panaccione R, O'Brien CD, Zhang H, Johanns J, et al. Ustekinumab as induction and maintenance therapy for ulcerative colitis. NEJM. 2019;381:1201-14.

15. Collaborative Group on Hormonal Factors in Breast Cancer. Type and timing of menopausal hormone therapy and breast cancer risk: Individual participant meta-analysis of the worldwide epidemiological evidence. Lancet. 2019;394:1159-68.

16. Stone GW, Kappetein AP, Sabik KF, Pocock SJ, Morice MC, Puskas J, et al. Five-Year Outcomes after PCI or CABG for Left Main Coronary Disease. N Engl J Med. 2019;381:1820-30.

17. Tardif JC, Kouz S, Waters DD, Bertrand OF, Diaz R, Maggioni AP, et al. Efficacy and safety of low-dose colchicine after myocardial infarction. N Engl J Med. 2019;381:2497-505.

18. Allegretti JR, Mullish BH, Kelly C, Fischer M. The evolution of the use of faecal microbiota transplantation and emerging therapeutic indications. Lancet. 2019;394:420-31.

19. Leon LJ, McCarthy FP, Direk K, Gonzalez-Izquierdo A, Prieto-Merino D, Casas JP, et al. Preeclampsia and Cardiovascular Disease in a Large UK Pregnancy Cohort of Linked Electronic Health Records: A CALIBER Study. Circulation. 2019;140:1050-60.

20. Enasa EA, Varkey B, Dharmarajan TS, Paree G, Bah VK. Lipoprotein(a): An independent, genetic, and causal factor for cardiovascular disease and acute myocardial infarction. Indian Heart J. 2019;71:99-112.

Section Editor: VK Bahl

Associate Editors: Gurpreet S Wander, Tiny Nair, Dinkar Bhasin

ARTICLE 1

Percutaneous coronary intervention versus coronary artery bypass grafting in patients with three-vessel or left main coronary artery disease: 10-year follow-up of the multicentre randomised controlled SYNTAX trial

Thuijs DJ, Kappetein AP, Serruys PW, Mohr FW, Morice MC, Mack MJ, et al. Percutaneous coronary intervention versus coronary artery bypass grafting in patients with three-vessel or left main coronary artery disease: 10-year follow-up of the multicentre randomised controlled SYNTAX trial.
Lancet. 2019;394:1325-34.

Abstract

Background: The SYNTAX (SYNergy between percutaneous coronary intervention with TAXus and Cardiac Surgery) trial was a noninferiority trial that compared percutaneous coronary intervention (PCI) using first-generation paclitaxel-eluting stents with coronary artery bypass grafting (CABG) in patients with de-novo three-vessel and left main coronary artery disease, and reported results up to 5 years. We now report 10-year all-cause death results.

Methods: The SYNTAX Extended Survival (SYNTAXES) study is an investigator-driven extension of follow-up of a multicenter, randomized controlled trial done in 85 hospitals across 18 North American and European countries. Patients with de-novo three-vessel and left main coronary artery disease were randomly assigned (1:1) to the PCI group or CABG group. Patients with a history of PCI or CABG, acute myocardial infarction, or an indication for concomitant cardiac surgery were excluded. The primary endpoint of the SYNTAXES study was 10-year all-cause death, which was assessed according to the intention-to-treat principle. Prespecified subgroup analyses were performed according to the presence or absence of left main coronary artery disease and diabetes, and according to coronary complexity defined by core laboratory SYNTAX score tertiles. This study is registered with ClinicalTrials.gov, NCT03417050.

Findings: From March, 2005 to April, 2007, 1,800 patients were randomly assigned to the PCI (n = 903) or CABG (n = 897) group. Vital status information at 10 years was complete for 841 (93%) patients in the PCI group and 848 (95%) patients in the CABG group. At 10 years, 248 (28%) patients had died after PCI and 212 (24%) after CABG {hazard ratio 1.19 [95% confidence interval (CI) 0.99–1.43]; p = 0.066}. Among patients with three-vessel disease, 153 (28%) of 546 had died after PCI versus 114 (21%) of 549 after CABG [hazard ratio 1.42 (95% CI 1.11–1.81)], and among patients with left main coronary artery disease, 95 (27%) of 357 had died after PCI versus 98 (28%) of 348 after CABG [0.92 (0.69–1.22), $p_{interaction}$ = 0.023]. There was no treatment-by-subgroup interaction with diabetes ($p_{interaction}$ = 0.60) and no linear trend across SYNTAX score tertiles (p_{trend} = 0.20).

Interpretation: At 10 years, no significant difference existed in all-cause death between PCI using first-generation paclitaxel-eluting stents and CABG. However, CABG provided a significant survival benefit in patients with three-vessel disease, but not in patients with left main coronary artery disease.

Funding: German Foundation of Heart Research (SYNTAXES study, 5–10-year follow-up) and Boston Scientific Corporation (SYNTAX study, 0–5-year follow-up).

"As to diseases, make a habit of two things — to help, or at least, to do no harm."

—**Hippocrates**

COMMENT

Despite the advanced knowledge and progress in the management of coronary artery disease (CAD), the role of percutaneous coronary intervention (PCI) on outcomes in patients with stable CAD continues to be debated. Several pivotal studies have shown that coronary artery bypass grafting (CABG) improves outcomes in patients with triple vessel disease and left main (LM) disease when compared to optimal medical therapy (OMT). The SYNTAX (SYNergy between percutaneous coronary intervention with TAXus and Cardiac Surgery) trial was a pivotal study that compared PCI with CABG for patients with LM disease or triple-vessel disease (TVD).[1] The study provided the SYNTAX score, based on anatomical characteristics of CAD, which is extensively used in clinical practice to decide the choice of revascularization, i.e., CABG or PCI, in decision-making regarding whether surgery or PCI will benefit the patients. PCI is preferred for patients with score ≤22, while CABG is preferred for patients with SYNTAX score ≥33. Patient with in between SYNTAX scores, PCI and CABG are comparable.

The SYNTAX Extended Survival study is a 10-year follow-up of the same cohort. The follow-up was complete in 94% of the patients but only survival data was available. There was no difference in all-cause mortality between the treatment modalities in the overall cohort. However, when patients were categorized on the basis of SYNTAX score, the survival advantage in patients with SYNTAX ≥33 was consistent. There was no difference in patients with LM disease irrespective of SYNTAX score. The presence or absence of diabetes mellitus (DM) did not influence outcomes. While a survival benefit with CABG was present in patients with TVD, subgroup analysis showed that this was significant only for patients with SYNTAX score >33.

Key Message

⊙ *While SYNTAX score acts as a good discriminatory tool for choice of revascularization, patients with SYNTAX score ≥33 should undergo CABG, while PCI should be preferred for SYNTAX score ≤22. However, the decision for revascularization should also consider other variables such as surgical risk, completeness of revascularization, and patient choice. The heart team approach is the most appropriate strategy to individualize the decision-making process for every patient.*

ARTICLE 2

Cardiovascular risk reduction with icosapent ethyl for hypertriglyceridemia

Bhatt DL, Steg PG, Miller M, Brinton EA, Jacobson TA, Ketchum SB, et al. Cardiovascular Risk Reduction with Icosapent Ethyl for Hypertriglyceridemia.
N Engl J Med. 2019;380:11-22.

Abstract*

Introduction: Increased levels of triglyceride expose patients to enhanced risk for ischemic events. Icosapent ethyl is a highly purified eicosapentaenoic acid ethyl ester that reduces the levels of triglyceride; however, there is a requirement of data for determining its effects on ischemic events.

Materials and methods: This multicenter, randomized, double-blind, placebo-controlled trial included patients who had previously known cardiovascular disease or with diabetes as well as other risk factors. The patients were on statin therapy and had fasting triglyceride level of 135–499 mg/dL (1.52–5.63 mmol/L) and low-density lipoprotein cholesterol level of 41–100 mg/dL (1.06–2.59 mmol/L). Randomization of the patients was done to receive either 2 g of icosapent ethyl twice daily (total daily dose was 4 g) or placebo. The primary endpoint considered in the study included a composite of nonfatal myocardial infarction, coronary revascularization, nonfatal stroke, unstable angina, or cardiovascular death. The key secondary endpoint in the study was a composite of nonfatal stroke, cardiovascular death, or nonfatal myocardial infarction.

Results: Total 8,179 patients were included in the study; out of these, 70.7% patients were for secondary prevention of cardiovascular events. Median duration of follow-up was 4.9 years. In comparison to the placebo group patients, primary endpoint event was noted in significantly less number of patients in the icosapent ethyl group {17.2% vs. 22.0%; [hazard ratio 0.75; 95% confidence interval (CI): 0.68–0.83; p < 0.001]}, and key secondary endpoint was also present in significantly less number of patients in the icosapent ethyl group (11.2% vs. 14.8%; hazard ratio 0.74; 95% CI 0.65–0.83; p < 0.001). As compared to placebo, icosapent ethyl group had significantly lower rates of additional ischemic endpoints (evaluated as per a prespecified hierarchical schema) (4.3% vs. 5.2%; hazard ratio 0.80; 95% CI 0.66–0.98; p = 0.03). Hospitalization rates for atrial fibrillation or flutter were significantly more in icosapent ethyl group than placebo group (3.1% vs. 2.1%, p = 0.004). Serious bleeding events were present in significantly more patients in the icosapent ethyl group (2.7% vs. 2.1%, p = 0.06) than the placebo group.

Conclusion: In spite of the use of statins in patients with increased triglyceride levels, the risk of ischemic events (consisting of cardiovascular death) was found to be significantly lower in individuals who received 2 g icosapent ethyl twice daily as compared to those who received placebo. (Funded by Amarin Pharma; REDUCE-IT ClinicalTrials.gov number, NCT01492361.) *Redrafted abstract

"The physician should not treat the disease, but the patient who is suffering from it."
—**Moses Maimonides**

COMMENT

Elevated low-density lipoprotein (LDL) cholesterol has been established as risk factor for atherosclerotic cardiovascular disease. Intensive statin therapy reduces this risk in proportion to the reduction of LDL levels. Several studies have shown that the elevated triglyceride (TG) levels also increased risk of atherosclerotic cardiovascular disease (ASCVD) independent of LDL levels. Further, in patients who have achieved target LDL levels on therapy, persistently elevated TGs have been associated with residual risk. However, previous trials evaluating TG-reducing agents, such as fibrates and niacin, have not shown any improvement in cardiovascular outcomes.

The REDUCTE-IT trial studied the role of icosapent ethyl, an ethyl ester of icosapentaenoic acid, in reducing cardiovascular outcomes on patients on optimal medical therapy but persistently elevated TG levels. In this study, over 8,000 patients with ASCVD or presence of diabetes with one additional risk factor for coronary artery disease (CAD), who were receiving statin therapy and had fasting TG levels between 135 and 499 mg/dL, were randomized to receive 2 g of icosapent ethyl twice a day or placebo of mineral oil. The primary composite outcome included death from cardiovascular (CV) causes, cerebrovascular accident (CVA), myocardial infarction, unstable angina, or revascularization for CAD. After a median follow-up for 5 years, there was a significant reduction in the primary endpoint in patients receiving icosapent ethyl (28.3% vs. 23.0%; p < 0.001). There was reduction in components of secondary outcome including death from CV causes (4.3% vs. 5.2%; p = 0.03), CVA (2.4% vs. 3.3%; p = 0.01) and MI (6.1% vs. 8.7%; p < 0.001). There was no difference in all-cause mortality. The number needed to treat to prevent one event over 5 years was 21. Interestingly, the benefit with icosapent ethyl was consistent irrespective of the baseline TG levels and or the TG levels achieved. There was an unexplained increase in incidence of atrial fibrillation (AF) in the interventions group.

The limitations of this study include use of mineral oil placebo agent, which could have influenced the lipid parameters in the placebo arm. Further, the mechanism of action of icosapent ethyl is unclear. It has been postulated to have pleiotropic effects such as plaque stabilization, anti-platelet activity, and anti-inflammatory action.

Key Message

⊙ *Icospent ethyl is a new agent, which can improve CV outcomes in patients with dyslipidemia. The target population comprises patients with elevated CV risk who have well-controlled LDL cholesterol levels but elevated TG levels.*

ARTICLE 3

Early or delayed cardioversion in recent-onset atrial fibrillation

Pluymaekers NAHA, Dudink EAMP, Luermans JGLM, Meeder JG, Lenderink T, Widdershoven J, et al. Early or Delayed Cardioversion in Recent-Onset Atrial Fibrillation.
N Engl J Med. 2019;380:1499-508.

Abstract*

Introduction: Generally, in patients who have recent-onset atrial fibrillation, immediate restoration of sinus rhythm is done by pharmacologic or electrical cardioversion. It is still not known whether immediate restoration of sinus rhythm is essential or not, because atrial fibrillation usually terminates spontaneously.

Materials and methods: This multicenter, randomized, open-label, noninferiority trial included patients with hemodynamically stable, recent-onset (<36 h), symptomatic atrial fibrillation who were admitted in the emergency department (ED). Patients were randomly assigned to be treated with early cardioversion or with a wait-and-see approach (i.e., delayed-cardioversion group). In the wait-and-see approach, initial treatment was given with rate-control medication only, and delayed cardioversion if the atrial fibrillation did not resolve within 48 hours. Presence of sinus rhythm at 4 weeks was considered as the primary endpoint. Noninferiority was demonstrated, if the lower limit of the 95% confidence interval (CI) for the between-group difference in the primary endpoint in percentage points was more than −10.

Results: As compared to the early-cardioversion group, presence of sinus rhythm at 4 weeks was present in significantly less number of patients of the delayed-cardioversion group [91% (193/212) vs. 94% (202/215); between-group difference −2.9 percentage points; 95% CI −8.2 to 2.2; p = 0.005 for noninferiority]. Conversion to sinus rhythm within 48 hours occurred spontaneously in more number of patients [69% (150/218) vs. 28% (n = 61)]. Conversion to sinus rhythm occurred spontaneously prior to the initiation of cardioversion in 16% (36/219) patients of the early-cardioversion group and 78% (n = 171) in delayed cardioversion group patients. In the patients who completed remote monitoring during 4 weeks of follow-up, a recurrence of atrial fibrillation was noted in 30% (49/164) patients in the delayed-cardioversion group and in 29% (50/171) in the early-cardioversion group. Within 4 weeks following randomization, cardiovascular complications were observed in 10 patients in the delayed-cardioversion group and 8 patients in the early-cardioversion group.

Conclusion: Among patients who presented to the ED with recent-onset, symptomatic atrial fibrillation, wait-and-see approach was found to be noninferior as compared to early cardioversion in attaining a return to sinus rhythm at 4 weeks. (Funded by the Netherlands Organization for Health Research and Development and others; RACE 7 ACWAS ClinicalTrials.gov number, NCT02248753.) *Redrafted abstract

"The more you learn, the more you understand how little you truly know."

—Sasha Scarr Graham

COMMENT

Guidelines recommend immediate cardioversion in patients with recent-onset atrial fibrillation (AF), either pharmacological or electrical. However, studies have shown that many patients with recent-onset AF undergo spontaneous cardioversion. The RACE 7 ACWAS was designed to evaluate a conservative approach to management of recent-onset AF.

In this study, over 200 patients with symptomatic, recent-onset AF (onset within 36 h), and hemodynamically stable, were randomized to immediate cardioversion or conservative management. Cardioversion using flecainide was successful in nearly half of the patients and electrical cardioversion was reserved for the remaining who did not respond to flecainide. In the conservative management group, rate control agents were used to target a heart rate <110 beat/min and the patients were discharged when stable. Patients were re-evaluated at 48 hours and if AF was present, cardioversion was done. The primary outcome measure was presence of normal sinus rhythm (NSR) after 4 weeks. In the conservative management group, 69% of the patients had spontaneous reversion to NSR, and 28% subsequently required cardioversion at 48 hours. In the immediate cardioversion group, 16% patients had spontaneous resolution to NSR while 78% underwent cardioversion. At the end of 4 weeks of follow-up, the conservative approach was noninferior to immediate cardioversion strategy (91% vs. 94%; p = 0.005 for noninferiority). There was no difference in the rate of recurrence of AF between the two groups.

Key Message

⊙ *This is a practice-changing trial, which has shown that symptomatic patients with recent-onset AF need not necessarily undergo immediate cardioversion. Waiting up to 48 hours for spontaneous reversion to NSR may be prudent. If not, delayed cardioversion can be opted for. Immediate cardioversion should be reserved for hemodynamically unstable patients.*

ARTICLE 4

Transcatheter aortic-valve replacement with a balloon-expandable valve in low-risk patients

Mack MJ, Leon MB, Thourani VH, Makkar R, Kodali SK, Russo M, et al. Transcatheter aortic-valve replacement with a balloon-expandable valve in low-risk patients.
N Engl J Med. 2019;380:1695-705.

Abstract*

Introduction: In patients who have aortic stenosis and at intermediate or high-risk for mortality with surgery, major outcomes are reported to be comparable with surgical aortic valve replacement and transcatheter aortic valve replacement (TAVR). There is scarcity of data comparing these two procedures among patients who are at low risk.

Materials and methods: This study included patients who had severe aortic stenosis and low surgical risk; patients were randomized to undergo either surgery or TAVR with transfemoral placement of a balloon-expandable valve. The primary endpoint considered in the study was a composite of stroke, rehospitalization at 1 year, or death. In the as-treated participants, noninferiority testing (with a prespecified margin of 6 percentage points) and superiority testing were done.

Results: Randomization was done in 1,000 patients at 71 centers; mean age was 73 years. The mean Society of Thoracic Surgeons risk score was 1.9% (range of scores: 0–100%; higher scores suggested higher risk of death within 30 days following the procedure). As compared to the surgery group, TAVR group had significantly lower Kaplan–Meier estimate of the rate of the primary composite endpoint at 1 year [8.5% vs. 15.1%; absolute difference −6.6 percentage points; 95% confidence interval (CI) −10.8 to −2.5; p < 0.001 for noninferiority; hazard ratio 0.54; 95% CI 0.37–0.79; p = 0.001 for superiority]. At 30 days, when compared with surgery, TAVR led to a lesser rate of stroke (p = 0.02), and lesser rates of stroke or death (p = 0.01) and new-onset atrial fibrillation (p < 0.001). At 30 days, in comparison with surgery, TAVR showed significantly shorter index hospitalization and significantly lower risk of a poor treatment outcome (low Kansas City Cardiomyopathy Questionnaire score or death) (p < 0.001). Major vascular complications, moderate or severe paravalvular regurgitation, and new permanent pacemaker insertions were comparable between groups.

Conclusion: In patients who had severe aortic stenosis and who were at low surgical risk, TAVR resulted in significantly lower rate of the composite of stroke, rehospitalization at 1 year, or death when compared with surgery. (Funded by Edwards Lifesciences; PARTNER 3 ClinicalTrials.gov number, NCT02675114.)
*Redrafted abstract

"Leap and the net will appear."

—Zen Saying

COMMENT

Transcatheter aortic valve replacement (TAVR) was started as a procedure for patients with prohibitive risk of surgical aortic valve replacement (SAVR). However, an increasing number of studies have established the safety of this procedure in a wide variety of patients with aortic stenosis (AS) who are candidates for bioprosthetic aortic valve. The PARTNER studies have established the safety and efficacy of balloon-expandable valve in patients with high and intermediate risk of surgery. There have been concerns that TAVR is associated with excess risk of complications such as significant paravalvular leak, complete heart block requiring pacemaker implantation, and stroke. Hence, use of TAVR in low-risk patients has been controversial.

The PARTNER 3 study evaluated the role of TAVR in patients at low-operative risk. In this study, 1,000 patients with severe AS and Society for Thoracic Surgery risk score <4% were randomized to either therapy. The primary outcome was a composite of all-cause death, repeat hospitalization, and cerebrovascular accident. After a median follow-up of 1 year, there was a significant reduction in the primary outcome (8.5% vs. 15.1%; p < 0.001). There was significant reduction in risk for cerebrovascular accident (CVA) (1.2% vs. 3.1%; p = 0.04), major bleeding (7.7% vs. 25.9%; p < 0.001) and atrial fibrillation (AF) (5% vs. 29.5%; p < 0.001) with TAVR. While minor paravalvular leak was more with TAVR, there was no difference in the rates of moderate paravalvular leak (0.6% vs. 0.5%; p = 1.0). Rates of pacemaker implantation were also not significantly different in the two groups (6.5% vs. 4.0%; p = 0.09).

This study, however, also has its limitations. The median age of the patients in the study was 73 years. The primary outcome was driven by a reduction in repeat hospitalizations. Data on long-term durability of the valve is limited.

Key Message

⊙ *Transcatheter aortic valve replacement is a feasible and safe option for low-risk patients with AS who are candidates for bioprosthetic valve. But, the generalizability of results is not clear. The median age of the population in the PARTNER 3 study was 73 years. Further, given the high cost of the procedure, surgery still remains the preferred treatment modality in the Indian setting.*

ARTICLE 5

Angiotensin–neprilysin inhibition in acute decompensated heart failure

Velazquez EJ, Morrow DA, DeVore AD, Duffy CI, Ambrosy AP, McCague K, et al.; PIONEER-HF Investigators. Angiotensin–Neprilysin Inhibition in Acute Decompensated Heart Failure.
N Engl J Med. 2019;380(6):539-48.

Abstract*

Background: In the United States, acute decompensated heart failure is responsible for >1 million hospitalizations annually. In patients hospitalized for acute decompensated heart failure, it is still not known whether initiating sacubitril–valsartan therapy is safe and effective or not.

Materials and methods: Patients who have heart failure with reduced ejection fraction and were hospitalized for acute decompensated heart failure at 129 sites in the United States were enrolled in the study. Randomization of the patients was done after hemodynamic stabilization; patients were randomly assigned to receive either sacubitril–valsartan (target dose was 97 mg of sacubitril plus 103 mg of valsartan twice daily) or enalapril (target dose was 10 mg twice daily). The primary efficacy outcome considered in the study was the time-averaged proportional change in the concentration of NT-proBNP (N-terminal pro-B-type natriuretic peptide) from baseline through weeks 4 and 8. The key safety outcomes included the rates of worsening renal function, symptomatic hypotension, hyperkalemia, and angioedema.

Results: Out of total 881 patients, 440 were randomly assigned to sacubitril–valsartan group and 441 patients to enalapril group. As compared to the enalapril group, the time-averaged decrease in the NT-proBNP concentration was significantly higher in the sacubitril–valsartan. In the sacubitril–valsartan group, the ratio of the geometric mean of values obtained at weeks 4 and 8 to the baseline value was 0.53 in comparison to 0.75 in the enalapril group [percent change −46.7% vs. −25.3%; ratio of change with sacubitril–valsartan vs. enalapril 0.71; 95% confidence interval (CI) 0.63–0.81; p < 0.001]. The higher decrease in the concentration of NT-proBNP with sacubitril–valsartan as compared with enalapril was evident as early as week 1 (ratio of change 0.76; 95% CI 0.69–0.85). There was no significant difference in the rates of worsening renal function, symptomatic hypotension, hyperkalemia, and angioedema between the two groups.

Conclusion: The initiation of sacubitril–valsartan therapy in patients with heart failure with reduced ejection fraction, who were hospitalized for acute decompensated heart failure, resulted in more reduction in the concentration of NT-proBNP as compared to enalapril therapy. No significant difference was noted in the rates of worsening renal function, symptomatic hypotension, hyperkalemia, and angioedema between the two groups. (Funded by Novartis; PIONEER-HF ClinicalTrials.gov number, NCT02554890.) *Redrafted abstract

"Angiotensin receptor–neprilysin inhibitors can now be used in acute heart failure also."

COMMENT

Angiotensin receptor-neprilysin inhibitors (ARNIs) are a class of drugs approved in 2015 for the treatment of chronic heart failure after the landmark PARADIGM-HF trial, which was published in New England Journal of Medicine (NEJM). This was one of the largest heart failure trials, which was stopped prematurely since a combination of sacubitril/valsartan (ARNI) in a dose of 200 mg twice daily was found to be better than standard angiotensin-converting enzyme (ACE) inhibitor, enalapril in dose of 10 mg twice daily. In 2016, the American College of Cardiology/American Heart Association (ACC/AHA) guidelines on chronic congestive heart failure (CHF) were upgraded and this agent was recommended as class-1 agent. It was suggested either of the three—ACE inhibitor, angiotensin receptor blocker (ARB), or an ARNI can be used as class-1 agent. In spite of good data, the percentage of patients with chronic CHF getting ARNI is less mainly due to the cost factor.

Neurohormonal activation occurs in heart failure as a compensatory mechanism to maintain blood pressure. However, it proves detrimental since it causes vasoconstriction, salt and water retention, and worsening cardiac remodeling. Blockage of this neurohormonal activation of the renin–angiotensin–aldosterone system (RAAS) is done with ACEIs or ARBs. The excessive activation of sympathetic nervous system is blocked with β-blockers. The third group of agents—aldosterone antagonists are used as blockers. Thus ACEIs/ARBs, β-blockers, and spironolactone, an aldosterone blocker, are used mostly in combination to improve the ejection fraction and survival of these patients. Along with these three neurohormonal systems, which need to be blocked, there are some beneficial neurohormones such as natriuretic peptides, prostaglandins, bradykinin, and adrenomedullin, which are also activated. Neprilysin, which is an endopeptidase, blocks these beneficial hormonal systems. Neprilysin inhibition along with angiotensin inhibition when done together by the ARNI class of drugs offers greater benefits than with ACEIs/ARBs. Patients who are on ACEIs/ARBs and who are not improving should be switched over to ARNIs.

In the present PIONEER-HF study, the ARNIs have been used in acute decompensated heart failure. It shows that this drug is well tolerated in acute heart failure patients who are hospitalized. Thus, after publication of this study, the ARNIs can be used in acute heart failure patients also. This helps to initiate these drugs in the hospital and then they can be continued on a long-term basis. The PIONEER-HF study shows that sacubitril/valsartan (ARNI) is well tolerated and reduces NT-proBNP (N-terminal pro B-type natriuretic peptide) to a greater extent than enalapril.

Key Messages

- *The PARADIGM-HF trial in 2015 showed us that ARNIs are better than ACE inhibitors in chronic heart failure.*
- *The PIONEER-HF study in 2019 now shows us that ARNIs can be started in hospitalized patients with acute heart failure. They are well tolerated and reduce NT-proBNP more than enalapril.*

ARTICLE 6

Large-scale assessment of a smartwatch to identify atrial fibrillation

Perez MV, Mahaffey KW, Hedlin H, Rumsfeld JS, Garcia A, Ferris T, et al. Large-scale assessment of a smartwatch to identify atrial fibrillation.
N Engl J Med. 2019;381:1909-17.

Abstract*

Introduction: Irregular pulses can be detected by use of optical sensors on wearable devices. The proficiency of a smartwatch application (app) for recognizing atrial fibrillation at the time of typical use is still not known.

Material and methods: A smartphone (e.g., Apple iPhone) app was used by participants without atrial fibrillation (as revealed by the participants) who consented to monitoring. In the case when possible atrial fibrillation was recognized by a smartwatch-based irregular pulse notification algorithm, a telemedicine visit was started. Also, an electrocardiography (ECG) patch that was required to be worn for up to 7 days was mailed to the participants. Administration of surveys was done 90 days after the irregular pulse was notified and at the end of the study. The main objectives of the study included estimation of— (1) The number of notified participants who had atrial fibrillation as demonstrated by an ECG patch and (2) The positive predictive value (PPV) of irregular pulse intervals along with a targeted confidence interval (CI) width of 0.10.

Results: Total 419,297 participants were included over 8 months. Monitoring was done for a median of 117 days; notifications of irregular pulse were sent to 0.52% (n = 2,161) participants. By 450 participants, ECG patches were returned consisting of data that could be evaluated, which was applied on an average of 13 days after notification; in these participants, atrial fibrillation was noted in 34% (97.5% CI 29–39) of overall participants and in 35% (97.5% CI 27–43) of participants who were ≥65 years of age. In the participants who were notified of an irregular pulse, the PPV was 0.84 (95% CI 0.76–0.92) for noting atrial fibrillation on the ECG simultaneously with a subsequent irregular pulse notification, and PPV was 0.71 (97.5% CI 0.69–0.74) for noting atrial fibrillation on the ECG simultaneously with a subsequent irregular tachogram. The 90-day survey was returned by 1,376 participants; out of these, 57% participants made contact with healthcare providers outside the study. Serious app-related adverse events were not reported.

Conclusion: Findings showed low probability of receiving an irregular pulse notification. In participants who obtained notification of an irregular pulse, atrial fibrillation on subsequent ECG patch readings was present in 34%; 84% of notifications were found to be concordant with atrial fibrillation. In this siteless (as there was no requirement of on-site visits by the participants) pragmatic study design, a foundation is offered for conducting large-scale pragmatic studies in which adherence or outcomes can be evaluated reliably with devices owned by users. (Funded by Apple; Apple Heart Study ClinicalTrials.gov number, NCT03335800.)
*Redrafted abstract

*"It is not the strongest of the species that survives, nor the most intelligent,
but the one most responsive to change."*

—Charles Darwin

COMMENT

Atrial fibrillation (AF) remains a major cause of stroke worldwide. However, AF is often diagnosed after stroke and significant disability has ensued. There has been a focus toward diagnosing asymptomatic AF or paroxysmal AF in high-risk patients and instituting anticoagulation therapy before stroke occurs. Several studies have shown that opportunistic screening with 12-lead electrocardiography (ECG) and 24-hour Holter have poor utility for paroxysmal AF. While implantable loop recorders have the highest diagnostic yield, such an approach for asymptomatic patients may not be reasonable.

The Apple Heart Study was unique in its design more than its results. In this study, over 400,000 volunteers using Apple Watch and compatible iPhones enrolled themselves when they downloaded the Heart Study application on their phones. The Apple Watch contains an optical sensor that can detect the pulse waveform and generate a graph called tachogram. By comparing the timing of the pulse waves, it can detect irregular beats. Presence of 5 or more of such irregular tachograms in a 48-hour duration generated an alert notification which required the participant to contact a doctor who determined the need for further monitoring. If required, patients were provided ECG patches to be worn for 7 days for diagnosis of AF.

After a median follow-up of 117 days, only 0.52% of the participant received an irregular pulse notification. Of these patients, 658 were provided ECG patches and 450 returned them. Of these, AF was detected in 34%. The limitations of this study include a small number of elderly patients with only 6% patients being aged ≥65 years. Of those who were notified for irregular pulse, only 57% contacted healthcare professionals.

Key Message

⊙ *While it is difficult to generalize the results of the Apple Heart Study, it is remarkable for its design and novelty. Wearable devices generate a large amount of health-related data, which when analyzed at a population level can provide insight into several health practices. This study may usher in the era of "Big Data" into health sciences.*

ARTICLE 7

Dapagliflozin in patients with heart failure and reduced ejection fraction

McMurray JJV, Solomon SD, Inzucchi SE, Køber L, Kosiborod MN, Martinez FA, et al. Dapagliflozin in patients with heart failure and reduced ejection fraction.
N Engl J Med. 2019;381:1995-2008.

Abstract*

Introduction: Among the patients who have type 2 diabetes mellitus (T2DM), sodium-glucose cotransporter-2 (SGLT-2) inhibitors are reported to decrease the risk of a first hospitalization for heart failure (HF), probably via glucose-independent mechanisms. There is a requirement of more data related to the effects of inhibitors of SGLT-2 among patients who have established HF as well as a reduced ejection fraction, irrespective of the absence or presence of T2DM.

Materials and methods: This phase-3, placebo-controlled trial included 4,744 patients with New York Heart Association class II, III, or IV HF as well as an ejection fraction of ≤40%. Patients were randomly assigned to receive either dapagliflozin (dose: 10 mg once daily) or placebo, along with recommended therapy. The primary outcome considered in the study was a composite of worsening HF (hospitalization or an urgent visit leading to intravenous therapy for HF) or cardiovascular death.

Results: In a median duration of 18.2 months, the primary outcome was noted in significantly less number of patients in the dapagliflozin group as compared to that of the placebo group [16.3% (386/2373) vs. 21.2% (502/2371); hazard ratio (HR) 0.74; 95% confidence interval (CI) 0.65–0.85; p < 0.001]. A first worsening HF event was present in 10.0% patients (n = 237) in the dapagliflozin group and in 13.7% patients (n = 326) in the placebo group (HR 0.70; 95% CI 0.59–0.83). Death from cardiovascular causes was present in 9.6% patients (n = 227) in the dapagliflozin group and in 11.5% patients (n = 273) in the placebo group (HR 0.82; 95% CI 0.69–0.98); 11.6% patients (n = 276) and 13.9% patients (n = 329), respectively, died from any cause (HR 0.83; 95% CI 0.71–0.97). There was no significant difference in findings in patients with diabetes compared to those without diabetes. The frequency of adverse events associated with volume depletion, hypoglycemia, and renal dysfunction was comparable among treatment groups.

Conclusion: In patients who have HF as well as a reduced ejection fraction, the risk of worsening HF or death from cardiovascular causes was found to be lesser in patients who received dapagliflozin as compared to those who received placebo, irrespective of the absence or presence of diabetes. (Funded by AstraZeneca; DAPA-HF ClinicalTrials.gov number, NCT03036124.) *Redrafted abstract

"Cure sometimes, treat often, and comfort always."

—**Hippocrates**

COMMENT

Drug approval agencies have required that all anti-diabetic agents be tested for cardiovascular safety. Recently, a group of trials on sodium–glucose cotransporter-2 (SGLT-2) inhibitors showed that these agents are not only safe but also improve outcomes in diabetic patients. The composite data suggests that SGLT-2 inhibitors decrease heart failure (HF) hospitalizations in patients with type 2 diabetes mellitus (T2DM) by reducing incidence of new HF. This benefit appears early after institution of therapy.

The DAPA-HF study was designed to evaluate the role of dapagliflozin as a therapeutic agent for HF irrespective of presence of diabetes. In this study, over 4,500 symptomatic patients with HF with reduced ejection fraction (HFrEF) were randomized to receive 10 mg of dapagliflozin daily or placebo. The median duration of follow-up was 18 months. The primary composite outcome included death from cardiovascular causes or HF exacerbation event (hospitalization for HF or hospital visit requiring use of intravenous agents for HF). The mean age of the population was 66 years. At the end of the follow-up period, there was 26% reduction in the primary outcome (11% vs. 15.6%; HR 0.74; p < 0.001). There was reduction in the individual component of the primary outcome. Further, there was a reduction in all-cause mortality (11.6% vs. 13.9%; HR 0.83; 95% CI 0.71–0.97) and overall symptom status of the patients receiving dapagliflozin. This benefit was consistent irrespective of status of DM, age, and initial health condition. Other benefits noted with SGLT-2 inhibitor therapy in this study were reduction in serum creatinine levels, blood pressure, and body weight. There was no difference in incidence of adverse effects between the two groups including dehydration, hypoglycemic episodes, renal complications, or bone fractures. The limitations of this study include a low rate of use of angiotensin-receptor neprilysin inhibitors (ARNIs) and only a small number of patients had advanced HF.

Key Message

⊙ *Use of dapagliflozin in patients with HFrEF is associated with improvement of cardiovascular outcomes irrespective of the presence of diabetes. The drug is safe and is a new class of agents in the armamentarium against HF.*

ARTICLE 8

Withdrawal of pharmacological treatment for heart failure in patients with recovered dilated cardiomyopathy (TRED-HF): an open-label, pilot, randomised trial

halliday BP, Wassall R, Lota AS, Khalique Z, Gregson J, Newsome S, et al. Withdrawal of pharmacological treatment for heart failure in patients with recovered dilated cardiomyopathy (TRED-HF): an open-label, pilot, randomised trial. *Lancet. 2019;393(10166):61-73.*

Abstract

Background: Patients with dilated cardiomyopathy whose symptoms and cardiac function have recovered often ask whether their medications can be stopped. The safety of withdrawing treatment in this situation is unknown.

Methods: We did an open-label, pilot, randomized trial to examine the effect of phased withdrawal of heart failure medications in patients with previous dilated cardiomyopathy who were now asymptomatic, whose left ventricular ejection fraction (LVEF) had improved from <40 to 50% or greater, whose left ventricular end-diastolic volume (LVEDV) had normalized, and who had an N-terminal pro-B-type natriuretic peptide (NT-pro-BNP) concentration <250 ng/L. Patients were recruited from a network of hospitals in the UK, assessed at one center (Royal Brompton and Harefield NHS Foundation Trust, London, UK), and randomly assigned (1:1) to phased withdrawal or continuation of treatment. After 6 months, patients in the continued treatment group had treatment withdrawn by the same method. The primary endpoint was a relapse of dilated cardiomyopathy within 6 months, defined by a reduction in LVEF of >10% and to <50%, an increase in LVEDV by >10% and to higher than the normal range, a two-fold rise in NT-pro-BNP concentration and to >400 ng/L, or clinical evidence of heart failure, at which point treatments were re-established. The primary analysis was by intention to treat. This trial is registered with ClinicalTrials.gov, number NCT02859311.

Findings: Between April 21, 2016 and August 22, 2017, 51 patients were enrolled. Around 25 were randomly assigned to the treatment withdrawal group and 26 to continue treatment. Over the first 6 months, 11 (44%) patients randomly assigned to treatment withdrawal met the primary endpoint of relapse compared with none of those assigned to continue treatment [Kaplan–Meier estimate of event rate 45.7% (95% CI 28.5–67.2); p = 0.0001]. After 6 months, 25 (96%) of 26 patients assigned initially to continue treatment attempted its withdrawal. During the following 6 months, nine patients met the primary endpoint of relapse [Kaplan–Meier estimate of event rate 36.0% (95% CI 20.6–57.8)]. No deaths were reported in either group and three serious adverse events were reported in the treatment withdrawal group: Hospital admissions for noncardiac chest pain, sepsis, and an elective procedure.

Interpretation: Many patients deemed to have recovered from dilated cardiomyopathy will relapse following treatment withdrawal. Until robust predictors of relapse are defined, treatment should continue indefinitely.

"Medicine heals doubts as well as diseases."

—**Karl Marx**

COMMENT

Many patients of dilated cardiomyopathy (DCM) respond well to medical therapy; in some, the symptoms disappear and left ventricle (LV) function improves to near-normal levels. Most of such patients are on polypharmacy including diuretics, mineralocorticoid receptor antagonist (MRA), beta-blockers (BB), and angiotensin-converting enzyme inhibitors (ACEIs) or angiotensin receptor blockers (ARBs). These drugs incur cost and can have long-term side effects. The safety of stopping or downgrading therapy in such patient population is unknown.

The TRED-HF trial tried to look into this unknown, but clinically relevant area. Around 51 cases of DCM with heart failure (HF) who had improved [left ventricular ejection fraction (LVEF) >50%, left ventricular end-diastolic volume (LVEDV) normalized, and NT-pro-BNP normalized] were randomized to gradual downgrading of therapy in a graded method. The primary endpoint was reduction of LVEF by 10% or LVEF going below 50%, LVEDV increase by >10%, 2 times increase in NT-pro-BNP to reaching to >400 pg/mL or development of clinical HF. Of the 51 patients, half (n = 25) were withdrawn from therapy while the other half (n = 26) continued on usual treatment. The withdrawal was done in a graded manner. Diuretics were reduced first, followed by MRA, then beta-blockers and lastly ACEI/ARB. After 6 months, post-exposure prophylaxis (PEP) (relapse) was noted in 44% of "withdrawal" group compared to none in continued group. After 6 months, those in the "continued treatment" arm were put on withdrawal. On follow-up, 36% of those newly downtitrated, again went for PEP (relapse).

This data, though small, conclusively supports continuation of treatment for patients of dilated cardiomyopathy with HF who have stabilized with therapy, since chance of relapse is very high on therapy withdrawal.

This data has significant implications, especially in clinical management of HF in India, where patients ask regarding reduction of pills since they are feeling fine. The physician asks for a battery of tests (echocardiogram and NT-pro-BNP). If these tests too show good control, the physician is in a dilemma as to whether he should curtail therapy or not. The economic burden on the exchequer, insurance company, and the family of the patient pressurizes him in trying to lower the pills since some of them are very expensive.

This trial clearly proves that reduction of medication result in a high and unacceptable rate of relapse in those patients controlled on therapy.

Key Message

⊙ *Despite reduction of symptoms and normalization of echocardiographic parameters and NT-pro-BNP, therapy (beta-blockers, MRA, ACEI, and ARB) in dilated cardiomyopathy should not be withdrawn in the long run. Withdrawal of therapy results in relapse in a substantial number of patients.*

ARTICLE 9

Efficacy and safety of statin therapy in older people: a meta-analysis of individual participant data from 28 randomised controlled trials

Cholesterol Treatment Trialists' Collaboration. Efficacy and safety of statin therapy in older people: A meta-analysis of individual participant data from 28 randomised controlled trials.
Lancet. 2019;393(10170):407-15.

Abstract

Background: Statin therapy has been shown to reduce major vascular events and vascular mortality in a wide range of individuals, but there is uncertainty about its efficacy and safety among older people. We undertook a meta-analysis of data from all large statin trials to compare the effects of statin therapy at different ages.

Methods: In this meta-analysis, randomized trials of statin therapy were eligible, if they aimed to recruit at least 1,000 participants with a scheduled treatment duration of at least 2 years. We analyzed individual participant data from 22 trials (n = 134,537) and detailed summary data from one trial (n = 12,705) of statin therapy versus control, plus individual participant data from five trials of more intensive versus less intensive statin therapy (n = 39,612). We subdivided participants into six age groups (55 years or younger, 56–60 years, 61–65 years, 66–70 years, 71–75 years, and older than 75 years). We estimated effects on major vascular events (i.e., major coronary events, strokes, and coronary revascularizations), cause-specific mortality, and cancer incidence as the rate ratio (RR) per 1.0 mmol/L reduction in low-density lipoprotein cholesterol (LDL-C). We compared proportional risk reductions in different age subgroups by use of standard χ^2 tests for heterogeneity when there were two groups, or trend when there were more than two groups.

Findings: Around 14,483 (8%) of 186,854 participants in the 28 trials were older than 75 years at randomization, and the median follow-up duration was 4.9 years. Overall, statin therapy or a more intensive statin regimen produced a 21% (RR 0.79; 95% CI 0.77–0.81) proportional reduction in major vascular events per 1.0 mmol/L reduction in LDL-C. We observed a significant reduction in major vascular events in all age groups. Although proportional reductions in major vascular events diminished slightly with age, this trend was not statistically significant (p_{trend} = 0.06). Overall, statin or more intensive therapy yielded a 24% (RR: 0.76; 95% CI: 0.73–0.79) proportional reduction in major coronary events per 1.0 mmol/L reduction in LDL cholesterol, and with increasing age, we observed a trend toward smaller proportional risk reductions in major coronary events (p_{trend} = 0.009). We observed a 25% (RR 0.75; 95% CI 0.73–0.78) proportional reduction in the risk of coronary revascularization procedures with statin therapy or a more intensive statin regimen per 1.0 mmol/L lower LDL-C, which did not differ significantly across age groups (p_{trend} = 0.6). Similarly, the proportional reductions in stroke of any type (RR 0.84; 95% CI 0.80–0.89) did not differ significantly across age groups (p_{trend} = 0.7). After exclusion of four trials, which enrolled only patients with heart failure or undergoing renal dialysis (among whom statin therapy has not been shown to be effective), the trend to smaller proportional risk reductions with increasing age persisted for major coronary events (p_{trend} = 0.01), and remained nonsignificant for major vascular events (p_{trend} = 0.3). The proportional reduction in major vascular events was similar, irrespective of age, among patients with pre-existing vascular disease (p_{trend} =0.2), but appeared smaller among older than among younger individuals not known to have vascular disease (p_{trend} = 0.05). We found a 12% (RR 0.88; 95% CI 0.85–0.91) proportional reduction in vascular mortality per 1.0 mmol/L reduction in LDL-C, with a trend toward smaller proportional reductions with older age (p_{trend} = 0.004), but this trend did not persist after exclusion of the heart failure or dialysis trials (p_{trend} = 0.2). Statin therapy had no effect at any age on nonvascular mortality, cancer death, or cancer incidence.

Interpretation: Statin therapy produces significant reductions in major vascular events irrespective of age, but there is less direct evidence of benefit among patients older than 75 years who do not already have evidence of occlusive vascular disease. This limitation is now being addressed by further trials.

"There is no need for fiction in medicine, for the facts will always beat anything you fancy."
—Sir Arthur Conan Doyle

COMMENT

There is always an inhibition in prescribing high-dose, intensive statin therapy, in elderly people; many physicians are not convinced about the long-term efficacy while worried about the safety of such therapy. This often results in prescription of subtherapeutic "small" doses of statin in this population.

In this meta-analysis, 28 trials (trials randomizing >1,000 patients with a minimum follow-up of 2 years) were included. Patients were stratified to age groups of <55 years, 56–60 years, 61–65 years, 66–70 years, 71–75 years, and >75 years; the primary endpoint was vascular events, which comprised of major coronary events, stroke, and coronary revascularization. The other endpoints were cause-specific mortality.

A total of 184,854 patients were eligible in these 28 trials, among whom 8% (14,483) were older than 75 years of age.

The results show that during a follow-up of an average 4.9 years, overall 1 mmol (40 mg/dL) reduction of low-density lipoprotein (LDL) resulted in 21% reduction of vascular events. Statins benefited patients by reduction of vascular events in every age group, including those above 75 years of age, but above the age of 75 years, the benefit tended to be lesser.

The interaction of age-related loss of benefit was noted; it persisted even when the data was reanalyzed after excluding four trials where heart failure and dialysis was included (areas where statin therapy had minimum benefit).

Analyzed individually, major coronary events reduction at age above 75 years was still significant, while coronary revascularization and stroke were not.

A further analysis showed that those (>75 years of age) with vascular disease benefited by 15% (substantial) while those without vascular disease had little benefit.

With increase in life expectancy and reduction of family size, Indian epidemiology is quickly progressing to society being overwhelmed by aging individuals, many of them are candidates for statin therapy by standard criteria. The physician's perception of lack of long-term benefit by statins in the age group above 75 years is of concern.

This study clearly shows that statins need to be prescribed to those who have a proper indication, and that clearly include elders above the age of 75 years. Those with pre-existing vascular disease benefit more as is expected, while decision in those without vascular disease needs to be individualized.

Key Message

⊙ *Elderly population with age >75 years benefit on exposure to intensive high-dose statin therapy, especially those with pre-existing vascular disease. Decision for statin therapy in elderly people with no vascular disease needs to be individualized.*

ARTICLE 10

Effect of ultra-short-term treatment of patients with iron deficiency or anaemia undergoing cardiac surgery: a prospective randomised trial

Spahn DR, Schoenrath F, Spahn GH, Seifert B, Stein P, Theusinger OM, et al. Effect of ultra-short-term treatment of patients with iron deficiency or anaemia undergoing cardiac surgery: a prospective randomised trial. *Lancet. 2019;393(10187):2201-12.*

Abstract

Background: Anemia and iron deficiency are frequent in patients scheduled for cardiac surgery. This study assessed whether immediate preoperative treatment could result in reduced perioperative red blood cell (RBC) transfusions and improved outcome.

Methods: In this single-center, randomized, double-blind, parallel-group controlled study, patients undergoing elective cardiac surgery with anemia [n = 253; hemoglobin (Hb) concentration <120 g/L in women and Hb <130 g/L in men] or isolated iron deficiency (n = 252; ferritin <100 µg/L, no anemia) were enrolled. Participants were randomly assigned (1:1) with the use of a computer-generated range minimization (allocation probability 0.8) to receive either placebo or combination treatment consisting of a slow infusion of 20 mg/kg ferric carboxymaltose, 40,000 U subcutaneous erythropoietin alpha, 1 mg subcutaneous vitamin B12, and 5 mg oral folic acid or placebo on the day before surgery. Primary outcome was the number of RBC transfusions during the first 7 days. This trial is registered with ClinicalTrials.gov, number NCT02031289.

Findings: Between January 9, 2014 and July 19, 2017, 1,006 patients were enrolled; 505 with anemia or isolated iron deficiency and 501 in the registry. The combination treatment significantly reduced RBC transfusions from a median of one unit in the placebo group (IQR 0–3) to zero units in the treatment group {0–2, during the first 7 days [odds ratio 0.70 (95% CI 0.50–0.98)] for each threshold of number of RBC transfusions, p = 0.036} and until postoperative day 90 (p = 0.018). Despite fewer RBC units transfused, patients in the treatment group had a higher hemoglobin concentration, higher reticulocyte count, and a higher reticulocyte hemoglobin content during the first 7 days (p ≤ 0.001). Combined allogeneic transfusions were less in the treatment group [0 (IQR 0–2)] versus the placebo group [1 (0–3)] during the first 7 days (p = 0.038) and until postoperative day 90 (p = 0.019). Around 73 (30%) serious adverse events were reported in the treatment group versus 79 (33%) in the placebo group.

Interpretation: An ultra-short-term combination treatment with intravenous iron, subcutaneous erythropoietin alpha, vitamin B12, and oral folic acid reduced RBC and total allogeneic blood product transfusions in patients with preoperative anemia or isolated iron deficiency undergoing elective cardiac surgery.

"Medicine is not merely a science but an art. The character of the physician may act more powerfully upon the patient than the drugs employed."

—**Paracelsus**

COMMENT

Cardiac surgery can be made safer by preoperative assessment and correction of comorbidities. Anemia and iron deficiency are common comorbidities that are often picked up for the first time prior to cardiac surgery. The choice then narrows down between postponing the procedure and correcting the underlying anemia and iron deficiency, or accept the procedure with an elevated risk.

In this trial, the authors have tried a "quick-fix" correction by a cocktail of iron supplement and vitamins and its effect on the procedure. Anemia was defined as hemoglobin level <12 g% in women and <13 g% in males. Iron deficiency was diagnosed by serum ferritin <100 µg/L.

253 cases of anemia and 252 cases of iron deficiency were identified and randomized. The primary endpoint was need for perioperative red blood cell (RBC) transfusion.

Patients were given a cocktail of IV ferric carboxymaltose 20 mg/kg slow IV infusion, 40,000 units of subcutaneous erythropoietin alpha, 1 mg of vitamin B12 by subcutaneous injection, 5 mg oral folic acid, on the day prior to surgery.

The treatment increased hemoglobin level, reticulocyte count, and reticulocyte hemoglobin and resulted in a reduction in the need for perioperative packed red cell transfusion in the first 7 days as well as till postoperative day 90.

India had a huge burden of chronic anemia, mostly iron deficiency, data indicate that around 45% of the population may be anemic. The outcome of cardiac surgery is often dependent on preoperative comorbidities.

Key Message

⊙ *A single dose of a preoperative cocktail of IV iron, subcutaneous erythropoietin, vitamin B12, and oral folic acid tends to normalize this deficiency and likely improves outcome of surgery, by reducing the need for RBC transfusion.*

ARTICLE 11

Irbesartan in marfan syndrome (AIMS): a double-blind, placebo-controlled randomised trial

Mullen M, Jin XY, Child A, Stuart AG, Dodd M, Aragon-Martin JA, et al. Irbesartan in Marfan syndrome (AIMS): a double-blind, placebo-controlled randomised trial.
Lancet. 2020;394(10216):2263-70.

Abstract

Background: Irbesartan, a long-acting selective angiotensin-1 receptor inhibitor, in Marfan syndrome might reduce aortic dilatation, which is associated with dissection and rupture. We aimed to determine the effects of irbesartan on the rate of aortic dilatation in children and adults with Marfan syndrome.

Methods: We did a placebo-controlled, double-blind randomized trial at 22 centers in the UK. Individuals aged 6–40 years with clinically confirmed Marfan syndrome were eligible for inclusion. Study participants were all given 75 mg open-label irbesartan once daily, then randomly assigned to 150 mg of irbesartan (increased to 300 mg as tolerated) or matching placebo. Aortic diameter was measured by echocardiography at baseline and then annually. All images were analyzed by a core laboratory blinded to treatment allocation. The primary endpoint was the rate of aortic root dilatation. This trial is registered with ISRCTN, number ISRCTN90011794.

Findings: Between March 14, 2012 and May 1, 2015, 192 participants were recruited and randomly assigned to irbesartan (n = 104) or placebo (n = 88), and all were followed for up to 5 years. Median age at recruitment was 18 years (IQR 12–28), 99 (52%) were female, mean blood pressure was 110/65 mm Hg (SDs 16 and 12), and 108 (56%) were taking β-blockers. Mean baseline aortic root diameter was 34.4 mm in the irbesartan group (SD 5.8) and placebo group (5.5). The mean rate of aortic root dilatation was 0.53 mm/year (95% CI 0.39–0.67) in the irbesartan group compared with 0.74 mm/year (0.60–0.89) in the placebo group, with a difference in means of −0.22 mm/year (−0.41 to −0.02; p = 0.030). The rate of change in aortic Z score was also reduced by irbesartan (difference in means −0.10/year, 95% CI −0.19 to −0.01; p = 0.035). Irbesartan was well tolerated with no observed differences in rates of serious adverse events.

Interpretation: Irbesartan is associated with a reduction in the rate of aortic dilatation in children and young adults with Marfan syndrome and can reduce the incidence of aortic complications.

"Research is a formalized curiosity. It is poking and prying with a purpose."
—**Zora Neale Hurston**

COMMENT

Marfan syndrome is an autosomal-dominant disease caused by mutation of *FBN1* gene. The main morbidity and mortality result from progressive dilatation of aortic root, leading to dissection and catastrophic aortic rupture. The standard therapy is to put them on beta-blockers to reduce wall stress and slow down the dilatation. It is theorized that excessive transforming growth factor (TGF)-beta is a causal factor for the aortic pathology, and institution of an angiotensin receptor blocker (ARB) might retard this process.

Irbesartan, an ARB, at a dose of 300 mg daily was pitted against placebo in this trial. Patients of confirmed Marfan syndrome were included. The average age was 6–40 years, and median age was 18 years. Patients went through a run-in phase with everyone receiving 75 mg daily dose of irbesartan for a week, after which it was up-titrated to 150 mg and then 300 mg of irbesartan (104 patients), while another 88 patients continued on placebo. The primary endpoint was dilatation of the aortic root as estimated by annual echocardiography.

Average age of patients was 18 years, half of them females and 56% received beta-blockers at baseline. The entry blood pressure was 110/65 mm Hg. The follow-up was for 5 years. The mean aortic root size at study entry was 34.4 mm.

At the end of follow-up, the irbesartan arm showed significantly slower rate of progression of aortic dilatation at 0.53 mm/year compared to 0.74 mm/year in the placebo arm. There were no excess adverse effects in the irbesartan arm. There were five interventions in the irbesartan arm versus four in the placebo arm (surgery/stenting), but this trial was not designed or powered to look into event rate. In a subset where TGF-beta was estimated, there was no significant difference between the irbesartan and placebo arm.

The traditional treatment of Marfan syndrome to prevent and slow down aortic root dilatation is beta-blockers. In this trial 56% patients were on beta-blockers. The benefits were not significantly different in the irbesartan arm in presence or absence of beta-blockers. Since the benefit was more in the beta-blocker (plus irbesartan) arm, it can be assumed that both beta-blockers and ARB benefit in prevention of catastrophic aortic root dissection and rupture by slowing down dilation rate as shown in this very important trial.

Key Message

⊙ *Aortic root dilatation, which is a precursor of catastrophic aortic dissection and aortic rupture, in Marfan syndrome, is slowed down by irbesartan and ARB. The effect is independent of beta-blockers.*

ARTICLE 12

Safety and efficacy of bempedoic acid to reduce LDL cholesterol

Ray KK, Bays HE, Catapano AL, Lalwani ND, Bloedon LT, Sterling LR, et al. Safety and efficacy of bempedoic acid to reduce LDL cholesterol.
N Engl J Med. 2019;380(11):1022-32.

Abstract*

Background: As reported in short-term studies, bempedoic acid [an inhibitor of adenosine triphosphate (ATP) citrate lyase] decreases low-density lipoprotein cholesterol LDL-C levels. There is scarcity of long-term studies related to the safety and efficacy of bempedoic acid treatment in patients with hypercholesterolemia and received guideline-recommended statin therapy.

Methods: This was a randomized, controlled trial that included patients who had atherosclerotic cardiovascular disease, heterozygous familial hypercholesterolemia, or both. Patients was required to have LDL-C level of minimum 70 mg/dL, while receiving maximally tolerated statin therapy with/without added lipid-lowering therapy. In the study, maximally tolerated statin therapy was defined as the highest intensity statin regimen, which a patient was able to maintain (as decided by the investigator). Patients were randomized in a 2:1 ratio to receive either bempedoic acid or placebo. The primary endpoint considered in the study was safety; the principal secondary endpoint (principal efficacy endpoint) was the percentage change in the level of LDL-C at week 12 of 52 weeks.

Results: Total 2,230 patients were included in the study that were randomized to bempedoic acid (n = 1,488) and placebo (n = 742).

At baseline, the mean (±SD) LDL-C level was 103.2 (±29.4) mg/dL. There was no significant difference in the incidence of adverse events [bempedoic acid vs. placebo, 78.5% (1167/1488) vs. 78.7% (584/742)] and serious adverse events [14.5% (216/1487) vs. 14.0% (104/742)] during the intervention period. However, as compared to placebo group, the incidence of adverse events resulting in discontinuation of the regimen was greater in the bempedoic acid group (10.9% vs. 7.1%) and incidence of gout was also higher in the bempedoic acid group (1.2% vs. 0.3%).

At week 12, bempedoic acid decreased the mean LDL-C level by 19.2 mg/dL, which represents a change of –16.5% from baseline (difference vs. placebo in change from baseline, –18.1 percentage points; 95% confidence interval –20.0 to –16.1; p < 0.001). A consistency in safety and efficacy findings was noted, irrespective of the intensity of background statin therapy.

Conclusion: This 52-week trial demonstrated that bempedoic acid added to maximally tolerated statin therapy did not result in an increased incidence of overall adverse events as compared to placebo and caused significantly reduced levels of LDL-C. (Funded by Esperion Therapeutics; CLEAR Harmony ClinicalTrials.gov number, NCT02666664.) *Redrafted abstract

"Half of science is putting forth the right questions."

—Francis Bacon

COMMENT

Since the understanding of the role of low-density lipoprotein (LDL) in development and progression of atherosclerotic vascular disease by Goldstein and Brown, efforts to lower it continue. Despite statins being a game changer, many subpopulations of poor responders to statins remain challenging.

Bempedoic acid is an inhibitor of adenosine triphosphate (ATP) citrate lyase, which lowers LDL. This study looked into the safety and efficacy of this new molecule.

Patients of atherosclerotic cardiovascular disease or heterozygous familial hypercholesterolemia or both with a LDL level of >70 mg%

despite maximally tolerated doses of statin therapy were included in this study. The primary endpoint was safety. The efficacy endpoint was percentage lowering of LDL.

Total 2,230 patients were randomized, 1,488 to bempedoic acid and 742 to placebo, on top of maximally tolerated statin therapy. Serious adverse effects were observed in around 14% patients in both groups (similar). Adverse effects needing to stoppage of bempedoic acid versus placebo were also similar (10.9 vs. 7.7%).

Efficacy endpoint was vastly different, with bempedoic acid ending up with an LDL lowering of 16.5% lower compared to the control group (lower by a mean level of 19.2 mg% of LDL).

The standard algorithm instructs physicians to first try maximally tolerated dose of statins (atorvastatin 80 mg or rosuvastatin 40 mg). If LDL is not reaching a goal level (70 mg% in ASCVD or very high-risk group), addition of Ezetimibe is advocated. If this fails, PCSK9 inhibitors are to be initiated as the next step. Despite such algorithm, it is often difficult to attain LDL goal in familial hypercholesterolemia.

Introduction of bempedoic acid, which acts on the same cholesterol synthesis pathway, is attractive new option in this background, since this study shows that it has an acceptable safety/efficacy profile.

Future studies may throw light on combination therapy of statins, bempedoic acid, and PCSK9 inhibitors in resistant cases of hypercholesterolemia.

Key Message

- ⊙ *Bempedoic acid is a new molecule, which lowers cholesterol on top of statin therapy. This study for the first time has shown its safety and efficacy in atherosclerotic coronary vascular disease and heterozygous familial hypercholesterolemia.*

ARTICLE 13

Coronary angiography after cardiac arrest without ST-segment elevation

Lemkes JS, Janssens GN, van der Hoeven NW, Jewbali LSD, Dubois EA, Meuwissen M, et al. Coronary angiography after cardiac arrest without ST-segment elevation.
N Engl J Med. 2019;380(15):1397-407.

Abstract*

Background: One of the main causes of out-of-hospital cardiac arrest is ischemic heart disease. In the treatment of patients who have been successfully resuscitated following a cardiac arrest [in the absence of ST-segment elevation myocardial infarction (STEMI)], the role of immediate coronary angiography and percutaneous coronary intervention (PCI) is still not certain.

Materials and methods: This was a multicenter trial in which randomization of 552 patients who had cardiac arrest (without signs of STEMI) was done to undergo either immediate coronary angiography or coronary angiography, which was delayed until after neurologic recovery. PCI was done in all patients, if indicated. The primary endpoint considered in the study was survival at 90 days. Secondary endpoints were survival at 90 days with good cerebral performance or mild/moderate disability, duration of catecholamine support, myocardial injury, recurrence of ventricular tachycardia, markers of shock, mechanical ventilation duration, major bleeding, occurrence of acute kidney injury, time to target temperature, requirement for renal replacement therapy, and neurologic status at discharge from the intensive care unit.

Results: At 90 days, 64.5% (176/273) patients of the immediate angiography group and 67.2% (178/265) patients of the delayed angiography group were alive [odds ratio 0.89; 95% confidence interval (CI) 0.62–1.27; p = 0.51]. The median time to target temperature in the immediate angiography group and the delayed angiography group was 5.4 hours and 4.7 hours, respectively (ratio of geometric means 1.19; 95% CI 1.04–1.36). Remaining secondary endpoints were comparable between both groups.

Conclusion: In patients who had been successfully resuscitated after out-of-hospital cardiac arrest and were without signs of STEMI, when compared to strategy of delayed angiography, strategy of immediate angiography was not found to be better in terms of overall survival at 90 days. (Funded by the Netherlands Heart Institute and others; COACT Netherlands Trial Register number, NTR4973.) *Redrafted abstract

"Treatment without prevention is simply unsustainable."

—**Bill Gates**

COMMENT

Out of hospital cardiac arrests most often have a bad outcome, many succumb before they can reach a hospital. Widespread global initiation and teaching and awareness of life support and resuscitation now enable a greater number of cases to get a bystander-initiated cardiopulmonary resuscitation (CPR) and subsequent hospitalization. Large percentage of out-of-hospital cardiac arrests occur secondary to coronary artery disease and acute coronary syndrome. Post-hospitalization, patients of ST-segment elevation myocardial infarction (STEMI) invariably go straight to cardiac catheterization laboratory, get a coronary angiogram done, and get their culprit lesions opened up by primary PCI.

But, the management strategy of those brought in with cardiac arrest with no clear evidence of STEMI in the electrocardiogram (ECG) remains controversial. While some get an immediate angiography done and the possible culprit lesion opened up, others wait till substantial neurologic recovery and get an angiogram done later.

This trial enrolled 552 cases of out-of-hospital cardiac arrest, with ECG showing no clear ST-elevation myocardial infarction (MI). They were randomized to either immediate angiography and necessary intervention or a delayed approach where angiography was planned after substantial neurologic recovery. While in the first group, angiogram was done in around 2.3 hours after hospital admission; in the delayed group, it was undertaken, on an average after 120 hours.

The primary endpoint was survival at 90 days. The secondary endpoints included a long list of survival at 90 days with good cerebral performance, mild or moderate disability, myocardial injury, duration of catecholamine support, markers of shock, recurrence of ventricular tachycardia (VT), duration of mechanical ventilation, major bleed, acute kidney injury, renal replacement therapy, time to target temperature, and neurological status at discharge.

Baseline data showed that the patients had an average age of 65 years, and 75% were males. Patients had substantial atherosclerotic vascular risk, 50% were hypertensives, 20% diabetic, 20% smokers, 25% dyslipidemia, previous coronary artery disease (CAD) in 40%, previous MI in 26%, cerebrovascular accident (CVA) in 6%, and revascularization in 40%. Overall, single vessel disease was found in 30% patients, 2-vessel disease in 20%, and 3-vessel disease in 15% patients. Around 36% patients had no significant lesions by angiogram.

In the immediate intervention arm, 97% had an angiogram done, 33% had PCI, 6% coronary artery bypass grafting (CABG) while in the conservative arm 65% had angiogram with 24% PCI and 9% CABG.

The results showed no substantial difference or benefit in the immediate angiogram arm compared to the delayed "conservative" arm in this trial.

In this study, patients were managed extremely well, before reaching the hospital. The time from cardiac arrest to initiation of CPR was 2 minutes and return of spontaneous circulation was 15 minutes. Despite that, the primary and secondary endpoints showed no benefit in the "rushed" angiogram group.

In India, where an angiogram and subsequent revascularization imparts substantial cost burden on the patient's family and most patients not being health insured, this area is challenging. Since most cardiac arrests come in an apparently normal people, the family wants all medical support including an angiogram and necessary revascularization, in the hope of a full recovery. Often, the neurologic recovery is suboptimal and with passage of time, in a substantially neurologically debilitated patient, the original decision of rushing into angiogram is questioned.

Key Message

⊚ *In the Indian scenario, out-of-hospital cardiac arrest with no clear STEMI in ECG should be monitored for neurologic recovery and a strategy of delayed angiogram pursued, rather than rushing through an angiogram and revascularization.*

ARTICLE 14

Antithrombotic therapy after acute coronary syndrome or PCI in atrial fibrillation

Lopes RD, Heizer G, Aronson R, Vora AN, Massaro T, Mehran R, et al. Antithrombotic therapy after acute coronary syndrome or PCI in atrial fibrillation.
N Engl J Med. 2019;380(16):1509-24.

Abstract*

Introduction: Appropriate antithrombotic regimens are still not clear for patients having atrial fibrillation with an acute coronary syndrome or who underwent percutaneous coronary intervention (PCI).

Materials and methods: This was an international trial with a two-by-two factorial design, in which randomization was done of patients who had atrial fibrillation with an acute coronary syndrome or who underwent PCI and were planning to receive a P2Y12 inhibitor to take apixaban or a vitamin K antagonist and to take aspirin or matching placebo for 6 months. The primary outcome considered in the study was major or clinically relevant nonmajor bleeding. Secondary outcomes were hospitalization, composite of ischemic events, and death.

Results: Total 4,614 patients from 33 countries were included. No significant interactions were noted between the two randomization factors on the primary or secondary outcomes. As compared to patients who received vitamin K antagonist, patients who received apixaban had significantly less major or clinically relevant nonmajor bleeding (10.5% vs. 14.7%) [hazard ratio (HR) 0.69; 95% confidence interval (CI) 0.58–0.81; $p < 0.001$ for both noninferiority and superiority]. Major or clinically relevant nonmajor bleeding was present in 16.1% of the patients who received aspirin, in comparison to 9.0% of the patients who received placebo (HR 1.89; 95% CI 1.59–2.24; $p < 0.001$). As compared to the vitamin K antagonist group, apixaban group had a lower incidence of death or hospitalization (23.5% vs. 27.4%; HR 0.83; 95% CI 0.74–0.93; $p = 0.002$) and comparable incidence of ischemic events. The incidence of death or hospitalization and of ischemic events was comparable between the aspirin and placebo groups.

Conclusion: Among the patients who had atrial fibrillation and a recent acute coronary syndrome or PCI and were treated with a P2Y12 inhibitor (an antithrombotic regimen that included apixaban), without aspirin, led to reduced bleeding and less number of hospitalizations; however, no significant differences were observed in the incidence of ischemic events than regimens that consisted of a vitamin K antagonist, aspirin, or both. (Funded by Bristol-Myers Squibb and Pfizer; AUGUSTUS ClinicalTrials.gov number, NCT02415400.)
*Redrafted abstract

"Knowledge is the acquiring of facts, understanding is the interpreting of the facts, wisdom the application."

—Edwin Louis Cole

COMMENT

Atrial fibrillation (AF) and acute coronary syndrome (ACS) both occur commonly in cardiology practice. A large number of ACS patients also end up getting a percutaneous procedure (PCI) done. The major concern in AF is stroke and needs an oral anticoagulant (OAC) either a vitamin K antagonists (VKA) or novel oral anticoagulants (NOACS) to prevent stroke. ACS/PCI needs dual antiplatelet (DAP) therapy to prevent ischemic events especially stent thrombosis. OACs or NOACS do not prevent stent thrombosis, and DAP has little effect on stroke prevention in AF.

This has led to the logic of combining an OAC with DAP. But, this strategy has resulted in excess bleeding. The attempt to hit the sweet spot of maximum efficacy in terms of prevention of ischemic events, stent thrombosis and stroke with least bleeding are still elusive.

This makes the AUGUSTUS trial so important and clinically relevant.

Total 4,614 patients of AF developing an ACS or undergoing PCI (or both) were randomized, within 14 days of index event of ACS or PCI (mean 6.6 days) in a 2 × 2 factorial design to either apixaban (NOAC) or warfarin (VKA); or aspirin or placebo. Patients of severe renal insufficiency, recent intracranial hemorrhage, major bleeding, or planned coronary artery bypass grafting (CABG) were excluded. The primary outcome was bleeding (major or clinically relevant nonmajor bleeding). The secondary endpoint was death, hospital admission, as well as composite ischemic events, which included myocardial infarction (MI), stroke, stent thrombosis, or urgent revascularization.

Results indicated overwhelming safety of NOAC-based therapy compared to VKA (primary event occurrence of apixaban 10.5%; warfarin 14.7%) and as expected placebo over aspirin. Death, hospitalization, and ischemic events also had a lower incidence in the apixaban group compared to VKA. When primary event occurrence (bleeding) was analyzed as event rate per 100 patient years, combination therapy with the apixaban with placebo (on top of P2Y12) was the best (16.8), while warfarin plus placebo (26.7) and apixaban plus aspirin (33.6) progressively worse with warfarin + aspirin the worst (49.1).

It is important to understand that all these were on top of background P2Y12 inhibitor therapy, and in AUGUSTUS, the P2Y12 was clopidogrel in 92.6% cases.

With the data available from PIONEER AF PCI testing of rivaroxaban and REDUAL PCI trial looking at dabigatran bringing out results on similar lines, the faith in NOACS is bolstered in AUGUSTUS. This trial highlights the safety and efficacy of clopidogrel with apixaban in patients with AF with ACS especially those undergoing PCI.

The dose of apixaban was 5 mg twice daily. It was reduced to 2.5 mg twice daily in presence of any two of the three conditions age >80 years, body weight <60 kg, and a serum creatinine >1.5 mg%.

Key Message

⦿ *In patients of ACS with PCI, with AF, combination of P2Y12 (Clopidogrel) with NOACs (apixaban) resulted in lowest bleeding episodes with best efficacy in prevention of ischemic and thromboembolic events.*

ARTICLE 15

A fully magnetically levitated left ventricular assist device—final report

Mehra MR, Uriel N, Naka Y, Cleveland JC Jr, Yuzefpolskaya M, Salerno CT, et al.; MOMENTUM 3 Investigators. A Fully Magnetically Levitated Left Ventricular Assist Device—Final Report.
N Engl J Med. 2019;380(17):1618-27.

Abstract*

Introduction: In two interim analyses of this trial, patients who had advanced heart failure and treated with a fully magnetically levitated centrifugal-flow left-ventricular assist device (LVAD) were less expected to have nondisabling stroke or pump thrombosis as compared to patients who were treated with a mechanical-bearing axial-flow LVAD.

Materials and methods: Patients with advanced heart failure were randomly assigned to receive either the centrifugal-flow pump or the axial-flow pump regardless of the intended goal of use (destination therapy or bridge to transplantation). The composite primary endpoint considered in the study was survival at 2 years free of disabling stroke or reoperation to remove/replace a malfunctioning device. Pump replacement at 2 years was the principal secondary endpoint.

Results: Total 1,028 patients were enrolled; patients in the centrifugal-flow pump group and the axial-flow pump group were 516 and 512, respectively. In the analysis of the primary endpoint, at 2 years, 76.9% patients (n = 397) in the centrifugal-flow pump group, in comparison to 64.8% (n = 332) in the axial-flow pump group, were alive and free of disabling stroke or reoperation to remove/replace a malfunctioning device [relative risk (RR) 0.84; 95% confidence interval (CI) 0.78–0.91; p < 0.001 for superiority]. As compared to the axial-flow pump group, pump replacement was found to be less common in the centrifugal-flow pump group [12 patients (2.3%) vs. 57 patients (11.3%); RR 0.21; 95% CI 0.11–0.38; p < 0.001]. In comparison with the axial-flow pump group, numbers of events per patient-year for stroke of any severity, gastrointestinal hemorrhage, and major bleeding were lower in the centrifugal-flow pump group.

Conclusion: In advanced heart failure patients, a fully magnetically levitated centrifugal-flow LVAD was found to be associated with less frequent requirement for pump replacement as compared to an axial-flow device and was superior in terms of survival free of disabling stroke or reoperation to remove/replace a malfunctioning device. (Funded by Abbott; MOMENTUM 3 ClinicalTrials.gov number, NCT02224755.)
*Redrafted abstract

"New left ventricular assist device (LVAD) HeartMate 3 is better than earlier devices."

COMMENT

Patients with end-stage congestive heart failure due to ischemic heart disease or dilated cardiomyopathy can only be saved by left ventricular assist devices (LVADs) or heart transplantation. Patients with ejection fraction <20% who are not responding to other mode of therapy are candidates for this. LVADs have been in use for last 15 years. The LVAD provides assistance to left ventricle and pumps blood to aorta from left ventricle (LV). Earlier pump were pulsatile. Recent devices are continuous flow pumps. The heart M2 is an axial continuous flow pump that requires thoracoabdominal replacement. This is the most commonly used LVAD. There are many others LVADs available. Initially, these were used as "bridge to transplant" for patients who needed support, till suitable organ was available from a cadaver for transplantation. Recently, LVAD has been used as "destination therapy." Since patient can live long, even up to 10 years. LVADs are expensive and cost around 40–70 lakhs in India. However for end-stage heart failure, these are the only form of therapy that can prolong life. The LVAD has problems of bleeding, stroke, infection, and device failure. These are not totally internal devices and there is a control belt which the patient has to wear. The portal of entry can be source of infection. More recently, a newer advance model called HeartMate 3 has been developed by same company. This is a magnetically levitated centrifugal flow intrathoracic device. In the present study, HeartMate 3 has been compared with HeartMate 2 in one thousand patients. In this study, 2-year survival free of stroke or reoperation was 77% with HeartMate 3 and 65% with HeartMate 2. This shows that the new magnetically levitated centrifugal flow pump works better than the earlier axial flow pump. LVAD is used as bridge to transplant in younger patients and destination therapy in those >65 years. More than 5,000 such devices have been implanted even in India, many centers are now doing LVAD implantation and heart transplantation. Patients with right ventricle (RV) dysfunction require right ventricular assist device (RVAD) for biventricular assist device (BVAD). However, these are used less frequently. Patients on LVAD have to be on lifelong anticoagulation. Since these are continuous flow devices, patient's pulse and blood pressure are to be recorded with special devices. The long-term success with the HeartMate 3 will further increase their usage. There are devices from many other companies also in use. Long-term LVADs are used in chronic patients; for patients in intensive coronary care unit (ICCU), who need short-term support, the assist devices include from the most simple intra-aortic balloon pump to Impella and extracorporeal membrane oxygenation (ECMO).

Key Messages

⊙ *Patients with end-stage heart failure can be offered LVAD or heart transplantation as a last resort.*

⊙ *The results with newer LVADs are promising and patients can live for many years with close follow-up. However, these devices are expensive.*

ARTICLE 16

Influenza vaccine in heart failure

Modin D, Jørgensen ME, Gislason G, Jensen JS, Køber L, Claggett B, et al. Influenza Vaccine in Heart Failure. *Circulation. 2019;139(5):575-86.*

Abstract*

Introduction: In patients with heart failure (HF), influenza infection is considered to be a serious event. There is scarcity of knowledge related to association between influenza vaccination and outcome in patients who have HF. This study aimed at determining whether there is an association between influenza vaccination and improved long-term survival in patients who have newly diagnosed HF.

Materials and methods: This was a nationwide cohort study that included 134,048 patients of >18 years of age with HF in Denmark during the period of January 1st, 2003 to June 1st, 2015. Linked data was collected from nationwide registries. The vaccination status, number as well as frequency during the follow-up were considered as time-varying covariates in the time-dependent Cox regression.

Results: Follow-up was 99.8%; the median follow-up time was 3.7 years (interquartile range 1.7–6.8 years). During the study period, the vaccination coverage of the study cohort was in the range of 16–54%. In unadjusted analysis, receiving more than one 1 vaccinations during follow-up was found to be associated with greater risk of death. After adjusting for inclusion date, medications, comorbidities, education level, and household income, receiving >1 vaccinations was observed to be associated with an 18% reduced risk of death [all-cause: hazard ratio (HR) 0.82; 95% confidence interval (CI) 0.81–0.84; p < 0.001; cardiovascular causes: HR 0.82; 95% CI 0.81–0.84; p < 0.001]. Vaccination early in the year (i.e., September to October), annual vaccination, and higher cumulative number of vaccinations were associated with greater reductions in the risk of death in comparison to intermittent vaccination.

Conclusion: Among patients who have HF, after extensive adjustment for confounders, influenza vaccination was noted to be associated with a decreased risk of both all-cause and cardiovascular death. When compared to intermittent and late vaccination, frequent vaccination and vaccination earlier in the year were associated with greater reductions in the risk of death. *Redrafted abstract

"Annual influenza vaccine reduces mortality in heart failure patients."

COMMENT

In chronic congestive heart failure (CHF), acute worsening can be precipitated by infections especially respiratory, arrhythmias, anemia, or poor drug compliance. Respiratory infections can be caused by influenza or pneumococcus. 50% of decompensation in CHF is due to respiratory infections. Influenza infection causes heart failure (HF) worsening due to the inflammatory action, progress in atherosclerosis, and production of cytokines which can have myocardial depressant effect. Influenza also causes a hypercoagulable state and is known to precipitate acute coronary syndromes.

Influenza vaccination is recommended by American College of Cardiology/American Heart Association (ACC/AHA) and European Society of Cardiology (ESC) guidelines for patients with ischemic heart disease and HF. Most patients with HF are aged >65 years and are frail. The increased metabolic demand of infection precipitates HF in these patients. Although annual influenza vaccination has been recommended in most guidelines, its clinical utilization has been suboptimal. In the present study from Denmark, where healthcare is universal and vaccination is provided free to patients with HF. The penetration of influenza vaccination was from 15–55%. In the PARADIGM-HF trial, influenza vaccination was found in only 0–15% of subjects from Asia, Eastern Europe, and South America. This low penetration is primarily due to physician inertia, lack of planning, and regular protocols in hospitals. The present study analyzed 130,000 subjects and observed a 20% reduction in all cause mortality in matched subjects who were given vaccination. It

was also observed that regular annual vaccination and vaccination early in September or October imparted greater benefits. This is a safe and effective therapy, which is not very expensive. Every patient >60 years of age with coronary artery disease (CAD) or HF should be administered annual influenza vaccine. Along with this, pneumococcal vaccine is to be given every 5 years.

Influenza infection has been shown to increase metabolic demand, cause hypoxia, and there is an adrenergic surge. All these three things precipitate HF. Infection is associated with hypercoagulable state, which precipitates acute coronary syndrome. Thirdly, infection also causes myocarditis and myocardial necrosis. All these three mechanisms are also seen in corona virus infections these days. The present pandemic of COVID-19 has highlighted the need for preventing infections in vulnerable subjects. We have a trivalent and a tetravalent vaccine for influenza. The two above-mentioned vaccines are being evaluated in a large randomized double-blind trial by National Institutes of Health (NIH) called the INVESTED study. The results of this will be available after few years. Meanwhile, the present study from Denmark is the largest ever study, showing prophylactic influenza vaccine in patients of HF. In fact, the 20% reduction in all-cause mortality is similar to that with the use of β-blockers and angiotensin-converting enzyme (ACE) inhibitors respectively. In the COVID-19 times, occurrence of influenza will cause even more confusion in the patients and hence this vaccination is of great value in all subjects early in September to prevent infections in the winter months. Till the time we have a COVID vaccine when we will start using both, we should use the influenza vaccine in all our patients with CAD, HF, and all post-percutaneous coronary intervention (PCI) and post-coronary artery bypass graft (CABG) subjects.

Key Messages

- *Patients of HF and CAD should have annual influenza vaccine in early September or October. This will reduce mortality by 20% in these high-risk subjects.*

- *In the present COVID-19 pandemic, influenza vaccination becomes even more important for these vulnerable subjects.*

ARTICLE 17

Adjunctive intermittent pneumatic compression for venous thromboprophylaxis

Arabi YM, Al-Hameed F, Burns KEA, Mehta S, Alsolamy SJ, Alshahrani MS, et al.; Saudi Critical Care Trials Group. Adjunctive Intermittent Pneumatic Compression for Venous Thromboprophylaxis.
N Engl J Med. 2019;380(14):1305-15.

Abstract*

Introduction: In critically ill patients receiving pharmacologic thromboprophylaxis, it is still not certain whether adjunctive intermittent pneumatic compression would lead to a reduced incidence of deep-vein thrombosis (DVT) as compared to pharmacologic thromboprophylaxis alone.

Material and methods: Randomization of the patients [considered as adults as per the local standards at the participating sites (age of ≥14, ≥16, or ≥18 years)] was done within 48 hours following admission to an intensive care unit (ICU) for receiving either intermittent pneumatic compression for minimum 18 hours each day along with pharmacologic thromboprophylaxis with unfractionated or low-molecular-weight heparin (i.e., pneumatic compression group) or pharmacologic thromboprophylaxis alone (i.e., control group). The primary outcome considered in the study was incident (new) proximal lower-limb DVT, as found on twice-weekly lower-limb ultrasonography after the 3rd calendar day since randomization until the time of ICU discharge, death, achievement of full mobility, or trial day 28, whichever happened firstly.

Results: Total 2,003 patients were included; out of these, 991 patients were assigned to the pneumatic compression group and 1,012 patients to the control group. Application of intermittent pneumatic compression was done for a median of 22 hours [interquartile range (IQR) 21–23] daily for a median of 7 days (IQR 4–13). The primary outcome was noted in 3.9% (37/957) patients in the pneumatic compression group and in 4.2% (41/985) patients in the control group [relative risk (RR) 0.93; 95% confidence interval (CI) 0.60–1.44; p = 0.74]. Venous thromboembolism (i.e., lower-limb DVT or pulmonary embolism) was found in 10.4% (103/991) patients in the pneumatic compression group and in 9.4% (95/1,012) patients in the control group (RR 1.11; 95% CI 0.85–1.44), and death from any cause at 90 days occurred in 26.1% (258/990) patients and 26.7% (270/1,011) patients, respectively (RR, 0.98; 95% CI 0.84–1.13).

Conclusion: In critically ill patients receiving pharmacologic thromboprophylaxis, adjunctive intermittent pneumatic compression did not lead to a significantly reduced incidence of proximal lower-limb DVT as compared to pharmacologic thromboprophylaxis alone. (Funded by King Abdulaziz City for Science and Technology and King Abdullah International Medical Research Center; PREVENT ClinicalTrials.gov number, NCT02040103; Current Controlled Trials number, ISRCTN44653506.) *Redrafted abstract

"Immobilized intensive care unit (ICU) patients, especially on ventilators, need thromboprophylaxis (LMWH)."

COMMENT

Venous thromboembolism (VT) develops in hospitalized patients who are immobilized. The Virchow's triad of stasis, vessel wall injury, and hypercoagulability favors thrombus formation. Deep vein thrombosis (DVT) of the leg can be in calf region or it can be proximal in ileo/femoral area. Patients of heart failure, those who are in intensive care unit (ICU), on ventilator, or those who are immobilized after major surgery are at risk of DVT. These individuals need DVT prophylaxis during hospitalization. The prophylaxis can be pharmacological with unfractionated heparin (UFH) or low-molecular weight heparin (LMWH). It can be mechanical prophylaxis with intermittent pneumatic compression or with graduated compression elastic stockings. In pharmacological prophylaxis, LMWH is preferred over UFH, since it can be administered once a day subcutaneously. In mechanical prophylaxis, intermittent compression is better than elastic stockings. Generally, patients who are obese, age >60 years, or with cancer or stroke are at higher risk. It has been seen, if DVT prophylaxis is not given, DVT leg can develop in 20–30% patients. This is reduced to 5% with pharmacological prophylaxis. Major surgeries, knee and hip replacement, are especially high risk for development of DVT. Often DVT can be missed and results in significant mortality in these hospitalized patients due to embolization and consequently pulmonary thromboembolism (PTE). In surgical patients, this prophylaxis causes significant reduction in mortality. In ICU setting, it reduces incidence of PTE.

The present PREVENT trial is from Saudi Arabia. It is a nonindustry-driven investigator initiated study. Hence, its credibility is high. In ICU setting, pharmacological thromboprophylaxis is standard of care in patients who are on ventilators and at high risk of DVT. The investigators here evaluated whether additional mechanical thromboprophylaxis was beneficial in addition to the LMWH. They did not find any additional benefit of mechanical compression in addition to the pharmacological prophylaxis.

As in ICU patients which have been evaluated in this trial, postoperative patients also benefit from LMWH for DVT prophylaxis. This is especially required in those who have prolonged immobilization, paraplegia, or knee and hip surgery. LMWH is to be given to all these subjects. Patients who have transurethral resection of the prostate (TURP) for prostate or cerebral surgery can be subjected to mechanical thromboprophylaxis.

In hip replacement surgery, aspirin, an antiplatelet agent, has also been used and found effective. However, in all other situations, the pharmacological agent used is LMWH. The inferior vena cava (IVC) filters, which were used earlier, have no place for prevention of PTE and are hence not recommended. More recently, a synthetic pentasaccharide, fondaparinux, which is a factor Xa inhibitor and is used once a day can also be used. Recently, newer oral anticoagulants (NOAC) have also been used and found to be better than LMWH in postoperative patients. Short-term thromboprophylaxis is for 2 weeks and long term is for 3 weeks. The duration depends on underlying disease and risk of thrombosis and bleeding. This study done in ICU setting shows LMWH alone is sufficient for these patients. However, in patients where there is contraindication to use of anticoagulation, we must use mechanical prophylaxis.

Key Messages

- *Patients of heart failure, paraplegia, after orthopedic surgery or other major surgery and those in ICU for prolonged time need thromboprophylaxis. Pharmacological (LMWH) and mechanical (compression devices) thromboprophylaxis both are available. The risk of thrombosis and bleeding is to be evaluated and these preventive therapies used accordingly.*

- *In ICU patients, LMWH alone can be used. Additional mechanical compression does not offer added advantage as shown in the PREVENT trial.*

ARTICLE 18

Infective endocarditis hospitalizations and antibiotic prophylaxis rates before and after the 2007 American Heart Association guideline revision

Garg P, Ko DT, Jenkyn KMB, Li L, Shariff SZ. Infective Endocarditis Hospitalizations and Antibiotic Prophylaxis Rates Before and After the 2007 American Heart Association Guideline Revision.
Circulation. 2019;140(3):170-80.

Abstract*

Background: According to the American Heart Association recommendations in 2007, for the prevention of infective endocarditis (IE), antibiotic prophylaxis is recommended for only the highest-risk patients. It is still not certain whether this change affected the antibiotic prophylaxis use and the incidence of IE.

Materials and methods: Identification of IE-related hospitalizations from 2002 to 2014 was done in all adults and those who were at high and moderate risk for IE, stratified by age. From the Ontario Drug Benefit database, prescriptions for antibiotic prophylaxis were collected for adults 65 years or more of age. Outcomes considered in the study included incidence of IE-related hospitalization and antibiotic prophylaxis prescription rates. Analysis of trends in patient and pathogen characteristics was done. Time series analyses were done with segmented regression and change-point analyses.

Results: There was a substantial reduction in the prescriptions for antibiotic prophylaxis in the moderate-risk cohort following the guideline revision [mean quarterly prescriptions, 30,680 vs. 17,954 (level change: −6,481; p = 0.0004) per 1 million population] with a minimal, yet significant, reduction followed by a slow increase in the high-risk group. In 6,884 adults more than or equal to 18 years of age, there were 7,551 IE-related hospitalizations. In adults 65 years or more of age, increase in the mean IE rate was from 872 to 1,385 and 229 to 283 per 1 million population at risk per quarter in the high- and moderate-risk groups, respectively. Change-point analyses showed that this increase was present in the second half of 2010 in adults 65 years or more of age, 3 years after revision of the American Heart Association guideline. For all IE, *Staphylococcus aureus* and streptococcal species were responsible for 30.3% and 26.4% of the cases, with a reduction in the streptococcal infections over time.

Conclusion: A significant reduction was present in the antibiotic prophylaxis in the moderate-risk group with minimum change in the high-risk group after revision of the American Heart Association guideline in 2007. There was an increase in the IE-related hospitalizations in high- as well as moderate-risk patients 3 years after the revision. This study supports the cessation of antibiotic prophylaxis in the case of moderate-risk population. *Redrafted abstract

"Infective endocarditis prophylaxis is required only in high-risk individuals."

COMMENT

Infective endocarditis (IE) occurs in subjects with underlying heart disease such as valvular regurgitation and stenosis, prosthetic valves, mitral valve prolapse, and congenital heart disease. Any condition with turbulent flow in the heart can increase risk of endocarditis. Traditionally, it was believed that dental procedures, gastrointestinal (GI), and genitourinary invasive procedures cause transient bacteremia during these procedures, which can result in increased risk of endocarditis. 1997 American College of Cardiology/American Heart Association (ACC/AHA) guidelines suggested antibiotics for dental and other above mentioned procedures. However, in 2007, the AHA revised the guidelines for IE prophylaxis. This very major change was made because it was realized that daily activities such as brushing or eating cause bacteremia similar to tooth extraction. Also, there were no randomized trials showing benefit of using antibiotics 1 hour before and 8 hours after these procedures. So in 2007 guidelines, it was suggested that only very high-risk subjects including those with prosthetic valves, with past history of endocarditis, and with incomplete repair of congenital heart disease, these three subgroups require IE prophylaxis. All other subjects including mitral valve prolapse, rheumatic heart disease, and hypertrophic cardiomyopathy do not need prophylaxis. Thus, the use of periprocedural antibiotics has been limited to these three situations only. This was endorsed by European society of cardiology in 2009 and by the NICE guidelines of UK in 2008. This was a major change from the previous practices.

The present study in circulation looks at the impact of these guidelines on the practices in USA. They looked at data from 2002 to 2014. They observed that in compliance with the guidelines, use of periprocedural prophylactic antibiotics reduced significantly after 2008. There was no significant increase in endocarditis, which could be attributed to the revised guidelines. Thus, the authors of the article and of an editorial published along with both feel that 2007 guidelines should be followed by us presently also.

Infective endocarditis is an uncommon complication but carries a mortality of 20–25%. Its prevalence is increasing in the population at risk. Also, IV mainliners are a special group in which we see right-sided endocarditis. The guidelines suggest good oro-dental hygiene to be maintained by at risk individuals. The bacteremias related to the procedures are not responsible for most episodes of IE.

Key Messages

- *The patients with prosthetic valves, history of IE, and incompletely repaired congenital heart disease are the only high-risk subjects who need IE prophylaxis with single dose of antibiotic administered orally or parenterally 30–60 minutes before the procedure.*

- *For moderate-risk subjects, such as mitral valve prolapse, hypertrophic obstructive cardiomyopathy (HOCM), aortic stenosis, and mitral stenosis, periprocedural antibiotic prophylaxis is not recommended by any national guidelines at present.*

ARTICLE 19

Prevalence of familial hypercholesterolemia in premature coronary artery disease patients admitted to a tertiary care hospital in North India

Sawhney JPS, Prasad SR, Sharma M, Madan K, Mohanty A, Passey R, et al. Prevalence of familial hypercholesterolemia in premature coronary artery disease patients admitted to a tertiary care hospital in North India.
Indian Heart J. 2019;71(2):118-22.

Abstract

Aims: The prevalence of premature coronary artery disease (CAD) in India is two to three times more than other ethnic groups. Untreated heterozygous familial hypercholesterolemia (FH) is one of the important causes for premature CAD. As the age advances, these patients without treatment have 100 times increased risk of cardiovascular (CV) mortality resulting from myocardial infarction (MI). Recent evidence suggests that one in 250 individuals may be affected by FH (nearly 40 million people globally). It is indicated that the true global prevalence of FH is underestimated. The true prevalence of FH in India remains unknown.

Methods: A total of 635 patients with premature CAD were assessed for FH using the Dutch Lipid Clinical Network (DLCN) criteria. Based on scores, patients were diagnosed as definite, probable, possible, or no FH. Other CV risk factors known to cause CAD such as smoking, diabetes mellitus, and hypertension were also recorded.

Results: Of total 635 patients, 25 (4%) were diagnosed as definite, 70 (11%) as probable, 238 (37%) as possible, and 302 (48%) without FH, suggesting the prevalence of potential (definite + probable) FH of about 15% in the North Indian population. FH is more common in younger patients, and they have lesser incidence of common CV risk factors such as diabetes, hypertension, and smoking than the younger MI patients without FH (26.32% vs. 42.59%; 17.89% vs. 29.44%; 22.11% vs. 40.74%).

Conclusion: FH prevalence is high among patients with premature CAD admitted to a cardiac unit. To detect patients with FH, routine screening with simple criteria such as family history of premature CAD combined with hypercholesterolemia and a DLCN criteria score >5 may be effectively used.

"Familial hypocholesterolemia—suspect when low-density lipoprotein (LDL) >190 and premature CAD."

COMMENT

Dyslipidemia indicates abnormality in one of the lipids, cholesterol, or triglycerides. Lipids are carried in the blood by protein molecules called lipoproteins. A lipid profile normally includes cholesterol, triglycerides, high-density lipoproteins (HDL), low-density lipoprotein (LDL), and very low-density lipoprotein (VLDL). Earlier, we used to do fasting lipid profiles since triglycerides get elevated in nonfasting state. All International and Indian guidelines now advise us to do nonfasting lipid profiles. It is convenient for the patient.

Yes, cholesterol is carried in blood mainly by LDL and HDL. LDL is bad cholesterol and HDL is good cholesterol. Triglycerides are carried mainly by chylomicrons and VLDL. High cholesterol and LDL are a risk factor for coronary artery disease (CAD). Most lipid abnormalities are polygenic in origin. Multiple genes determine the lipid levels of an individual. However, there are some monogenic dyslipidemias. Familial hypercholesterolemia (FH) is the most common and most significant single gene abnormality. It is autosomal-dominant and affects 1:250 individuals in general population. Michael Brown and Goldstein won the noble prize for discovering the LDL receptors on hepatocytes.

Genetically, it can be due to abnormalities in LDL receptor (LDL-R), apoB mutation, or *PCSK9* gene abnormality. LDL-R abnormality is responsible for 80% cases. FH causes premature CAD. It should be suspected when LDL is >160–190 and there is history of premature CAD. The most commonly used diagnostic criteria are—the Dutch lipid clinic network criteria. This includes family history of CAD, patient with CAD <55 years, arcus cornealis or tendinous xanthomata, and mutation in LDL-R on DNA analysis. In every patient with premature CAD (<50 years) and high LDL >160, one should suspect this condition. On clinical examination, look for arcus cornealis in eye and tendon xanthomata.

In this study, the prevalence of FH was found to be 15% in patients of premature CAD. This is the first Indian study and incidence is same as in other races.

Dyslipidemia were traditionally classified by Fredrickson's classification. It has five varieties—Type 1 is increased chylomicrons, Type 2 A is FH which is most common and is what we are discussing, Type 3 is intermittent density lipoproteins (IDL), and 2b, 4, and 5 have high VLDL. These days, this classification based on lipoproteins is used less commonly. Genetic classification is used more commonly. The message from the above study is—we should suspect FH in all patients with premature CAD, look for arcus and xanthoma, and wherever possible, get genetic testing for LDL-R mutation. All family members, first-degree relatives of these suspected patients (with LDL >190), should have nonfasting lipid profiles done. This is called as cascade testing. This will help to diagnose other relatives at high risk of premature CAD.

Key Messages

- *Familial hypercholesterolemia is the most common inherited single gene disorder. It causes premature CAD.*
- *Cascade screening, nonfasting lipid profiles of all first-degree relatives of such patients, should be done.*

ARTICLE 20

Mitral valve calcium assessment: an independent predictor of balloon valvuloplasty results

Sarmiento RA, Solernó R, Blanco R, Giachello F, Hauqui A, Oscos M, et al. Mitral valve calcium assessment: an independent predictor of balloon valvuloplasty results.
Indian Heart J. 2019;71(6):454-8.

Abstract

Objective: Percutaneous mitral valvuloplasty (PMV) is an effective treatment for patients with mitral valve stenosis. Echocardiographic score (ES) is a useful predictor of outcomes. However, mitral valve calcification (MVC) has been shown to predict immediate results even in patients with otherwise low ES. We sought to evaluate the usefulness of MVC assessment as a predictor of immediate and long-term out comes after PMV.

Methods: PMV was performed in 168 consecutive patients. Clinical and echocardiographic variables were analyzed. Patients were classified into 2 groups: group 1—minimal MVC and group 2—moderate-to-severe MVC. Primary success was defined as post-PMV mitral valve area (MVA) $\geq$1.5 cm^2 in the absence of major complications. Restenosis (RE) was defined as a decrease in MVA >50% of initial gain or a final MVA <1.5 cm^2.

Results: Mean age was 46.5 $\pm$ 11 years, and 86.9% (146) were women. Forty-two patients (25%) had mild MVC (group 1), and 75% of the patients had moderate-to-severe MVC (group 2). Procedural success was achieved in 95.2% and 76.2% for groups 1 and 2, respectively, p = 0.01. MVA after PMV was 1.82 cm^2 [interquartile range (IQR) 25–75 = 1.60–2.00] in group 1 and 1.67 cm^2 (IQR 25–75 = 1.44–1.97) in group 2, p = 0.02. After 48 months, 28.2% of patients presented with RE. Multivariate analysis identified the presence of MVC as an independent predictor of poor immediate results [hazard ratio (HR) 0.12, 95% confidence interval (CI) 0.03–0.91] and RE (HR 1.94, 95% CI 1.02–5.21).

Conclusion: Our study shows that the presence of MVC may predict immediate and long-term outcomes after PMV.

"Mitral valve (MV): The treatment of choice for severe mitral stenosis."

COMMENT

Severe mitral stenosis is common in India. Mostly patients present in second or third decade. The treatment of choice for severe mitral stenosis is percutaneous transvenous mitral commissurotomy (PTMC). It is also called balloon mitral valvotomy (BMV). Mitral stenosis is graded as mild when mitral valve area (MVA) is >1.5 cm^2, moderate when MVA is 1.0–1.5 cm^2, and severe when MVA is <1 cm^2. Severe mitral stenosis when isolated is amenable to BMV. The only cause of mitral stenosis in adults is chronic rheumatic heart disease. When mitral valve disease is mixed, i.e., mitral stenosis with mitral regurgitation, then BMV cannot be done in the presence of significant regurgitation. These patients have to be subjected to mitral valve replacement, if they are symptomatic.

Balloon mitral valvotomy is now the treatment of choice for severe isolated mitral stenosis. Before 1994, a surgical procedure called closed mitral valvotomy (CMV) was done in which the surgeon opened the chest and using a dilator and the finger, valve was dilated. Now BMV procedure is nonsurgical and can be done by femoral vein puncture from the right groin. The Inoue balloon is introduced and by atrial puncture taken from right atrium to left atrium and then across mitral valve, where it is inflated. The inflation of balloon causes commissural splitting and so MVA increases. On echocardiography, a Wilkins score is calculated, which looks at four things—leaflet thickening, calcification, mobility, and subvalvular fusion. A maximum score of 16 can be there with 4 for each of the four items. When score is <8, the patient is suitable for BMV. It means when the valve is not markedly thickened, not calcified, still mobile, and there is not much subvalvular fusion. Contraindications to BMV are heavily calcified valve, which is markedly thickened and having subvalvular fusion. A good BMV will increase MVA to 2 cm^2. Patients get significant relief in symptoms for a period of 7–10 years. After 10 years, mitral valve restenosis occurs and these patients have to get repeat procedures.

In this study, the authors have shown that out of these four parameters, valve calcification is most important. Whenever there is more calcification, the chances of success of the procedure are reduced, complications are increased, and long-term benefits are not achieved. The procedure of BMV is routinely done in most hospitals of India since rheumatic heart disease is still very common with us. The procedure costs almost 1/4th the cost of mitral valve replacement and is the procedure of choice for severe mitral stenosis with a suitable valve morphology. Highly calcified valves with associated mitral regurgitations and/or subvalvular fusion will have to be subjected to mitral valve replacement.

Key Messages

◉ *The Wilkins echo scoring is done for assessing suitability of valve for BMV in patients of severe mitral stenosis.*

◉ *Leaflet thickening, calcification, mobility, and valvular fusion are the factors evaluated for this scoring on echocardiography.*

ARTICLE 21

Angiotensin-neprilysin inhibition in heart failure with preserved ejection fraction

Solomon SD, McMurray JJV, Anand IS, Ge J, Lam CSP, Maggioni AP, et al. Angiotensin-neprilysin inhibition in heart failure with preserved ejection fraction.
N Engl J Med. 2019;381:1609-20.

Abstract*

Background: In patients who have heart failure and reduced ejection fraction, the angiotensin receptor–neprilysin inhibitor (ARNI) sacubitril–valsartan resulted in a decreased risk of hospitalization for heart failure or death due to cardiovascular causes. The impact of ARNI among patients who have heart failure with preserved ejection fraction (HFpEF) is still not clear.

Materials and methods: Total 4,822 patients who have New York Heart Association (NYHA) class II to IV heart failure, ejection fraction of ≥45%, increased natriuretic peptides level, and structural heart disease were included. Patients were randomly assigned to receive either sacubitril–valsartan (target dose: 97 mg sacubitril with 103 mg valsartan twice daily) or valsartan (target dose: 160 mg twice daily). The primary outcome considered in the study was a composite of total hospitalizations for heart failure and death due to cardiovascular causes. Assessment of primary outcome components, secondary outcomes [consisting of NYHA class change, worsening renal function, and change in Kansas City Cardiomyopathy Questionnaire (KCCQ) clinical summary score (scale: 0–100; higher scores suggested fewer symptoms as well as physical limitations)], and safety was done.

Results: Primary events in the sacubitril–valsartan group were 894, and in the valsartan group, there were 1,009 primary events [rate ratio (RR) 0.87; 95% confidence interval (CI) 0.75–1.01; p = 0.06]. The incidences of death because of cardiovascular causes in the sacubitril–valsartan group and valsartan group were 8.5% and 8.9%, respectively (hazard ratio (HR) 0.95; 95% CI 0.79–1.16); total hospitalizations for heart failure were 690 and 797, respectively (RR 0.85; 95% CI 0.72–1.00). Improvement of NYHA class was present in 15.0% of the patients in the sacubitril-valsartan group and in 12.6% in the valsartan group (odds ratio 1.45; 95% CI 1.13–1.86); worsening of renal function occurred in 1.4% and 2.7%, respectively (HR 0.50; 95% CI 0.33–0.77). At 8 months, the mean change in the KCCQ clinical summary score was found to be 1.0 point (95% CI 0.0–2.1) higher in the sacubitril–valsartan group.

As compared to patients of valsartan group, there was a greater incidence of hypotension and angioedema and lesser incidence of hyperkalemia in the sacubitril–valsartan group. In patients with lower ejection fraction and in women, in 12 prespecified subgroups, heterogeneity was suggested with possible benefit with sacubitril–valsartan.

Conclusion: In patients who have heart failure and an ejection fraction of ≥45%, use of sacubitril–valsartan did not led to a significantly lesser rate of total hospitalizations for heart failure and death due to cardiovascular causes. (Funded by Novartis; PARAGON-HF ClinicalTrials.gov number, NCT01920711.)
*Redrafted abstract

"Research is a way of taking calculated risks to bring about incalculable consequences."
—Celia Green

COMMENT

Heart failure with preserved ejection fraction (HFpEF) remains an enigmatic entity with very few therapies available to improve outcome. Management relies on symptomatic improvement with diuretic therapy and management of comorbidities. There has been an unmet need of new drugs for this condition. The angiotensin-neprilysin inhibitor sacubitril–valsartan has proven efficacy in improving cardiovascular outcomes in patients with heart failure with reduced ejection fraction (HFrEF) with significant reduction in composite outcome of heart failure hospitalization and cardiovascular death. A recent study demonstrated that use of this agent results in larger reduction of N-terminal pro-b-type natriuretic peptide (NT-pro-BNP) levels and improvement of functional status in patient with HFpEF when compared to valsartan alone.

The PARAGON-HF trial was designed to assess the role of angiotensin receptor–neprilysin inhibitor (ARNI) on outcomes in patient with HFpEF. In this study, over 4,000 symptomatic patients with HFpEF were randomized to 200 mg of sacubitril–valsartan or placebo. The primary outcome was a composite of cardiovascular death or HF hospitalization. After a median follow-up of 18 months, there was no significant difference in the primary outcome (14.6% vs. 12.8%; RR 0.87; 95% CI 0.75–1.01) or its individual component. However, ARNI was associated with an improvement in NYHA class (OR 1.45; 95% CI 1.13–1.86) and renal outcomes (1.4% vs. 2.7%; RR 0.50; 95% CI 0.33–0.77). Subgroup analysis showed that women and patient with ejection fraction in the range of 45–57% had improvement in primary outcome, but these findings are only hypothesis generating. ARNI was associated with more frequent hypotension and angioedema. The limitations of this study include a lower event rate than expected and potential beneficial effect of valsartan used in the comparison arm, which may have reduced the difference between the groups.

Key Message

- *Unlike HFrEF, ARNIs do not improve cardiovascular outcomes in patients with HFpEF. This may be attributable to the lesser degree of neurohormonal activation in these patients compared to HFrEF. In absence of disease-modifying agents for this condition, therapy should focus on symptom relief and management of comorbidities.*

Section 2: Chest and Critical Care

Section Editor: Surinder K Jindal

Associate Editors: Aditya Jindal, Uma M Krishnaswamy, Uma Devaraj, Kavitha V

Interstitial Lung Disease

ARTICLE 1

Effect of pulmonary rehabilitation (PR) program in patients with interstitial lung disease (ILD)–Indian scenario

Devani P, Pinto N, Jain P, Prabhudesai P, Pandey A. Effect of Pulmonary Rehabilitation (PR) Program in Patients with Interstitial Lung Disease (ILD)–Indian scenario.
J Assoc Physicians India. 2019;67:28-33.

Abstract

Introduction: Interstitial lung diseases (ILDs) are group of disorders wherein due to varied etiologies, interstitium goes into progressive inflammation or fibrosis. Although the awareness has improved but, the therapy is still facing challenges. Pulmonary rehabilitation (PR) is a worthy modality, which not only supports but also imparts evident benefits in these patients.

Materials and methods: The study is a retrospective observational study conducted over a period of 2 years at "pulmonary rehabilitation center", a private clinic setup on patients with different restrictive lung diseases such as ILDs, neuromuscular disorders, and postsurgical patients. A total of 100 patients were enrolled, out of which 21 patients were lost to follow-up. The study population included 34% males and 66% females with a mean age of 56.3 ± 14.2 years. Around 24 patients required oxygen support (where SpO_2 <90% at baseline). Outcome measures were assessed in these patients at the time of enrollment into the program (0 week) and at the end of the program (8 weeks). Effect of PR program was then analyzed with appropriate statistical methods.

Results: Overall, statistically significant benefits were noted in 6-minute walk distance (6MWD), muscle strength, dyspnea, and quality of life with 8 weeks. The mean 6 MWTD was 297.9 m pre-PR, which improved to 359.7 m at the completion of 8 weeks post PR. Mean difference was 61.8 m, which was found to be statistically significant (p value < 0.001). Improvement in muscle strength of different upper and lower limb muscle groups were noted. Also, significant improvement in comprehensive score of chronic respiratory diseases questionnaire (CRDQ) scores was documented. Statistically significant improvement was found in the dyspnea, fatigue, and emotional components. However, mastery components did not show statistically significant change.

Conclusion: Pulmonary rehabilitation has proven to be a very useful modality in the management of restrictive lung diseases, especially with the known limitations of pharmacological options to treat this disabling chronic lung diseases, even with those with evident type I respiratory failure at the beginning.

"Nothing is to be found that can substitute for exercise in any way....Exercise is only one of the components of rehabilitation."

COMMENT

Pulmonary rehabilitation (PR) is a supervised and structured program that involves a multi-disciplinary approach in the management of certain chronic lung conditions. PR consists of exercise training and breathing techniques, health education, nutrition and psychological supports. PR is beneficial in that it helps to decrease the symptoms (dyspnea and fatigue) as well as to improve quality of life and exercise tolerance. In addition, it causes reduction of healthcare utilization (particularly bed-days) and increase in physical activity. Benefits of PR in cases of chronic obstructive pulmonary disease (COPD) have been shown in several studies in the past; therefore, PR constitutes an essential component of its management.

Unlike in case of COPD, there is much less experience with PR in patients with chronic interstitial lung diseases (ILDs) who suffer from progressive breathlessness and respiratory disability. Nonetheless, the limited data from a few studies support its role to improve both short-term and long-term outcomes in these patients. In a Cochrane Library Systematic Data Review, the authors found low-to-moderate quality of evidence in favor of PR as safe for patients with ILD causing improvements in functional exercise capacity, dyspnea, and quality of life.[1] But, there was little evidence regarding longer-term benefits.

There are very few reports from India on PR in different diseases. It is generally considered as a labor-intensive and time-consuming method of management. The authors of this study analyzed their retrospective data of 100 patients with restrictive lung disease seen in a 2-year period. Final data were available in only 79 patients since 21 were lost to follow-up. After 8 weeks of PR, there was significant improvement in 6-minute walk distance (6MWD), muscle strength, and quality of life. The authors also report improvement of symptoms such as dyspnea, fatigue, and emotional components.

The present study included patients with restrictive diseases such as neuromuscular disorders and postsurgical patients with generally healthy lungs. These disorders do not necessarily behave like parenchymal ILD with progressive fibrosis. Therefore, the benefit cannot be directly applied to different kinds of ILDs. Importantly, however, the authors have taken a step toward the institution of a regular program of PR in patients with different diseases. Such a step should significantly help in the development of similar programs in other chronic pulmonary disorders.

Key Messages

- *Pulmonary rehabilitation caused significant improvement in 6-minute walk distance (6MWD), muscle strength, and quality of life in patients with restrictive lung disease.*

- *Pulmonary rehabilitation also causes symptomatic improvement of dyspnea, fatigue, and emotional components.*

ARTICLE 2

The natural history of progressive fibrosing interstitial lung diseases

Kolb M, Vašáková M. The natural history of progressive fibrosing interstitial lung diseases. *Respir Res. 2019;20:57.*

Abstract

A proportion of patients with certain types of interstitial lung disease (ILD), including chronic hypersensitivity pneumonitis and ILDs associated with autoimmune diseases, develop a progressive fibrosing phenotype that shows similarities in clinical course to idiopathic pulmonary fibrosis (IPF). Irrespective of the clinical diagnosis, these progressive fibrosing ILDs show commonalities in the underlying pathogenetic mechanisms that drive a self-sustaining process of pulmonary fibrosis. The natural history of progressive fibrosing ILDs is characterized by decline in lung function, worsening of symptoms and health-related quality of life, and early mortality. Greater impairment in forced vital capacity (FVC) or diffusion capacity of the lungs for carbon monoxide and a greater extent of fibrotic changes on a computed tomography scan are predictors of mortality in patients with fibrosing ILDs. However, the course of these diseases is heterogenous and cannot accurately be predicted for an individual patient. Data from ongoing clinical trials and patient registries will provide a better understanding of the clinical course and impact of progressive fibrosing ILDs.

"All pulmonary fibrosis is not idiopathic pulmonary fibrosis (IPF)."

COMMENT

After nearly 2 decades of characterizing idiopathic interstitial pneumonias into distinct histopathological entities and determining specific treatment protocols for these subtypes, we are beginning to understand that up to 40% of interstitial lung diseases (ILDs) with histological features other than usual interstitial pneumonia (UIP) can evolve into the so-called "progressive fibrosing ILDs (PF-ILD), whose disease behavior mirrors that of UIP. Some ILDs known to progress thus include connective tissue disease-related ILDs (rheumatoid arthritis, systemic sclerosis, and polymyositis/dermatomyositis), chronic sarcoidosis, chronic hypersensitivity pneumonitis, idiopathic nonspecific interstitial pneumonia, and some unclassifiable ILDs. The possible pathogenetic mechanisms contributing to PF-ILD include recurrent epithelial and vascular injury resulting in an unregulated fibroblast migration and proliferation, and fibrosis.

In this review, Kolb and Vasakova have reviewed literature pertaining to the natural history of PF-ILDs. The authors discuss various physiological indicators, serum biomarkers, and genetic variations in PF-ILD and their relation to rate of disease progression and mortality (**Fig. 1**).

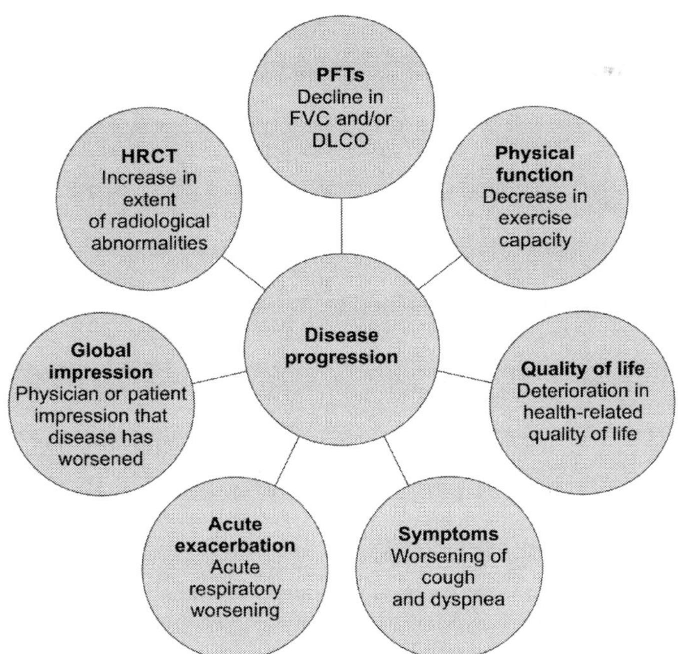

(DLCO: diffusing capacity of the lungs for carbon monoxide; FVC: forced vital capacity; HRCT: high-resolution computed tomography; PFT: pulmonary function test)

FIG. 1: Factors affecting progression of various nonidiopathic pulmonary fibrosis interstitial lung diseases (IPF ILDs).
Courtesy: Adapted from the article under discussion.

Most of the studies reviewed in this article pertain to individual categories of ILD and thus the statistical figures are heterogenous. However, a common theme that emerges is that a poorer pulmonary function at diagnosis [forced vital capacity (FVC) and diffusing capacity of the lungs for carbon monoxide (DLCO)], increased rate of decline of FVC (>10%) and DLCO, a greater degree of fibrosis on CT, and propensity for exacerbations characterizes this subset of patients and determines mortality. Besides, serum biomarkers of progression to fibrosis such as KL-6 (Kerbs von den Lungen-6 protein), Matrix metalloproteinase-7, surfactant protein-D and serum collagen degradation products are being evaluated as prognostic indicators. Certain genetic changes reported in idiopathic pulmonary fibrosis (IPF) such as the *MUCB* single nucleotide polymorphisms and short telomere length have been reported with rheumatoid arthritis-related interstitial lung disease (RA-ILD) and chronic hypersensitivity pneumonitis respectively.

This review summarizes the available diverse literature on PF-ILD and drives home the point that initial histological radiological characterization does not predict progression of non-UIP ILD and that identification of indicators of progression is important at diagnosis and during follow-up. There is also an emerging indication for the use of antifibrotic agents in the subset of patients who evolve to PF-ILD.

■ FURTHER READING

1. Collins BF, Raghu G. Eur Respir Rev. 2019;28(153):190022.
2. Cottin V, Wollin L, Fischer A, Quaresma M, Stowasser S, Harari S. Fibrosing interstitial lung diseases: knowns and unknowns. Eur Respir Rev. 2019;28:180100.

Key Messages

⊙ *Although histopathological and radiological characterization of ILD can help prognostication, emerging evidence indicates that many categories of non-UIP ILD can progress to the fibrosing phenotype.*

⊙ *It is very important to assess disease progression using spirometric, radiological, and possibly serological markers during follow-up for early identification of progression to PF-ILD.*

ARTICLE 3

Clinical effectiveness of antifibrotic medications for idiopathic pulmonary fibrosis

Dempsey TM, Sangaralingham LR, Yao X, Sanghavi D, Shah ND, Limper AH. Clinical effectiveness of antifibrotic medications for idiopathic pulmonary fibrosis.
Am J Respir Crit Care Med. 2019;200:168-74.

Abstract

Rationale: Since their approval, there has been no real-world or randomized trial evidence evaluating the effect of the antifibrotic medications pirfenidone and nintedanib on clinically important outcomes such as mortality and hospitalizations.

Objectives: To evaluate the clinical effectiveness of the antifibrotic medications pirfenidone and nintedanib in patients with idiopathic pulmonary fibrosis (IPF).

Methods: Using a large US insurance database, we identified 8,098 patients with IPF between October 1, 2014 and March 1, 2018. A one-to-one propensity score-matched cohort was created to compare patients treated with antifibrotic medications (n = 1,255) with those not on treatment (n = 1,255). The primary outcome was all-cause mortality. The secondary outcome was acute hospitalizations. Subgroup analyses were performed to evaluate mortality differences by drug.

Measurements and main results: The use of antifibrotic medications was associated with a decreased risk of all-cause mortality [hazard ratio (HR) 0.77; 95% confidence interval (CI) 0.62–0.98; p value = 0.034]. However, this association was present only through the first 2 years of treatment. There was also a decrease in acute hospitalizations in the treated cohort (HR 0.70; 95% CI 0.61–0.80; p value < 0.001). There was no significant difference in all-cause mortality between patients receiving pirfenidone and those on nintedanib (HR 1.14; 95% CI 0.79–1.65; p = 0.471).

Conclusions: Among patients with IPF, antifibrotic agents may be associated with a lower risk of all-cause mortality and hospitalization compared with no treatment. Future research should test the hypothesis that these treatments reduce early, but not long-term, mortality as demonstrated in our study.

"Antifibrotics in IPF: Does it buy time?"

COMMENT

Idiopathic pulmonary fibrosis (IPF) is a progressive and irreversible lung disease with a median survival of 3–5 years. In this article, the authors have attempted to unravel an unanswered aspect in treatment of IPF; namely, the mortality benefit and reduction in hospitalization among patients treated with pirfenidone or nintedanib. A retrospective cohort was built from a large private insurance database from 2014 to 2018; propensity score-matching yielded 1,255 pairs of patients with IPF who were treated or untreated.

All-cause mortality was reduced both in the pirfenidone and nintedanib group with hazard ratio (HR) of 0.77; hospitalization was also reduced by 30% in the treated group. Pirfenidone showed better mortality benefit than nintedanib, although this was statistically insignificant. Nevertheless, nintedanib reduced the risk of acute exacerbation. However, the mortality benefit with either antifibrotic did not extend beyond 2 years of therapy.

This study adds a silver lining to patients diagnosed with a progressive and fatal disease, for whom no treatment existed or was harmful, prior to the advent of antifibrotics. Prior CAPACITY (Clinical Studies Assessing Pirfenidone in IPF: Research of Efficacy and Safety Outcomes) and ASCEND (Assessment of Pirfenidone to Confirm Efficacy and Safety in IPF) studies, evaluating pirfenidone, have shown reduction in risk of death or disease progression by 38%. The INPULSIS-1 and -2 studies have also proven fall in forced vital capacity (FVC) of 125 mL/year in patients treated with nintedanib as opposed to 236 mL/year in untreated patients.

Although unmeasured confounders could account for some of the observed effect in this type of observational study, newer evidences, such as the INSIGHTS-IPF (INvestigating SIGnificant Health TrendS in Idiopathic Pulmonary Fibrosis) registry from Germany and the French National Health System claim data, also support the benefits from treatment with antifibrotics. Many trials such as INJOURNEY™ have explored the safety and tolerability of combined therapy with pirfenidone and nintedanib.

The important aspect of reduced mortality and acute exacerbations addressed by the antifibrotics are proven in a clinical setting in this study. This finding raises pertinent questions for further research pathways as shown in **Figure 1**. Large multicentric randomized controlled trials (RCTs) with multiple collaborators and funding are needed to address these issues.

■ FURTHER READING

1. Behr J, Prasse A, Wirtz H, Koschel D, Pittrow D, Held M, et al. Survival and course of lung function in the presence or absence of antifibrotic treatment in patients with idiopathic pulmonary fibrosis: long-term results of the INSIGHTS-IPF registry. Eur Respir J. 2020:1902279. [online ahead of print].

2. Torrisi SE, Pavone M, Vancheri A, Vancheri C. When to start and when to stop antifibrotic therapies. Eur Respir Rev. 2017;26:170053.

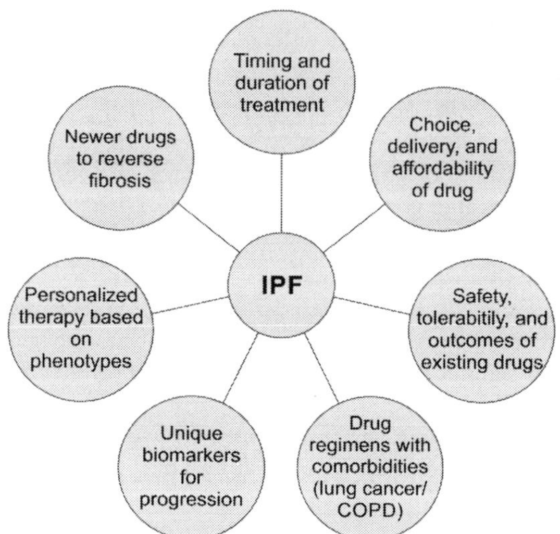

(COPD: chronic obstructive pulmonary disease)

FIG. 1: Future directions in idiopathic pulmonary fibrosis (IPF) management.

Key Message

⊙ *The antifibrotics, either pirfenidone or nintedanib, used in treatment for IPF reduce the risk of all-cause mortality and acute hospitalizations.*

ARTICLE 4

Nintedanib in progressive fibrosing interstitial lung diseases

Flaherty KR, Wells AU, Cottin V, Devaraj A, Walsh SLF, Inoue Y, et al. Nintedanib in progressive fibrosing interstitial lung diseases. *N Engl J Med. 2019;381:1718-27.*

Abstract*

Background: Nintedanib, an intracellular inhibitor of tyrosine kinases, is known to slow down the progression of lung fibrosis. Although its efficacy has been shown in idiopathic pulmonary fibrosis (IPF), it is not known if shows the same effect across a broad range of fibrosing lung diseases.

Methods: A double-blind, placebo-controlled, randomized phase 3 trial was conducted in 15 countries in which patients with fibrosing lung disease affecting >10% of lung volume on high-resolution computed tomography (CT) received either nintedanib at a dose of 150 mg twice daily or placebo. All the patients met criteria for progression of interstitial lung disease in the past 24 months despite treatment and had a forced vital capacity (FVC) of at least 45% of the predicted value and a diffusing capacity of the lung for carbon monoxide ranging from 30 to 80% of the predicted value. Stratified randomization according to the fibrotic pattern [a pattern of usual interstitial pneumonia (UIP) or other fibrotic patterns] on high-resolution CT was done. The annual rate of decline in the FVC assessed over a 52-week period was the primary outcome which was observed in the overall population and patients with a UIP-like fibrotic pattern.

Results: A total of 663 patients were treated. In the overall population, the adjusted rate of decline in the FVC was −80.8 mL/year and −187.8 mL/year with nintedanib and placebo, respectively. The between-group difference was 107.0 mL/year [95% confidence interval (CI) 65.4–148.5; p <0.001). In patients with a UIP-like fibrotic pattern, the adjusted rate of decline in the FVC was −82.9 mL/year and −211.1 mL/year with nintedanib and placebo, respectively. Here, the between-group difference was 128.2 mL (95% CI 70.8–185.6; p <0.001). Diarrhea was reported in 66.9% and 23.9% of patients treated with nintedanib and placebo, respectively. Also, nintedanib group was more commonly associated with abnormalities on liver-function testing.

Conclusion: Nintedanibin is associated with lower annual rate of decline in FVC of patients with progressive fibrosing interstitial lung diseases, as compared to placebo. Diarrhea was a common adverse event. *Redrafted abstract

"The person who takes medicine must recover twice, once from the disease and once from the medicine."

—**William Osler**

COMMENT

Treatment of interstitial lung disease (ILD) has undergone a sea change in the last decade with the addition of new antifibrotics such as pirfenidone and nintedanib while older combinations of medicines such as N-acetyl cysteine and immunosuppressant combinations becoming discredited.[2] However, most of the newer studies have targeted patients suffering from idiopathic pulmonary fibrosis (IPF), while other ILDs were mostly ignored.

A new paradigm in the treatment of ILDs has been the description of the phenotype of "progressive fibrosing ILDs (PF-ILD)". Conceptually, it suggests that all ILDs, regardless of cause, enter a final common phase characterized by progressive fibrosis and respiratory failure with common pathophysiological mechanisms of progression. At this stage, the individual aspects of the ILD are diluted down and symptoms are mainly due to progressive fibrosis. Therefore, treatment with antifibrotic medication should be effective in any ILD which has reached this phase.[3] One of the main trials in this area was the SENSCIS™ (The Safety and Efficacy of Nintedanib in SystemIc Sclerosis) trial, in which patients with systemic sclerosis associated ILD were treated with nintedanib and showed a favorable outcome.[4]

The INBUILD trial builds on the aforementioned concept where patients diagnosed to have PF-ILD were treated for nintedanib for 1 year. It was a multicenter, double-blind, placebo-controlled, phase 3 randomized control trial. A total of 663 patients were randomized to either placebo (n = 331) or nintedanib (n = 332) 150 mg twice a day daily for 1 year. The inclusion criteria for the study population included patients who, in the past 2 years, had (i) a relative decline in the FVC of at least 10% of the predicted value, or (ii) a relative decline in the FVC of 5% to <10% of the predicted value and worsening of respiratory symptoms or an increased extent of fibrosis on high-resolution CT, or (iii) worsening of respiratory symptoms and an increased extent of fibrosis on high-resolution CT. Patients were allowed to take immunosuppressant medications for up to 4 weeks before start of trial by were excluded if they had taken nintedanib or pirfenidone previously. The study included mild-to-moderate patients of ILD.

The results were studied in four groups—placebo group, treatment effect in patients with usual interstitial pneumonia (UIP) pattern on CT, treatment effect in patients with non-UIP pattern, and in the overall population. The primary study endpoint was the rate of decline of forced vital capacity (FVC) at 1 year while the secondary endpoints were the change in K-BILD score (a respiratory questionnaire for quality of life), acute exacerbation, and death rates. It was found that use of nintedanib for 1 year led to a reduction of the decline of FVC in the treatment group as compared to the placebo groups. The difference in the overall population was −80.8 mL/year with nintedanib and –187.8 mL/year with placebo, while in patients with a UIP-like fibrotic pattern it was –82.9 mL/year with nintedanib and –211.1 mL/year with placebo, for a difference of 128.2 mL. In patients with a non-UIP-like fibrotic pattern it was –79.0 mL/year in the nintedanib group and –154.2 mL/year in the placebo group (between-group difference, 75.3 mL). The hazard ratios for acute exacerbations and death were also better with nintedanib. Adverse effects were on expected lines with diarrhea and liver function test abnormalities being associated with nintedanib use.

This trial is the first study to show usefulness of nintedanib in non-IPF-ILDs with a progressive fibrosing phenotype. The place of nintedanib in these patients would be probably after the initial, nonfibrotic phase of illness which has not responded to conventional treatment. The results are significant and if the reduction of the rate of decline of FVC persists with use beyond 1 year it would translate to a significant benefit over time. However, we have to wait for long-term data to trickle in before making any conclusion. For the time being, it can be said that a new weapon has been added to the armamentarium!

Key Message

⊙ *Nintedanib is also useful for non-IPF patients who show a progressing fibrosing phenotype.*

Airway Disease

ARTICLE 5

Association of indoor air pollution with allergic respiratory diseases in paediatric population residing in national capital region

Kumar R, Singh K, Nagar JK, Mavi AK, Kumar M, Kumar D. Association of indoor air pollution with allergic respiratory diseases in paediatric population residing in national capital region.
Indian J Chest Dis Allied Sci. 2019;61:181-97.

Abstract

Background: World Health Organization (WHO) has observed that around seven million people died every year globally due to indoor air pollution. The purpose of this study is to evaluate the effect of indoor air pollution on respiratory health [bronchial asthma (BA) and/or allergic rhinitis (AR)] in a pediatric population in the National Capital Region (NCR) of Delhi, India.

Methods: A cross-sectional study to assess the factors responsible for respiratory diseases (BA and/or AR) in homes in rural areas of National Capital Region (NCR), India, was done. Around 61 households where at least one child who had symptoms of BA/AR (case households; Group A) and another 61 households with children without any symptom of BA/AR (Group B) were selected for the study. A standard questionnaire was used to collect the information about the health status of children and pollution levels in these homes.

Results: A total of 95 (43.8%) children in Group A households were found to have history of allergic respiratory diseases (n = 43–BA, n = 19–AR) while 33 children had both BA and AR. There was a statistically significant difference in the 24-hour particulate matter concentration (24 h) PM2.5 (p = 0.01) and 6-hour concentration of PM10 (p = 0.02) in Group A households as compared to Group B households. The 6-hour concentration of PM2.5 and PM1 and 12-hour concentration of volatile organic compounds (VOCs) was found to be higher in households of Group A. Group A households also had a higher number of smokers and usage of kerosene oil for lighting of lamps.

Conclusions: Tobacco smoking, use of kerosene oil for lighting and combustion of solid fuel for cooking results in an increased level of particulate matter, and VOCs in indoor air are the major contributing factors for respiratory illness in the pediatric population.

"Respiratory disease is the index of air we breathe—more so in children."

COMMENT

Most people, particularly the children, spend 12–18 hours every day in their homes. This is about half to two-thirds of their daily indoor time. Therefore, the indoor air is far more important for health. Indoor air pollution (IAP) these days is better referred to as household air pollution (HAP) because of the continuous exchange of indoor and outdoor air. World-over, HAP is an important issue in being responsible for adverse health effects for both children and adults. The list of diseases caused by IAP or HAP is rather large. In particular, the burden of cardiorespiratory illnesses caused and/or aggravated by exposure to HAP is quite significant.[5] There is proven association of HAP with presence of general respiratory symptoms, infections, and chronic obstructive pulmonary disease. There is also some evidence to suggest its relationship with exacerbations of asthma necessitating increased healthcare utilization. But, there is ambiguity whether HAP is also responsible for an increased prevalence of respiratory allergies including allergic rhinitis (AR) and bronchial asthma (BA).

Kumar and colleagues in this paper have studied the factors responsible for IAP in homes in rural areas of National Capital Region (NCR). They selected 61 households with presence of at least one child with history of respiratory diseases (BA and/or AR) and 61 households with children without any symptom of BA/AR. They found higher 6-hour concentrations of particulate matter (PM2.5 and PM1) and 12-hour concentration of volatile organic compounds (VOCs) in households with presence of children with respiratory allergies. The number of smokers and usage of kerosene oil for lighting of lamps was also higher in these households. The evidence suggests a causal relationship of indoor pollutants with AR and asthma.

The study is rather small for an epidemiological interpretation. But, the authors have measured and compared the concentrations of particulate pollutants and VOCs in households with and without children suffering from nasobronchial allergies. They have convincingly shown a higher prevalence of respiratory allergies in households with higher levels of HAP. This is a significant addition to our existing knowledge about the possible adverse effects of IAP or HAP on respiratory disease. Both AR and BA are responsible for an enormous morbidity. This is particularly so in children in whom it is responsible for ill health, school absenteeism, and poor development of lung function. The observations raise the need to study the subject in larger samples among different populations.

Key Messages

- *Households with children suffering from nasobronchial allergies had higher concentrations of indoor air-pollutants.*
- *Increased levels of particulate matter and VOCs in indoor air are the major contributing factors for respiratory illness in the pediatric population.*

ARTICLE 6

Diffusing capacity of carbon monoxide in assessment of COPD

Balasubramanian A, MacIntyre NR, Henderson RJ, Jensen RL, Kinney G, Stringer WW, et al. Diffusing capacity of carbon monoxide in assessment of COPD.
Chest. 2019;156:1111-9.

Abstract

Background: Diffusing capacity of the lung for carbon monoxide (DLCO) is inconsistently obtained in patients with chronic obstructive pulmonary disease (COPD), and the added benefit of DLCO testing beyond that of more common tools is unknown.

Objective: The goal of this study was to determine whether lower DLCO is associated with increased COPD morbidity independent of emphysema assessed via spirometry and CT imaging.

Methods: Data for 1,806 participants with COPD from the genetic epidemiology of COPD (COPDgene) study 5-year visit were analyzed including pulmonary function testing, quality of life (QoL), symptoms, exercise performance, and exacerbation rates. DLCO% predicted was primarily analyzed as a continuous variable and additionally categorized into four groups: (1) DLCO and forced expiratory volume in 1 second (FEV1) >50%; (2) only DLCO ≤50%; (3) only FEV1 ≤50%; and (4) both ≤50% predicted. Outcomes were modeled by using multivariable linear and negative binomial regression including emphysema and FEV1% predicted among other confounders.

Results: In multivariable analyses, every 10% predicted decrease in DLCO was associated with symptoms and QoL [COPD assessment test: 0.53 (p < 0.001); St George's respiratory questionnaire: 1.67 (p < 0.001); Medical Outcomes Study Short Form 36 Physical Function: –0.89 (p < 0.001)], exercise performance (6-minute walk distance: –45.35 feet; p < 0.001), and severe exacerbation rate (rate ratio: 1.14; p < 0.001). When categorized, severe impairment in DLCO alone, FEV1 alone, or both DLCO and FEV1 were associated with significantly worse morbidity compared with the reference group (p < 0.05 for all outcomes).

Conclusions: Impairment in DLCO was associated with increased COPD symptoms, reduced exercise performance, and severe exacerbation risk even after accounting for spirometry and CT evidence of emphysema. These findings suggest that DLCO should be considered for inclusion in future multidimensional tools assessing COPD.

Trial registration: ClinicalTrials.gov NCT00608764.

"The missing link in chronic obstructive pulmonary disease (COPD) profiling?"

COMMENT

Chronic obstructive pulmonary disease (COPD) has been conventionally diagnosed with a combination of pertinent clinical history and spirometry. With the expansion of knowledge on diverse disease behavior, multidimensional profiling of COPD is becoming the norm with spirometry, effort tolerance, and quality of life (QoL) measures being included as part of the standard workup for COPD. Although serum biomarkers and additional pulmonary function measurements are being studied as indicators of disease progression and frequent exacerbations, they have not found widespread use in COPD phenotype profiling (**Fig. 1**).

Among the pulmonary function parameters, diffusing capacity of the lung for carbon monoxide (DLCO) is a sparingly used modality to prognosticate COPD except in the context of patients with emphysema, where impaired DLCO has been demonstrated and has been postulated

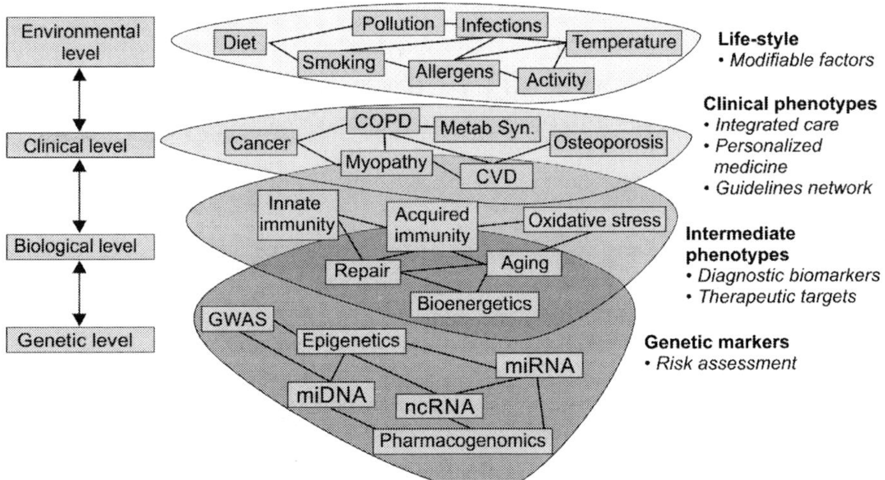

(CVD: cardiovascular disease; GWAS: genome-wide association studies; miDNA: mitochondrial deoxyribonucleic acid; miRNA: micro ribonucleic acid; ncRNA: noncoding ribonucleic acid)

FIG. 1: A model for phenotypes and endotypes in chronic obstructive pulmonary disease (COPD).

Source: Adapted from Agusti A, Vestbo J. Current controversies and future perspectives in chronic obstructive pulmonary disease. Am J Respir Crit Care Med. 2011;184:507-13.

to result from destruction of the airspace and capillary membrane. However, the association of impaired DLCO with QoL and exacerbations independent of emphysema has not been studied.

In this study, Balasubramaniam et al. have hypothesized that DLCO, independent of forced expiratory volume in 1 second (FEV1) and quantitative CT measures of emphysema, is associated with worse COPD morbidity. They classified 1,806 patients from the COPDgene cohort into four subgroups based on FEV1 and DLCO (DLCO and FEV1 >50%, only DLCO <50%, only FEV1 <50%, and both <50% predicted) and analyzed the association between isolated and combined impairment of these parameters with morbidity indicators such as symptoms, QoL, exercise performance, and exacerbations. On multivariate analysis, they found that a lower predicted DLCO alone was associated with increased COPD morbidity, independent of

FEV1 values and the presence of emphysema on quantitative CT.

This study raises the interesting possibility of including DLCO as a standard of care test in the initial assessment as well as follow-up of patients with COPD as it can be used as a predictor of worsening symptoms, effort tolerance, and development of acute exacerbations. An improvement in DLCO can also be used as a predictor of the efficacy of pulmonary rehabilitation.

■ FURTHER READING

1. Boutou AK, Shrikrishna D, Tanner RJ, Smith C, Kelly JL, Ward SP, et al. Lung function indices for predicting mortality in COPD. Eur Respir J. 2013;42(3):616-25.
2. Nambu A, Zach J, Schroeder J, Jin GY, Kim SS, Kim YI, et al. Relationships between diffusing capacity for carbon monoxide (DLCO), and quantitative computed tomography measurements and visual assessment for chronic obstructive pulmonary disease. Eur J Radiol. 2015;84(5):980-5.

Key Messages

⊙ *As precision medicine is being increasingly employed in the management of chronic respiratory diseases, sparingly used diagnostic tests have come to the forefront as markers of disease severity and progression.*

⊙ *Diffusing capacity of the lung for carbon monoxide is one among these tests, which can be used at baseline and at follow-up to assess progression as well as response to treatment.*

ARTICLE 7

Low and high blood eosinophil counts as biomarkers in hospitalized acute exacerbations of COPD

MacDonald MI, Osadnik CR, Bulfin L, Hamza K, Leong P, Wong A, et al. Low and high blood eosinophil counts as biomarkers in hospitalized acute exacerbations of COPD.
Chest. 2019;156:92-100.

Abstract

Background: Characterizing acute exacerbations of chronic obstructive pulmonary disease (AECOPD) and individualizing therapy is challenging. Key exacerbation therapies include antibiotics and systemic corticosteroids. Blood eosinophils, when either low or high, may offer a simple and inexpensive distinction to predict beneficial responses to these therapies.

Methods: We conducted derivation (n = 242) and validation (n = 99) cohort studies of patients hospitalized for AECOPD. Patients who received oral corticosteroids before emergency department (ED) presentation were excluded. The derivation cohort was identified by individual case file review. The validation cohort was prospectively recruited during hospital admission. Exacerbations were grouped according to blood eosinophil count as low (<50/µL), normal (50–150/µL), or high (>150/µL). Exacerbations were classified as being associated with infection if either virus testing was positive or C-reactive protein was ≥20 mg/L. Associations of eosinophil groups with infection, hospital length of stay, and 12-month survival were compared using appropriate statistical methods.

Results: There were no significant differences in baseline characteristics between patients with low, normal, or high-blood eosinophils in either cohort. Eosinophil counts <50/µL were more strongly associated with infection (91 vs. 51.9%, p = 0.001), distinguished patients with longer median hospital stays (7 vs. 4 days, p < 0.001), and were associated with lower 12-month survival (82.4 vs. 90.7%, p = 0.028; pooled data of both cohorts) than eosinophil counts >150/µL.

Conclusions: Low and high blood eosinophil counts in hospitalized patients with AECOPD provide a practical clinical distinction that can potentially be used to inform management strategies. Prospective studies are needed to evaluate if this strategy can guide discriminate use of antibiotics and/or corticosteroids.

"Blood eosinopenia in acute exacerbations of chronic obstructive pulmonary disease (AECOPD): A new phenotype?"

COMMENT

Chronic obstructive pulmonary disease (COPD) is a disease where fixed airway obstruction is the common denominator, but varied symptomatology and response to existing therapies contribute to its heterogeneity and variable disease trajectory.

Approximately 15–40% of COPD exacerbations are eosinophil driven with no evidence of infection. The GOLD (Global initiative for chronic Obstructive Lung Disease) guidelines have incorporated the role of inhaled corticosteroids (ICS) in patients with >3% (>300 cells/mL) eosinophils and in frequent exacerbators.

The authors have used eosinophil count as a simple biomarker to help in decision making in the treatment of acute exacerbation of chronic obstructive pulmonary disease (AECOPD). A retrospective derivation cohort of 242 subjects with AECOPD was followed up with a prospective validation cohort of 99 subjects with AECOPD. Associations between eosinopenia (<50/mm^3), high eosinophil counts (>150/mm^3) and clinical outcomes were evaluated. Infective or noninfective causes of the AECOPD were based on results of viral polymerase chain reaction (PCR) and C-reactive

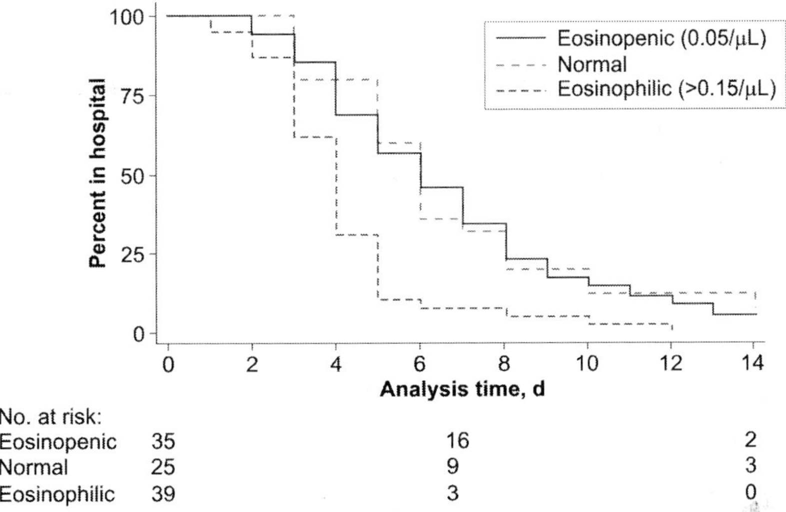

FIG. 1: Length of hospital stay according to blood eosinophil group. Kaplan–Meier analysis of length of hospital stay in validation cohort.

Courtesy: Adapted from the GOLD study.

protein (CRP) measurements. Eosinopenia was associated with longer hospital stay and higher mortality at 1-year follow-up (**Fig. 1**).

Although the proportion of exacerbation was similar across the different eosinophil groups and majority of them had infective etiology, a significant drop in infection rates was observed in the increasing blood eosinophil groups (<50/mL, 90.6% vs. >150/mL, 51.9%). Around 89% of the eosinophilic subjects were discharged from hospital within 5 days versus 42% in the eosinopenic group.

The role of airway eosinophil count of >3% has been widely studied and incorporated into treatment guidelines. A higher eosinophil count denotes better response to steroids in AECOPD and a better clinical outcome. This study further refines our understanding of the role of eosinophils in COPD. A lower blood eosinophil count may similarly portend an infective etiology and steroids may be avoided, as it can increase viral replication and delay cure. This revelation of low eosinophil association with neutrophil predominant infection in AECOPD raises the possibility of an emerging phenotype, where specific therapies may be beneficial. A 55% reduction in the exacerbation rate was seen with losmapimod, a p38 mitogen-activated protein kinase (MAPK) inhibitor, in COPD subjects with <2% eosinophils as compared to no such effect in subjects with >2% eosinophils.

As management strategies move toward individualized treatment, fine tuning of the description of phenotypes and clear categorization will be the game changers in COPD management. Simple biomarkers, such as eosinopenia and eosinophilia, fit the bill very well and can be widely used in deciding management pathways.

■ FURTHER READING

1. Marks-Konczalika J, Costaa M, Robertson J, McKieb E, Yang S, Pascoec S. A post-hoc subgroup analysis of data from a six month clinical trial comparing the efficacy and safety of losmapimod in moderate-severe COPD patients with ≤2% and >2% blood eosinophils. Respir Med. 2015;109:860-9.

2. Sidhaye VK, Nishida K, Martinez FJ. Precision medicine in COPD: where are we and where do we need to go? Eur Respir Rev. 2018;27:180022.

Key Message

⊙ *Stratifying blood eosinophil count as a biomarker in hospitalized AECOPD may be useful to guide management algorithms to target populations for receiving antibiotics and/or corticosteroids.*

Budesonide-formoterol reliever therapy versus maintenance budesonide plus terbutaline reliever therapy in adults with mild to moderate asthma (PRACTICAL): a 52-week, open-label, multicentre, superiority, randomised controlled trial

Hardy J, Baggott C, Fingleton J, Reddel HK, Hancox RJ, Harwood M, et al. Budesonide-formoterol Reliever Therapy versus Maintenance Budesonide plus Terbutaline Reliever Therapy in Adults with Mild to Moderate Asthma (PRACTICAL): a 52-week, Open-label, Multicentre, Superiority, Randomised Controlled Trial.
Lancet. 2019;394:919-28.

Abstract

Background: In adults with mild asthma, a combination of an inhaled corticosteroid with a fast-onset long-acting β-agonist (LABA) used as reliever monotherapy reduces severe exacerbations compared with short-acting β-agonist (SABA) reliever therapy. We investigated the efficacy of combination budesonide-formoterol reliever therapy compared with maintenance budesonide plus as-needed terbutaline.

Methods: We did a 52-week, open-label, parallel-group, multicenter, superiority, randomized controlled trial at 15 primary care or hospital-based clinical trials units and primary care practices in New Zealand. Participants were adults aged 18–75 years with a self-reported doctor's diagnosis of asthma who were using SABA for symptom relief with or without maintenance low-to-moderate doses of inhaled corticosteroids in the previous 12 weeks. We randomly assigned participants (1:1) to either reliever therapy with budesonide 200 µg-formoterol 6 µg Turbuhaler® (one inhalation as needed for relief of symptoms) or maintenance budesonide 200 µg Turbuhaler® (one inhalation twice daily) plus terbutaline 250 µg Turbuhaler® (two inhalations as needed). Participants and investigators were not masked to group assignment; the statistician was masked for analysis of the primary outcome. Six study visits were scheduled: Randomization, and weeks 4, 16, 28, 40, and 52. The primary outcome was the number of severe exacerbations per patient per year analyzed by intention to treat (severe exacerbations defined as use of systemic corticosteroids for at least 3 days because of asthma, or admission to hospital or an emergency department visit because of asthma requiring systemic corticosteroids). Safety analyses included all participants who had received at least one dose of study treatment. This trial is registered with the Australian New Zealand Clinical Trials Registry, number ACTRN12616000377437.

Findings: Between May 4, 2016, and December 22, 2017, we assigned 890 participants to treatment and included 885 eligible participants in the analysis: 437 assigned to budesonide-formoterol as needed and 448 to budesonide maintenance plus terbutaline as needed. Severe exacerbations per patient per year were lower with as-needed budesonide-formoterol than with maintenance budesonide plus terbutaline as needed (absolute rate per patient per year: 0.119 vs. 0.172; relative rate: 0.69; 95% CI 0.48–1.00; p = 0.049). Nasopharyngitis was the most common adverse event in both groups, occurring in 154 (35%) of 440 patients receiving as-needed budesonide-formoterol and 144 (32%) of 448 receiving maintenance budesonide plus terbutaline as needed.

Interpretation: In adults with mild-to-moderate asthma, budesonide-formoterol used as needed for symptom relief was more effective at preventing severe exacerbations than maintenance low-dose budesonide plus as-needed terbutaline. The findings support the 2019 Global Initiative for Asthma recommendation that inhaled corticosteroid-formoterol reliever therapy which is an alternative regimen to daily low-dose inhaled corticosteroid for patients with mild asthma.

"Scientific research is one of the most exciting and rewarding of occupations."

—Fredirick Sanger

COMMENT

Treatment of asthma has become more systematized in recent years with more and more evidence accumulating on the use of long-acting β-agonist (LABA) and inhaled corticosteroid (ICS) combination inhalers. The use of short-acting β-agonists (SABA) has been minimized and relegated to be used in acute exacerbations and in mild asthma for symptom control. The commonly used agents are salbutamol and terbutaline.

The use of the so-called SMART therapy—a combination of ICS-LABA with the properties of fast onset of action and long duration has come increased over the last decade. In this concept because of the combination of properties, the same inhaler can be used both as a reliever and for maintenance, freeing the patient from carrying and using two separate reliever and maintenance devices. The main benefit of using this approach, apart from convenience, has been a reduction in the amount of acute exacerbations.

In this randomized controlled study, the single inhaler concept was compared for as needed use in patients with mild asthma.

The test group was allowed to use a single puff of budesonide-formoterol on an as-needed basis while the control group was put on twice a day maintenance budesonide plus as-needed terbutaline. The amount of severe exacerbations per patient per year was lower with as-needed budesonide-formoterol than with maintenance budesonide plus terbutaline as needed (absolute rate per patient per year: 0.119 vs. 0.172). This led to the interpretation that budesonide-formoterol used as needed for symptom relief was more effective at preventing severe exacerbations than maintenance low-dose budesonide plus as-needed terbutaline.

However, one should consider that this patient population is not very prone to developing acute exacerbations, especially severe ones. This is borne out by the low rate of exacerbations in both groups. Other treatment outcomes such as number of emergency actuations of the inhalers, disease progression, quality of life, etc., might be more meaningful in this setting.

This study provides a useful alternate treatment guide for treatment of patients with mild asthma.

Key Message

- *Combination inhalation of budesonide-formoterol used as needed for symptom relief was more effective at preventing severe exacerbations than maintenance low-dose budesonide plus as-needed terbutaline in adults with mild-to-moderate asthma.*

ARTICLE 9

Single inhaler extrafine triple therapy in uncontrolled asthma (TRIMARAN and TRIGGER): two double-blind, parallel-group, randomised, controlled phase 3 trials

Virchow JC, Kuna P, Paggiaro P, Papi A, Singh D, Corre S, et al. Single inhaler extrafine triple therapy in uncontrolled asthma (TRIMARAN and TRIGGER): two double-blind, parallel-group, randomised, controlled phase 3 trials.
Lancet. 2019;394:1737-49.

Abstract

Background: To date, no studies have assessed the efficacy of single-inhaler triple therapy in asthma. Here we report on two studies that compared the single-inhaler extrafine combination of beclometasone dipropionate [BDP; inhaled corticosteroid (ICS)], formoterol fumarate [FF; long-acting β_2-agonist (LABA)], and glycopyrronium [G; long-acting muscarinic antagonist (LAMA)] with the combination of BDP with FF.

Methods: Two parallel-group, double-blind, randomized, active-controlled, phase 3 trials TRIMARAN (TRIple in asthMA with uncontRolled pAtient on medium streNgth of ICS + LABA) and TRIGGER (TRIple in asthma hiGh strenGth vErsus ICS/LABA HS and tiotRopium) recruited patients from 171 sites across 16 countries (TRIMARAN), and from 221 sites across 17 countries (TRIGGER). The sites were a mixture of secondary and tertiary care centers and specialized investigation units. Eligible patients were adults (aged 18–75 years) with uncontrolled asthma, a history of one or more exacerbations in the previous year, and previously treated with ICS (TRIMARAN: medium dose; TRIGGER: high dose) plus a long-acting β_2 agonist. Enrolled patients were initially treated with BDP/FF (TRIMARAN: 100 µg BDP and 6 µg FF; TRIGGER: 200 µg BDP and 6 µg FF) for 2 weeks, then randomly assigned to treatment using an interactive response technology system with a balanced block randomization scheme stratified by country. Patients, investigators, site staff, and sponsor staff were masked to BDP/FF/G and BDP/FF assignment. In TRIMARAN, patients were randomly assigned (1:1) to 52 weeks of BDP/FF/G (100 µg BDP, 6 µg FF, and 10 µg G) or BDP/FF (100 µg BDP and 6 µg FF), two inhalations twice daily. In TRIGGER, patients were randomly assigned (2:2:1) to 52 weeks of BDP/FF/G (200 µg BDP, 6 µg FF, and 10 µg G) or BDP/FF (200 BDP and 6 µg FF), both two inhalations twice daily, or open-label BDP/FF (200 µg BDP and 6 µg FF) two inhalations twice daily plus tiotropium 2.5 µg two inhalations once daily. Co-primary endpoints for both trials (BDP/FF/G vs. BDP/FF) were predose forced expiratory volume in 1 second (FEV1) at week 26 and rate of moderate and severe exacerbations over 52 weeks. Safety was assessed in all patients who received at least one dose of study treatment. These trials were registered with ClinicalTrials.gov, NCT02676076 (TRIMARAN), NCT02676089 (TRIGGER).

Findings: Between February 17, 2016, and May 17, 2018, 1,155 patients in TRIMARAN were given BDP/FF/G (n = 579) or BDP/FF (n = 576). Between April 6, 2016, and May 28, 2018, 1,437 patients in TRIGGER were given BDP/FF/G (n = 573), BDP/FF (n = 576), or BDP/FF plus tiotropium (n = 288). Compared with the BDP/FF group, week 26 predose FEV1 improved in the BDP/FF/G group by 57 mL [95% confidence interval (CI) 15–99; p = 0.0080] in TRIMARAN and by 73 mL (26–120; p = 0.0025) in TRIGGER with reductions in the rate of moderate and severe exacerbations of 15% (rate ratio 0.85, 95% CI 0.73–0.99; p = 0.033) in TRIMARAN and 12% (0.88, 0.75–1.03; p = 0.11) in TRIGGER. Four patients had treatment-related serious adverse events, one in TRIMARAN in the BDP/FF/G group and three in TRIGGER-one in the BDP/FF/G and two in the BDP/FF group. Three patients in the BDP/FF/G group in TRIMARAN and two patients in TRIGGER-one in the BDP/FF/G group and one in the BDP/FF group had adverse events leading to death. None of the deaths were considered as related to treatment.

Interpretation: In uncontrolled asthma, addition of a long-acting muscarinic antagonist to ICS plus long-acting β_2-agonist therapy improves lung function and reduces exacerbations.

"Individual curiosity, often working without practical ends in mind, has always been a driving force for innovation."

—**Frederick Seitz**

COMMENT

Combination of long-acting β-agonist (LABA) and inhaled corticosteroid (ICS) inhalers is the mainstay of treatment in asthma. However, in patients poorly controlled on these medications treatment options are limited. One step is to increase the dose of inhaled steroids while more severe disease requires addition of oral steroids or other agents. Use of long-acting muscarinic agents (LAMAs) was not initially thought to be useful.

However, use of triple agent therapy in uncontrolled or poorly controlled asthma is now gaining ground. Use of tiotropium as an add-on agent was tested and found to be useful in many trials in the last few years. In this context, these two trials were carried out to assess whether a single triple combination inhaler would be as effective as using separate ICS-LABA and LAMA inhalers.

Both the trial recruited patients with uncontrolled or poorly controlled asthma. In the TRIMARAN trial, the patients had been receiving medium dose of ICS while in the TRIGGER trial, they had received high dose of ICS. Co-primary endpoints for both trials were predose forced expiratory volume in 1 second (FEV1) at week 26 and rate of moderate and severe exacerbations over 52 weeks. In the TRIMARAN trial patients were randomly assigned (1:1) to 52 weeks of BDP/FF/G (beclomethasone dipropionate/formoterol fumarate/glycopyrronium) or BDP/FF. In the TRIGGER trial patients received either BDP/FF/G or BDP/FF or open-label BDP/FF plus tiotropium.

By week 26, predose FEV1 improved in the BDP/FF/G group by 57 mL in TRIMARAN and by 73 mL in TRIGGER with reductions in the rate of moderate and severe exacerbations of 15% in TRIMARAN and 12% in TRIGGER. There was no significant difference in side effects. The results show that addition of LAMAs to ICS-LABA combinations is effective in uncontrolled asthma and can be used as a single triple combination inhaler.

■ FURTHER READING

1. Adams KS, Lowe DK. Tiotropium for adults with inadequately controlled persistent asthma. Ann Pharmacother. 2013;47(1): 117-23.

Key Message

⊙ *Addition of a long-acting muscarinic antagonist to inhaled corticosteroid (ICS) plus long-acting β2-agonist (LABA) therapy is effective to improve lung function and reduce exacerbations in uncontrolled asthma.*

Tuberculosis

ARTICLE 10

Extrapulmonary drug-resistant tuberculosis at a drug-resistant tuberculosis center, Mumbai: our experience—hope in the midst of despair

Desai U, Joshi JM. Extrapulmonary drug-resistant tuberculosis at a drug-resistant tuberculosis center, Mumbai: our experience—Hope in the midst of despair.
Lung India. 2019:36:3-7.

Abstract

Background: Drug-resistant tuberculosis (DR-TB) is a global problem with only 52% reported cure rate. Extrapulmonary (EP) DR-TB poses a formidable diagnostic, therapeutic challenge. We aimed to study their clinical profile and treatment outcomes under the programmatic setting.

Materials and methods: This retrospective observational study included the database of consecutive EPDR-TB cases enrolled at the DR-TB center from 2012 to 2014. The demographic, clinical details, drug susceptibility tests (DSTs), follow-up, therapy, adverse events (AEs), and outcomes were reviewed. Statistical analysis was done using percentages and mean.

Results: Of total 1,743 DR-TB patients, 76 (4.4%) EPDR-TB cases were included. These consisted of 53 (69.7%) adults and 23 (30.3%) children, with female preponderance. The mean age in adults and children was 27.96 (9.63) and 12.56 (3.83), respectively. EP sites involved were lymph nodes in 39 (51.3%), spine in 15 (19.7%), other bones in 6 (7.9%), pleural effusion in 9 (11.9%), central nervous system in 2 (2.6%), and disseminated EP disease in 5 (6.6%) patients. Forty-one (53.9%) patients had multi-DR-TB (MDR-TB), 29 (38.2%) MDR-TB with fluoroquinolone resistance [pre-extensively DR-TB (pre-XDR-TB (FQ)], 1 (1.3%) MDR-TB with aminoglycoside resistance [pre-XDR-TB (AM)], and 5 (6.6%) extensively DR-TB (XDR-TB) on DST.

Thirteen (17.11%) patients had comorbidities. None had human immunodeficiency virus (HIV). Two (2.63%) had diabetes mellitus (DM). Patients were treated as per the revised TB control program–programmatic management of DR-TB guidelines. Duration of intensive (IP) was 6.55 (1.22) months. Ten (13.2%) patients received shorter regimens, wherein therapy was stopped at 12–18 months due to severe adverse drug reactions and treatment response. Sixty-two (81.6%) completed treatment, 8 (10.5%) defaulted, 3 (4%) died, 2 (2.6%) failed, and 1 (1.3%) patient was transferred out. Two-thirds of patients reported AE.

Conclusion: The prevalence of EP cases in DR-TB was 4.4%. Treatment completion rate was very high (81.6%). Shorter regimens were efficacious.

"The tubercle bacillus bore cheerfully a degree of medication which proved fatal to its host!"

—**Edward Trudeau**

COMMENT

There is an increased concern about drug-resistant tuberculosis (DR-TB) in view of the enormity of the problem. DR-TB is mostly described among patients of pulmonary TB with an extensive disease who had been treated with inadequate and erratic regimens. DR-TB, previously considered to be uncommon in extrapulmonary tuberculosis (EPTB), is now being seen with an increasing frequency in the last two decades especially after the recognition of human immunodeficiency virus (HIV) infection. The authors of this paper report 76 (4.4%) EPDR-TB cases among 1,743 DR-TB patients seen by them in Mumbai. Lymph nodes and spine were the two most common sites.

In the past, somewhat similar experience was described from the National Institute for Research in Tuberculosis (NIRT), Chennai.[6] Of 1,295 extrapulmonary specimens, 189 grew *Mycobacterium tuberculosis*, 37 (19%) cases were multidrug resistant (MDR) between 2005 and 2012. It would, therefore, seem that there is a significant number of MDR among EPTB patient population which mandates the need for a specific diagnostic and treatment strategy for these patients.

Dr Desai describes the pattern of drug resistance on drug-sensitivity tests: 41 (53.9%) suffering from multi-DR-TB (resistance to isoniazid and rifampicin with or without other first-line anti-tubercular drugs), 29 (38.2%) had MDR-TB with additional fluoroquinolone resistance, 1 (1.3%) with additional aminoglycoside resistance, and 5 (6.6%) with extensively DR-TB (i.e., MDR with additional resistance to at least one of fluoroquinolone and an injectable drug). Emergence of resistance to drugs such as fluoroquinolone and aminoglycosides is a serious challenge which immensely complicates the scene of tuberculosis control in India.

Tuberculosis control is a serious issue in this country with a huge burden and restrained health infrastructure. The Government of India has now modified the Revised National Tuberculosis Control Program (RNTCP) to National TB Elimination Program (NTEP) which aims to reduce the TB incidence to <1 case of infectious TB per million population or a prevalence of latent TB infection of <1%. This is tough goal to achieve especially in the light of an increased burden of drug-resistance.

Drug-resistance in EPTB is likely to pose several other clinical issues. It is generally to obtain clinical samples for microbiological demonstration of mycobacteria in cases of EPTB. Therefore, diagnosis of DR-EPTB will remain conjectural in a vast majority of cases. Moreover, the duration of treatment for several types of EPTB as well as DR-TB is longer than for pulmonary and some forms of EPTB. We do not know the duration of different drugs for management of EP-DRTB. It will be rather long before we find answers to the vexed questions.

Key Messages

⦿ *There was 4.4% prevalence of drug-resistance in patients of extrapulmonary tuberculosis.*

⦿ *Outcomes of treatment were satisfactory in DR-EPTB cases.*

ARTICLE 11

Effect of bronchial artery embolisation on the management of tuberculosis-related haemoptysis

Peng Y, Zhu Y, Ao G, Chen Z, Yuan X, Li Q, et al. Effect of bronchial artery embolisation on the management of tuberculosis-related haemoptysis.
Int J Tuberc Lung Dis. 2019;23:1269-76.

Abstract*

Objective: To analyze the outcome of bronchial arterial embolization (BAE) in tuberculosis (TB)-related hemoptysis and the risk factors influencing the outcome.

Methods: The clinical data of 207 patients who underwent BAE for TB-related hemoptysis between March, 2014 and March, 2018, were reviewed. Follow-up ranged from 24 to 1,749 days.

Results: Around 94.2% of the enrolled patients attained immediate hemostasis. Cumulative recurrence-free rates were 98.5%, 94.8%, 88.7%, 79.9%, 68.5%, 65.7%, and 62.7% for 1, 3, 6, 12, 24, 36, and 48 months, respectively. A total of 8 and 15 patients recovered from pneumonectomy and re-BAE, respectively. However, five patients required a third BAE. Aggressive pleural thickening (PT) (p = 0.000), diabetes mellitus (DM) (p = 0.018), and pulmonary fungal infection (PFI) (p = 0.001) were independent risk factors for recurrence, as derived by Cox regression analysis.

Conclusion: Bronchial arterial embolization is an effective strategy for treatment of TB-related hemoptysis in most cases. Aggressive PT, DM, and PFI, as independent risk factors, influence the outcome following BAE, and hence should be properly managed. *Redrafted abstract

"Pleural thickening in TB-related hemoptysis—Is it aggressive enough?"

COMMENT

Massive hemoptysis is a dreaded complication in patients with active tuberculosis and post-tubercular sequelae alike. Bronchial arterial embolization (BAE) is commonly performed either as a bridging procedure before definitive surgery or exclusively in poor surgical candidates to control hemoptysis.

The authors aimed to evaluate factors associated with recurrence of hemoptysis in patients with tuberculosis (TB) or TB sequelae who underwent BAE. The retrospective analysis of 207 patients presents a few interesting findings:

- Patients aged >50 years were more likely to have aggressive pleural thickening (PT) and pulmonary fungal infections (PFI).
- Patients with PT had more angiographically abnormal arteries.
- Presence of aggressive PT was an independent risk factor for failure of BAE [odds ratio (OR) 22.5; p < 0.001] and death (OR 8.14; p < 0.001).

Deaths were predominantly due to recurrence of massive hemoptysis.
- Aggressive PT, PFI, and diabetes were independent predictors of recurrence of hemoptysis; other risk factors being presence of cavity, destroyed lung, drug-resistant TB, and presence of shunts (**Table 1**).

TABLE 1: Independent factors of recurrence-free time after bronchial arterial embolization (BAE) in a multivariate analysis using a Cox's regression hazards model.*

Risk factors	Hazard ratio	OR (95% CI)	p value
Aggressive PT	2.501	1.843–3.394	0.000
PFI	2.686	1.547–4.664	0.000
Diabetes	1.865	1.089–3.194	0.023

(CI: confidence interval; OR: odds ratio, PFI: pulmonary fungal infection; PT: pleural thickening)

*Table from the index article.

Bronchial arterial embolization was successful in 94.2% of patients in whom immediate hemostasis was achieved with very few early recurrences indicative of the technical expertise of the team. Majority of recurrences occurred after 3–6 months of the procedure which is likely to be due to recanalization or recruitment of new arteries. No inadvertent systemic embolizations were reported which could be attributed to superselective catheterization and use of appropriately sized embolizing materials.

Presence of PT as a risk factor for recurrence has shown contradictory results in previous studies which looked at it as a dichotomous variable. The current study adds a new radiological dimension by further characterizing PT (pleural thickness >3 mm) as aggressive if spanning >2 ribs and local if limited to two ribs. Aggressive PT was significantly associated with poor outcomes. This could probably be due to recruitment of nonbronchial systemic collateral vessels which enter the pulmonary parenchyma from adjacent pleura.[7,8] PFI, which is probably a reference to the presence of an aspergilloma, has been identified as an important risk factor for recurrence of hemoptysis in previous studies also. The presence of aggressive PT or PFI may warrant consideration of definitive surgical procedures for hemoptysis to prevent untoward complications in such patients.

Key Messages

⦿ *Bronchial arterial embolization for tuberculosis-related hemoptysis is a safe procedure with high rates of immediate hemostasis.*

⦿ *However, presence of risk factors such as aggressive PT and PFI which are associated recurrence and death should prompt early consideration of definitive surgical procedures.*

ARTICLE 12

A trial of a shorter regimen for rifampin-resistant tuberculosis

Nunn AJ, Phillips PPJ, Meredith SK, Chiang CY, Conradie F, Dalai D, et al. A trial of a shorter regimen for rifampin-resistant tuberculosis.
N Engl J Med. 2019;380:1201-13.

Abstract*

Background: For treatment of multidrug-resistant tuberculosis (MDR-TB), the World Health Organization (WHO) in their guidelines released in 2011 recommended longer duration (20 months) of treatment with second-line antitubercular drugs. However, cohort studies conducted in Bangladesh has shown promising cure rates with shorter regimens.

Methods: A phase 3 noninferiority trial was conducted in participants with rifampin-resistant but fluoroquinolones and aminoglycosides susceptible tuberculosis. Participants were randomly assigned, in a 2:1 ratio, to receive a short regimen (9–11 months) that included high-dose moxifloxacin or a long regimen (20 months). The primary efficacy outcome was a favorable status at 132 weeks, defined by cultures negative for *Mycobacterium tuberculosis* at 132 weeks and at a previous occasion, with no intervening positive culture or previous unfavorable outcome. An upper 95% confidence limit for the between-group difference in favorable status that was 10% points or less was used to determine noninferiority.

Results: Of 424 participants who underwent randomization, 383 were included in the modified intention-to-treat population. Favorable status was reported in 79.8% of participants in the long-regimen group and in 78.8% of those in the short-regimen group—a difference, with adjustment for human immunodeficiency virus status, of 1.0% point [95% confidence interval (CI) –7.5 to 9.5; p = 0.02 for noninferiority]. Around

321 participants in the per-protocol population showed this consistent results with respect to noninferiority (adjusted difference –0.7% points; 95% CI –10.5 to 9.1). Around 45.4% of participants in the long-regimen group and in 48.2% in the short-regimen group had an adverse event of grade 3 or higher. Around 11.0% of participants in the short-regimen group as compared with 6.4% in the long-regimen group (p = 0.14) showed QT prolongation (calculated with Fridericia's formula). Close monitoring of these participants and medication adjustments for some of them were done. Around 8.5% of participants in the short-regimen group and in 6.4% in the long-regimen group died. Also, acquired resistance to fluoroquinolones or aminoglycosides was observed in 3.3% and 2.3%, respectively.

Conclusion: We concluded that a short regimen was noninferior and similar to the long regimen with respect to the primary efficacy outcome and safety, respectively in MDR-TB. *Redrafted abstract

"Research is to see what everyone else has seen, and to think what nobody else thought."
—Albert Szent-Gyorgyi

COMMENT

The term "multidrug-resistant tuberculosis (MDR-TB)" is used for a form of tuberculosis which is resistant to both isoniazid and rifampicin. It affects almost 500,000 individuals worldwide and had a higher morbidity and mortality than drug susceptible tuberculosis. Moreover, the treatment regimens required for treatment are extremely long, with an intensive period of 6–8 months and a maintenance phase of 18 months, leading to a total duration of 20 months or above. Despite the long and costly treatment, success rates are low.[9]

Efforts are ongoing in order to find newer drugs and regimens that would shorten the treatment duration in MDR-TB and improve the success rate. A trial of six treatment regimens conducted in Bangladesh showed efficacy for a shorter treatment regimen of 9 months.[10] The current study has used a similar protocol and tried to compare it with the standard regimen in randomized manner. The short regimen consisted of an intensive phase of ethambutol, pyrazinamide, high dose of moxifloxacin and clofazamine along with kanamycin, isoniazid, and prothionamide in the first 16 weeks followed by the first four drugs in the continuation phase for a total duration of 40 weeks.

Patients were randomized into treatment groups of the short and standard regimens in a ratio of 2:1 and also stratified according to human immunodeficiency virus (HIV) status. Approximately one-third of patients were HIV positive and 60% had cavitations on chest X-ray. Overall the short regimen was noninferior to standard regimen in terms of outcome and had similar safety. There was a significant difference in the duration of treatment; 40.1 weeks in the short regimen versus 82.7 weeks in the standard regimen. However, there was a trend toward unfavorable bacteriological outcomes in the short regimen (10.6%) as compared to the standard regimen (5.6%). A limited trend of increased mortality in the HIV co-infected patients was also noted in the short regimen.

Overall, this study demonstrated that short-course treatments for MDR-TB are possible without adding significantly to the cost and also without compromising on success rates. Further studies and new drugs are needed to further clarify the issue.

Key Message

⊛ *Short-course treatments for multidrug-resistant tuberculosis (MDR-TB) are possible without adding significantly to the cost and also without compromising on success rates provided the effective and prescribed regimens are followed.*

Infectious Diseases

ARTICLE 13

Comparative risks of chronic inhaled corticosteroids and macrolides for bronchiectasis

Henkle E, Curtis JR, Chen L, Chan B, Aksamit TR, Daley CL, et al. Comparative risks of chronic inhaled corticosteroids and macrolides for bronchiectasis.
Eur Respir J. 2019;54:1801896.

Abstract*

Introduction: An increased risk of respiratory infections has been observed with the chronic use of drugs especially corticosteroids for treatment of noncystic fibrosis (CF) bronchiectasis. This can be a guiding factor for deciding on the treatment regimen, but the data is scarce. Here, we compare the risks of respiratory infections associated with chronic use of inhaled corticosteroids (ICSs) and macrolide monotherapy.

Methods: The study was conducted on a cohort of the United States Medicare enrollees diagnosed with bronchiectasis (International Classification of Diseases, Ninth Revision, Clinical Modification code 494.0 or 494.1) between 2006 and 2014, excluding CF. Chronic new use was defined as the first ≥28-day prescription of ICS therapy or macrolide monotherapy. The characteristics of the exposure cohorts using standardized mean differences (SMDs) and computed a propensity score (PS) were compared. PS decile-adjusted Cox regression models were used to compare the risks of acute exacerbation, hospitalized respiratory infection, all-cause hospitalization, and mortality.

Results: Of the total 285,043 Medicare enrollees with bronchiectasis, 83,589 were new users of ICSs and 6,500 were new users of macrolides. The crude incidence of hospitalized respiratory infection was 12.6 (ICS therapy) and 10.3 (macrolide monotherapy) per 100 patient-years. The PS-adjusted hazard ratios (HRs) comparing ICS with macrolide new users were 1.39 (95% CI 1.23–1.57) for hospitalized respiratory infection, 1.56 (95% CI 1.49–1.64) for acute exacerbation, and 1.09 (95% CI 0.95–1.25) for mortality.

Interpretation: The use of ICSs was significantly associated with an increased risk of hospitalized respiratory infections compared with macrolide monotherapy. *Redrafted abstract

"Macrolides versus inhaled steroids in bronchiectasis: Doubts dispelled."

COMMENT

This article compares the effect of anti-inflammatory treatment with long-term macrolides and inhaled corticosteroids (ICS) in prevention of acute exacerbations in noncystic fibrosis (CF) bronchiectasis. Various meta-analysis and guidelines favor macrolide use, though proof of effectiveness is based on limited number of studies. In this study, macrolides have been pitted against ICS to evaluate not only hospitalized respiratory infection, but also reduction in exacerbation, all-cause hospitalization, and mortality.

The advantage of this study is the huge cohort, built from an insurance database of 618,303 patients with bronchiectasis, from which 83,589 ICS and 6,500 macrolide monotherapy new users were selected and matched by propensity score (PS). Patients taking ICS were 39% more likely to be hospitalized for respiratory infections and 56% more likely to have acute exacerbations in the adjusted models. Though exacerbations have been linked to increased mortality, surprisingly there was no difference in mortality [adjusted hazard ratio (HR) 1.09] between the two arms in this study (**Fig. 1**).

We now have emphatic evidence to back our understanding that long-term macrolides reduce respiratory infection and hospitalization. Not only

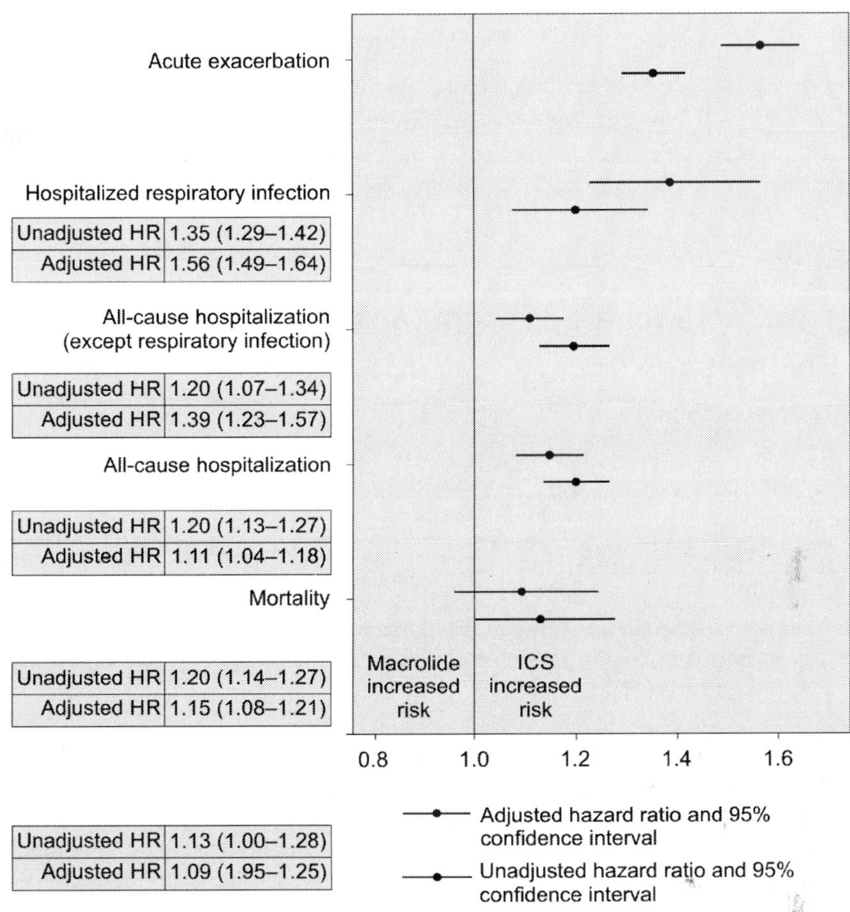

FIG. 1: Forest plot of unadjusted and adjusted* hazard ratio (HR) and 95% confidence interval of key outcomes comparing new use of inhaled corticosteroids (ICS) to macrolide monotherapy for bronchiectasis.

do macrolides lower bacterial load, but also have an immunomodulatory effect in the treatment of non-CF bronchiectasis. However, development of drug-resistant bacteria and cardiac adverse events secondary to the macrolide use should be weighed before starting therapy.

It was common practice to treat non-CF bronchiectasis with ICS, with/without bronchodilators, as there is an element of airway obstruction in this disease. However, ICS is not suitable for all types of patients as it increases the risk of nontuberculous mycobacteria (NTM), facilitates microbial overgrowth, and is not effective in predominant neutrophilic inflammation. The evidence from this study helps us to steer away from ICS in non-CF bronchiectasis, other than in those cases with coexistent asthma or chronic obstructive pulmonary disease (COPD).

Extrapolation of the findings in this study to our population should be carefully considered before choosing treatment as our population comprises younger patients with post-TB bronchiectasis as opposed to the study population, who were older and had a high proportion of COPD (80%).

Nevertheless, this study backed by robust data has helped in clearing the air and confirmed the benefits of macrolides in non-CF bronchiectasis.

■ FURTHER READING

1. Fan LC, Lu HW, Wei P, Ji XB, Liang S, Xu JF. Effects of long-term use of macrolides in patients with non-cystic fibrosis bronchiectasis: a meta-analysis of randomized controlled trials. BMC Infect Dis. 2015;15:160.
2. Kelly C, Chalmers JD, Crossingham I, Relph N, Felix LM, Evans DJ, et al. Macrolide antibiotics for bronchiectasis (Review). Cochrane Database Syst Rev. 2018;3:CD012406.

Key Message

⊙ *Macrolides may be a better choice than ICS to prevent hospitalized respiratory infections and acute respiratory infections in older bronchiectasis patients with frequent exacerbations.*

ARTICLE 14

Causes of severe pneumonia requiring hospital admission in children without HIV Infection from Africa and Asia: the PERCH multi-country case-control study

Pneumonia Etiology Research for Child Health (PERCH) Study Group. Causes of severe pneumonia requiring hospital admission in children without HIV infection from Africa and Asia: the PERCH Multi-Country Case-Control Study. *Lancet. 2019;394:757-79.*

Abstract

Background: Pneumonia is the leading cause of death among children younger than 5 years. In this study, we estimated causes of pneumonia in young African and Asian children, using novel analytical methods applied to clinical and microbiological findings.

Methods: We did a multisite, international case–control study in nine study sites in seven countries: Bangladesh, The Gambia, Kenya, Mali, South Africa, Thailand, and Zambia. All sites enrolled in the study for 24 months. Cases were children aged 1–59 months admitted to hospital with severe pneumonia. Controls were age-group-matched children randomly selected from communities surrounding study sites. Nasopharyngeal and oropharyngeal (NP-OP), urine, blood, induced sputum, lung aspirate, pleural fluid, and gastric aspirates were tested with cultures, multiplex polymerase chain reaction (PCR), or both. Primary analyses were restricted to cases without human immunodeficiency virus (HIV) infection and with abnormal chest X-rays and to controls without HIV infection. We applied a Bayesian, partial latent class analysis to estimate probabilities of etiological agents at the individual and population level, incorporating case and control data.

Findings: Between August 15, 2011, and January 30, 2014, we enrolled 4,232 cases and 5,119 community controls. The primary analysis group was comprised of 1,769 (41.8% of 4,232) cases without HIV infection and with positive chest X-rays and 5,102 (99.7% of 5,119) community controls without HIV infection. Wheezing was present in 555 (31.7%) cases out of 1,752 cases (range by site 10.6–97.3%). 30-day case-fatality ratio was 6.4% (114 of 1,769 cases). Blood cultures were positive in 56 (3.2%) of 1,749 cases, and *Streptococcus pneumoniae (S. pneumoniae)* was the most common bacteria isolated [19 (33.9%) of 56]. Almost all cases (98.9%) and controls (98.0%) had at least one pathogen detected by PCR in the NP-OP specimen. The detection of respiratory syncytial virus (RSV), parainfluenza virus, human metapneumovirus, influenza virus, *S. pneumoniae, Haemophilus influenzae (H. influenza)* type b (Hib), *H. influenzae* non-type b, and *Pneumocystis jirovecii (P. jirovecii)* in NP-OP specimens was associated with case status. The etiology analysis estimated that viruses accounted for 61.4% [95% credible interval (CrI) 57.3–65.6] of causes, whereas bacteria accounted for 27.3% (23.3–31.6), and *Mycobacterium tuberculosis (M. tuberculosis)* for 5.9% (3.9–8.3). Viruses were less common (54.5%, 95% CrI 47.4–61.5 vs. 68.0%, 62.7–72.7) and bacteria were more common (33.7%, 27.2–40.8 vs. 22.8%, 18.3–27.6) in very severe pneumonia cases than in severe cases. RSV had the greatest etiological fraction (31.1%, 95% CrI 28.4–34.2) of all pathogens. Human rhinovirus, human metapneumovirus A or B, human parainfluenza virus, *S. pneumoniae, M. tuberculosis,* and *H. influenzae* each accounted for 5% or more of the etiological distribution. We observed differences in etiological fraction by age for *Bordetella pertussis,* parainfluenza types 1 and 3, parechovirus-enterovirus, *P. jirovecii,*

RSV, rhinovirus, *Staphylococcus aureus (S. aureus)*, and *S. pneumoniae*, and differences by severity for RSV, *S. aureus*, *S. pneumoniae*, and parainfluenza type 3. The leading 10 pathogens of each site accounted for 79% or more of the site's etiological fraction.

Interpretation: In our study, a small set of pathogens accounted for most cases of pneumonia requiring hospital admission. Preventing and treating a subset of pathogens could substantially affect childhood pneumonia outcomes.

"In nothing do men more nearly approach the Gods, than in giving health to men."
—Marcus Tullius Cicero

COMMENT

Pneumonia remains among the main causes of mortality and morbidity in children <5 years of age, especially in the developing countries of Asia and Africa. Despite improvements resulting from economic progress, scientific advancements, more equitable distribution, and vaccination, the problem is still substantial. Problems include lack of etiological data, difficulty in diagnosis, coinfection with human immunodeficiency virus (HIV), lack of treatments, etc., among more mundane problems such as poverty and illiteracy.[11]

The Pneumonia Etiology Research for Child Health (PERCH) study sought to address some of these issues by trying to characterize the causes of severe childhood pneumonia (<5 years) requiring hospital admission in eight low-income countries in Asia and Africa. The study tried to integrate a combination of clinical criteria, radiological and standard microbiological investigations, such as chest X-rays, body fluid, and swab cultures, with 33 target multiplex quantitative polymerase chain reaction (PCR) for diagnosis of a wide variety (up to 30) etiological agents. A standardized common protocol was used at each site and inter-site comparison was also done. Additionally, most sites had a good prevalence of vaccination against respiratory pathogens such as *Streptococcus pneumoniae (S. pneumoniae)*, *Haemophilus influenzae (H. influenza)*, measles, etc.

The study threw up some interesting results. Viruses caused 61.4% of cases while bacteria were responsible for 27.3%; *Mycobacterium tuberculosis (M. tuberculosis)* contributed 5.9% of cases. Respiratory syncytial virus (RSV) was the most common pathogen at all sites accounting for some 30% of cases. Surprisingly, influenza A and B viruses were uncommon. Bacterial infections became progressively more common in cases with severe pneumonia. The most common 10 microbiological agents accounted for 79–80% of all cases across all sites and age groups.

Important inferences which can be drawn from this study are as follows. Firstly, as RSV is the most common pathogen overall, public health measures targeted at this agent might allow for a significant reduction in the number of cases. Secondly, bacterial infections still account for a significant proportion of childhood pneumonia, especially severe cases and proper treatment facilities including wider availability of antibiotics would help in further curbing this menace. Lastly, only about 60% of patients had a positive chest X-ray which implies that radiological screening alone will miss a significant number of cases.

More studies of this kind are needed from different parts of the world to further define and characterize etiological agents of pneumonia so that better public health and treatment strategies are available.

Key Messages

⊙ *Respiratory syncytial virus is the most common pathogen of childhood pneumonia.*

⊙ *Chest X-ray is positive for pneumonia in only about 60% of patient.*

ARTICLE 15

Balanced crystalloids versus saline in sepsis. A secondary analysis of the SMART clinical trial

brown RM, Wang L, Coston TD, Krishnan NI, Casey JD, Wanderer JP, et al. Balanced crystalloids versus saline in sepsis. a secondary analysis of the SMART clinical trial.
Am J Respir Crit Care Med. 2019;200(12):1487-95.

Abstract*

Introduction: The main therapy for sepsis is administration of intravenous crystalloid solutions; however, the impact of composition of crystalloid on patient outcomes is still not known. This study aimed to compare the effect of balanced crystalloids as compared to saline on 30-day in-hospital mortality in critically ill adults with sepsis.

Materials and methods: This study included patients from SMART (Isotonic Solutions and Major Adverse Renal Events Trial) who had an *International Classification of Diseases, 10th Edition, Clinical Modification System* code for sepsis and were admitted to the medical ICU. Secondary analysis was done by using multivariable regression to control for potential confounders. Total 15,802 patients were included in SMART; out of these, 1,641 patients had sepsis and were admitted to the medical ICU.

Results: In the balanced crystalloids group, 30-day in-hospital morality was noted in 26.3% (n = 217) patients in comparison to 31.2% (n = 255) patients in the saline group [adjusted odds ratio (aOR) 0.74; 95% confidence interval (CI) 0.59–0.93; p = 0.01]. In comparison to the saline group, patients in the balanced group had lower incidence of major adverse kidney events within 30 days (35.4% vs. 40.1%; aOR 0.78; 95% CI 0.63–0.97) and more vasopressor-free days (20 ± 12 vs. 19 ± 13; aOR 1.25; 95% CI 1.02–1.54) and renal replacement therapy-free days (20 ± 12 vs. 19 ± 13; aOR 1.35; 95% CI 1.08–1.69).

Conclusion: In this large randomized trial including patients with sepsis, use of balanced crystalloids was found to be associated with reduced 30-day in-hospital mortality in comparison to use of saline. Clinical trial registered with www.clinicaltrials.gov (NCT02444988). *Redrafted abstract

"Choice of resuscitation fluids in sepsis: Time to get SMART?"

COMMENT

The intravenous fluid of choice for resuscitation of critically ill patients has been a subject of debate. Although normal saline (NS) continues to be the most used fluid, presence of supraphysiologic concentration of chloride in NS is associated with adverse effects (**Table 1**).

Balanced crystalloids are solutions in which chloride ions are replaced with bicarbonate or buffers (lactate, acetate, or gluconate) to reduce acid–base imbalance resulting from administration of fluids.[12] The Surviving Sepsis guidelines do not favor the use of any particular for fluid resuscitations. Whether this choice has an impact on patient-centered outcomes is an important clinical question.

The SMART trial showed that in critically ill adults, administration of balanced salt solutions in comparison to NS decreased the composite outcome of death, new renal replacement therapy (RRT) or persistent renal dysfunction at 30 days.[13] Since the study population was from diverse ICUs, the authors conducted a secondary analysis of the

SMART dataset to evaluate the effectiveness of balanced crystalloids in patients with sepsis and septic shock.

Of the 824 patients randomized to balanced crystalloids, >90% received Ringer's lactate. The 30-day mortality was significantly lower in the balanced crystalloid group. This becomes significant in practice since the number needed to treat to avoid one mortality is just over 20 patients. The incidence of major adverse kidney events at 30 days, need for RRT and acute kidney injury were lower in the balanced crystalloid group. They also experienced more ventilator-free, vasopressor-free, and RRT free days than the saline group.

This study provides additional evidence that balanced crystalloids improve outcomes in adults with sepsis. However, being the secondary analysis of a single center study, the results cannot be generalized and need further evaluation for external validity. Given that the study had no patients with traumatic brain injury in whom use of balanced crystalloids may be counter-productive, the results cannot be applied to this population. Besides, as majority of study subjects in the balanced crystalloid group received Ringer's lactate, we cannot extrapolate these results to other balanced salt solutions. These questions may be answered by the ongoing PLUS and BaSICS studies.

Thus, it would be reasonable to choose balanced crystalloids over saline for resuscitating patients in sepsis. Future research should also focus on delineating the pathophysiological mechanisms to explain the benefits of balanced crystalloids.

TABLE 1: Detrimental effects of saline-induced metabolic acidosis preclinical and clinical research.

Acid-base balance	Hyperchloremic metabolic acidosis
Inflammation	• Higher inflammatory markers (IL-6)
Renal function	• Renal vasoconstriction • Decreased GFR • Increased incidence of AKI • Increased need for renal replacement therapy
Cardiovascular	• Vasodilatation • Hypotension • Decrease microcirculation • Increase vasopressor requirement

(AKI: acute kidney injury; GFR: glomerular filtration rate; IL: interleukin)
Source: Summarized from Semler MW, Kellum JA. Balanced Crystalloid Solutions. Am J Respir Crit Care Med. 2019;199(8):952-60.

Key Messages

⊙ *Selection of the right resuscitation fluid affects patient-centered outcomes in critically ill.*

⊙ *In adult patients with sepsis, balanced salt solutions are associated with better outcomes compared to saline.*

Sleep

ARTICLE 16

Mixed method model to assess CPAP adherence among patients with moderate to severe OSA

Ramachandran P, Devaraj U, Sandeepa HS, Kavitha V, Uma Maheswari K, D'Souza G. Mixed Method Model to Assess CPAP Adherence among Patients with Moderate to Severe OSA.
Indian J Chest Dis Allied Sci. 2019;61:119-22.

Abstract

Background: Continuous positive airway pressure (CPAP) is an effective therapy for obstructive sleep apnea (OSA). Despite proven benefits of CPAP in OSA, adherence has been suboptimal. The present study was designed to evaluate the compliance of CPAP therapy and factors affecting it in patients with moderate-to-severe OSA.

Methods: Patients diagnosed to have moderate/severe OSA [apnea-hypopnea index (AHI) >15] during the period April to December, 2015 were evaluated using a predefined questionnaire on the number of hours of usage, number of nights per week usage and challenges faced in using CPAP; Epworth Sleepiness Score was recorded. CPAP usage was documented from the downloaded data from their CPAP machines.

Results: Forty patients (mean age 50.6 ± 11.4 years; 29 men) were studied. Their average body mass index (BMI) was 33.2 kg/m². Of these, 31 had severe OSA (mean AHI 47.8/h). The objective usage of CPAP among patients with OSA was less by 89 minutes when compared with perceived duration (p = 0.001). Twenty patients had used the device for <4 h/night. Patients reported social factors, dryness of mouth, not reapplying machine after nocturia, power shut down, and reduced motivation as reasons for nonadherence to use CPAP.

Conclusions: Despite the recognized benefits of CPAP, the acceptance and adherence with therapy remains a considerable barrier. Objective assessment of CPAP compliance should be a part of routine follow-up in patients with OSA.

"Machine-on and mask-on times are not the same for measurement of compliance of CPAP use."

COMMENT

Obstructive sleep apnea (OSA) is common but frequently unrecognized. Even when the disease is diagnosed, people tend to ignore unless it is severe and complicated. The trend is similar all over the world but much more so in India. The prevalence in India, however, is same as elsewhere when it is specifically looked for. It is relevant here to mention that OSA is a progressive disease leading to serious complications such as hypertension, cardiovascular ischemia, arrhythmias, pulmonary artery hypertension, cerebrovascular atherosclerosis, and stroke. It is frequently accompanied with metabolic syndrome of uncontrolled diabetes, hyperlipidemia, and obesity.

Continuous positive airway pressure (CPAP) is the most effective therapy which is currently available. The compliance with CPAP therapy is poor. Patients do not want to sleep while tied down to a machine, mostly throughout their lives. Inability to buy a device was reported in an earlier study, as the most important barrier for CPAP use in India.[14] Other barriers included patients' behaviors and attitudes for the use of CPAP.

It is most crucial that CPAP therapy is used regularly and effectively for the best benefits.

It has been reported often that patients' perception about its use is generally erratic. It is therefore, important to keep a check on patient's compliance. Several methods are employed to assess the compliance of a patient with CPAP therapy. The authors of this study have used a mixed method model for this purpose. They used a predefined questionnaire to calculate the number of hours of usage and number of nights per week usage in patients diagnosed to have moderate/severe OSA [apnea-hypopnea index (AHI) >15]. They also documented the CPAP usage from the downloaded data from their CPAP machines. The objective assessment of CPAP use from the machine data was significantly less than the perceived usage. It is therefore, important to assess the compliance objectively for more meaningful interpretation. The observation is important in stressing that the treatment in most patients is suboptimal and inadequate.

Different methods have been recommended to improve CPAP compliance. Cheaper, noiseless, and comfortable devices are also being developed. Use of flexible bilevel airway pressure can also be shown to achieve improved compliance in patients previously noncompliant with CPAP. We believe that patient education is the most important step which must be considered.

Key Messages

- *The acceptance and adherence with CPAP therapy for OSA were poor despite the recognized benefits.*
- *Objective assessment of treatment compliance is important in patients with OSA.*

ARTICLE 17

Association of short sleep duration and atrial fibrillation

Genuardi MV, Ogilvie RP, Saand AR, DeSensi RS, Saul MI, Magnani JW, et al. Association of short sleep duration and atrial fibrillation.
Chest. 2019;156:544-52.

Abstract

Background: Short sleep may be a risk factor for atrial fibrillation. However, previous investigations have been limited by lack of objective sleep measurement and small sample size. We sought to determine the association between objectively measured sleep duration and atrial fibrillation.

Methods: All 31,079 adult patients undergoing diagnostic polysomnography (PSG) from 1999 to 2015 at multiple sites within a large hospital network were identified from electronic medical records. Prevalent atrial fibrillation was identified by continuous electrocardiogram (ECG) during PSG. Incident atrial fibrillation was identified by diagnostic codes and 12-lead ECGs. Logistic regression and Cox proportional hazards modeling were used to examine the association of sleep duration and atrial fibrillation prevalence and incidence, respectively, adjusting for age, sex, body mass index (BMI), hypertension, coronary artery disease, cerebrovascular disease, peripheral vascular disease, heart failure, and sleep apnea severity.

Results: We identified 404 cases of prevalent atrial fibrillation among 30,061 individuals (mean age ± SD, 51.0 ± 14.5 years; 51.6% women) undergoing PSG. After adjustment, each 1-hour reduction in sleep duration was associated with a 1.17-fold (95% CI 1.11–1.30) increased risk of prevalent atrial fibrillation. Among 27,589 patients without atrial fibrillation at baseline, we identified 1,820 cases of incident atrial fibrillation over 4.6 years median follow-up. After adjustment, each 1-hour reduction in sleep duration was associated with a 1.09-fold (95% CI 1.05–1.13) increased risk for incident atrial fibrillation.

Conclusions: Short sleep duration is independently associated with prevalent and incident atrial fibrillation. Further research is needed to determine whether interventions to extend sleep can lower atrial fibrillation risk.

"Too little sleep makes the heart erratic!"

COMMENT

Normal sleep is known to be associated with subtle alterations in cardiac rhythm related to autonomic fluctuations, as parasympathetic and sympathetic activity predominate in non-rapid eye movement (NREM) and rapid eye movement (REM) sleep, respectively. Benign arrhythmias reported during normal sleep include transient sinus pauses, bradycardia, and first-degree atrioventricular (AV) block, all of which occur in NREM sleep.

Arrhythmias have also been described with sleep disorders such as obstructive sleep apnea and insomnia. In the former, autonomic fluctuations, hypoxemia, and intrathoracic pressure changes occurring during apneic episodes predispose to atrial arrhythmias. Nocturnal arrhythmias have also been described with structural heart disease without an underlying sleep disorder.

Atrial fibrillation is a widely prevalent arrhythmia wherein no cause is identifiable in almost 30% of patients. Hence, the search for hitherto unrecognized risk factors is ongoing, of which sleep quality and disorders are putative risk factors. It has been reported in the "Health eHeart" and "Cardiovascular Health" studies that self-reported nocturnal awakening was associated with atrial fibrillation after adjusting for multiple confounding factors.

In the present study, Genuardi et al. have included 30,061 patients undergoing diagnostic polysomnography (PSG) to determine the association between sleep duration and atrial fibrillation detected on PSG (prevalent atrial fibrillation). Those patients without atrial fibrillation on PSG were followed up for a median of 4.6 years to determine incidence of atrial fibrillation.

After adjustment for age, sex, body mass index, cardiovascular disease, and sleep apnea, the authors report that a 1-hour reduction in sleep duration below 6 hours was associated with 17% increased odds of prevalent atrial fibrillation and 9% increase in incident atrial fibrillation on follow-up.

Although the authors concluded on the reduced sleep duration based on a single night PSG (which may have skewed the results due to the "first-night effect" wherein patients are not able to achieve adequate sleep duration and quality in a sleep laboratory), it is interesting to note that not only interrupted sleep, but also sleep duration plays a role in inducing atrial fibrillation. If this theory is proven in a better designed study, wherein overnight PSG data are corroborated with patient-maintained sleep diaries to determine sleep duration and quality, simple measures such as optimizing sleep duration may help in prevention of atrial fibrillation in a subset of patients.

■ FURTHER READING

1. Gula LJ, Krahn AD, Skanes AC, Yee R, Klein GJ. Clinical relevance of arrhythmias during sleep: guidance for clinicians. Heart. 2004;90(3):347-52.
2. Verrier RL, Josephson ME. Impact of sleep on arrhythmogenesis. Circ Arrhythm Electrophysiol. 2009;2(4):450-9.

Key Messages

- ⊙ *Disturbed sleep, short sleep duration, and sleep disorders can predispose to atrial fibrillation.*
- ⊙ *Ensuring good sleep hygiene practices and timely recognition and treatment of sleep disorders can help in prevention of atrial fibrillation.*

Critical Care

ARTICLE 18

Predictors and microbiology of ventilator-associated pneumonia among patients with exacerbation of chronic obstructive pulmonary disease

Khilnani GC, Dubey D, Hadda V, Sahu SR, Sood S, Madan K, et al. Predictors and microbiology of ventilator-associated pneumonia among patients with exacerbation of chronic obstructive pulmonary disease.
Lung India. 2019;36:506-11.

Abstract

Background: Understanding the risk factors and microbiology of ventilator-associated pneumonia (VAP) among patients with chronic obstructive pulmonary disease (COPD) is important for the application of preventive and therapeutic interventions. Therefore, this study was planned to assess the clinical predictors and microbiological features of VAP among COPD patients.

Materials and methods: This prospective study involved patients with exacerbation of COPD who required mechanical ventilation and admitted in respiratory intensive care unit at a tertiary care teaching hospital. Various baseline demographic and clinical features were compared between patients with VAP and without VAP. Univariate and multivariable analyses were done to assess the impact of demographic and clinical features on the development of VAP.

Results: The study included 100 intubated patients with age [mean ± standard deviation (SD)] of 62.45 ± 8.32 years, duration (median) of COPD of 6 years, and acute physiology, age, and chronic health evaluation score (mean ± SD) of 18.60 ± 4.30. In this cohort, 17 patients developed VAP. Multivariable analysis showed that sequential organ failure assessment (SOFA) score at admission, reintubation, and history of previous hospitalization were independent predictors of VAP with odds ratio (95% confidence interval) of 2.70 (1.24, 5.63; p = 0.012), 66.96 (4.86, 922.72; p = 0.002), and 35.92 (2.84, 454.63; p = 0.006), respectively. *Acinetobacter baumannii* was the most frequent organism (n = 8; 47%), followed by *Klebsiella pneumoniae* (n = 5; 29%), *Pseudomonas aeruginosa* (n = 1; 6%), and *Enterobacter* species (n = 1; 6%). All organisms were multidrug resistant (MDR).

Conclusions: Sequential organ failure assessment score at admission, reintubation, and history of previous hospitalization were independent predictors of VAP. Antimicrobial therapy for VAP should cover MDR gram-negative organism.

"Body invasion cannot be safe without consequences—not for long!"

COMMENT

Ventilator-associated pneumonia (VAP) is a dreaded complication seen by an intensivist working in any type of intensive care unit (ICU). The prevalence and pattern, however, vary significantly between postoperative, surgical, medical, and speciality ICUs. There are a large number of other factors which affect the occurrence and outcomes of VAPs. Presence of a pre-existing disease is one of the important variables, which determines the outcome. The occurrence of an infection especially the VAP prolongs the length and cost of ICU stay. Both the morbidity and mortality are significantly high.

There are very few studies on VAPs in respiratory or medical ICUs reported from India.[15] Incidence as high as 57.14% was reported in one study with *Acinetobacter* species and *Pseudomonas aeruginosa* as the most common pathogens.[15] In this study, the incidence of VAP was directly proportional to the duration of mechanical ventilation and a high fatality rate.[15] Khilnani and colleagues in their paper prospectively looked for VAP in 100 intubated patients of chronic obstructive pulmonary disease (COPD). They found VAP in 17% of their patients with multidrug-resistant (MDR) organisms such as *Acinetobacter baumannii* as the most frequent pathogen followed by *Klebsiella pneumoniae, Pseudomonas aeruginosa,* and *Enterobacter* species They also reported sequential organ failure assessment (SOFA) score at admission, reintubation, and history of previous hospitalization as independent predictors of VAP. It was recommended that antimicrobial therapy for VAP should cover MDR gram-negative organisms.

The high occurrence of VAP at most of the centres in India especially with MDR organisms is a worrisome phenomenon. While VAP is common all over the world, it is more so disturbing in the developing countries such as India where the ICU cost becomes enormous in an alarming proportion. Factually, the cost of ICU management goes beyond the means of an average Indian patient. VAP and sepsis is an ominous sign which is feared by every intensivist.

The authors of this paper have focused on patients with COPD who are likely to go for repeated ICU visits because of COPD exacerbations. Fortunately, many of them do well with noninvasive positive pressure ventilation without requiring intubation. Those who require intubation are sick with more severe disease. They are also more likely to suffer from infective episodes. Some of the important predictors of high mortality of VAP in COPD included old age, late onset VAP, reintubation, and prolonged use of antibiotics. The relationship between VAP and COPD was recently studied in an interesting paper which also reported higher mortality and longer duration of mechanical ventilation in these patients.[16]

Acinetobacter baumannii was the most common pathogen reported in the Indian study under discussion. This has been the experience of several other Indian centers although the causative organisms may differ from place-to-place depending upon the local epidemiology. This is a serious issue since the organism is resistant to most of the commonly used antibiotics. Prevention of the occurrence of VAP therefore, becomes an all-important issue in the ICU management.

Key Messages

- Ventilator-associated pneumonia with MDR organisms was diagnosed in 17% of intubated COPD patients.
- Antimicrobial therapy for VAP should cover MDR gram-negative organisms.

ARTICLE 19

Aetiology and predictors of outcome in patients presenting with acute respiratory failure requiring mechanical ventilation in a medical intensive care unit

Harikrishna J, Mohan A, Reddy PS, Sharma PS, Kumar PVA, Guntupalli KK, et al. Aetiology and predictors of outcome in patients presenting with acute respiratory failure requiring mechanical ventilation in a medical intensive care unit. *Indian J Chest Dis Allied Sci. 2019;61:7-11.*

Abstract

Background: Sparse published data are available regarding the etiology, course, complications, and outcome in patients presenting with acute respiratory failure requiring mechanical ventilation from India.

Methods: Retrospective study of 116 patients with acute respiratory failure requiring mechanical ventilatory support (AcRFMV) in the medical intensive care unit (ICU) at our tertiary care teaching hospital in South India.

Results: Patients with AcRFMV (mean age 44.5 ± 19.5 years; 52.6% females) constituted 23.9% of the 486 patients admitted to the medical ICU during the study period of 18 months. Etiological causes included sepsis syndrome (46.6%), acute deliberate self-poisoning (22.4%), acute exacerbation of chronic obstructive pulmonary disease (15.5%), snakebite and tuberculosis (5.2% each), and severe complicated malaria (3.4%) among others. The median [interquartile range (IQR)] duration (days) of mean hospital stay and medical ICU stay were 10 (4–13.8) and 7 (4–11), respectively. Median (IQR) duration of mechanical ventilator support was 5 (3–8) days. Complications observed during medical ICU stay were ventilator-associated pneumonia (13.8%), bed sore (7.8%), and pneumothorax (2.6%); 12.1% patients required tracheostomy. Fifty-eight (50%) patients died. On multivariable analysis using binary logistic regression (forward conditional method) shock at initial presentation [odds ratio (OR) 3; 95% confidence intervals (CI) 1.638–5.493, p < 0.001] emerged as independent predictor of death.

Conclusions: Acute respiratory failure requiring mechanical ventilatory support is an important cause of admission to medical ICU and is associated with high mortality. Intense search for and monitoring of predictor variables can help clinicians in reducing the mortality.

"The earlier you get out of mechanical respiratory supports, the better the outcome."

COMMENT

There is paucity of published literature on experience with mechanical ventilation in patients of acute respiratory failure. This is especially so with reference to the predictors of the outcome. The index paper analyzes data of 486 patients admitted over 18 month period in a tertiary level hospital in India. Of them, 116 patients were diagnosed with acute respiratory failure requiring mechanical ventilatory support. Sepsis syndrome was the most common cause while suicidal poisoning and chronic obstructive pulmonary disease were second and third among the list of causes. Shock at initial presentation was determined as an independent predictor of death. The mean hospital and medical intensive care unit (ICU) stay as well as the days of mechanical ventilation were important predictors of outcome of mechanical ventilation.

Mechanical ventilation for patients with acute respiratory failure is practiced in India for the past several decades. However, it is in the last few years that the practice has enormously expanded to centers in even the small towns. In an earlier report on 49 patients, acute respiratory failure due to sepsis was the most common cause; the median duration on mechanical ventilator and the median length of ICU stay were 20 days and 39 days, respectively.[17] Duration of vasopressor support and need for hemodialysis were significant independent predictors of unsuccessful weaning.[15]

This issue of a successful ICU stay and outcome has assumed great significance in the present era of severe acute respiratory syndrome coronavirus-2 (SARS-CoV-2) pandemic (COVID-19). Severe acute respiratory illness (SARI) is the most dreaded complication of COVID-19 which has been responsible for a general hue and cry. There has been a large scale demand for the ventilators and the intensive care beds including in the lay media. The study belongs to the pre-COVID era but relevant for all kinds of SARI patients with or without COVID infection. The different outcome variables listed by the authors are true for all kinds of patients of acute respiratory failure requiring mechanical ventilation.

Key Messages

⊛ *Sepsis syndrome was the most common cause of respiratory failure requiring mechanical ventilatory support.*

⊛ *Shock at initial presentation was an independent predictor of death.*

Pulmonary Vascular Disease

ARTICLE 20

Diagnosis of pulmonary embolism with D-dimer adjusted to clinical probability

Kearon C, de Wit K, Parpia S, Schulman S, Afilalo M, Hirsch A, et al. Diagnosis of pulmonary embolism with D-dimer adjusted to clinical probability.
N Engl J Med. 2019;381:2125-34.

Abstract*

Background: A D-dimer level of l ≤500/mL has a moderate clinical pretest probability (C-PTP) while ≤1,000 ng/mL has a low C-PTP for ruling out pulmonary embolism in patients.

Methods: A prospective study was conducted in outpatients wherein pulmonary embolism was ruled out without further testing when D-dimer level was <1,000 ng/mL with a low C-PTP and <500 ng/mL with a moderate C-PTP. Chest imaging (usually computed tomographic pulmonary angiography) was done and it was done for rest of the patients. No anticoagulant therapy was given, if pulmonary embolism was not diagnosed. Follow-up for 3 months was done to detect venous thromboembolism.

Results: Of 2,017 enrolled patients, 7.4% had pulmonary embolism on initial diagnostic testing. None of the patients who had a low C-PTP (1,285 patients) or moderate C-PTP (40 patients) and a negative D-dimer test i.e., <1,000 ng/mL or <500 ng/mL, respectively, developed venous thromboembolism during follow-up [95% confidence interval (CI) 0.00–0.29%]. These included 315 patients who had a low C-PTP and a D-dimer level of 500–999 ng/mL (95% CI 0.00–1.20%). There was only 1 patient out of 1,863 patients who was not diagnosed pulmonary embolism initially and did not receive anticoagulant therapy (0.05%; 95% CI 0.01–0.30), but developed venous thromboembolism. The use of chest imaging was done in 34.3% of patients as per our diagnostic strategy, whereas a strategy in which pulmonary embolism is considered to be ruled out with a low C-PTP and a D-dimer level of <500 ng/mL would result in the use of chest imaging in 51.9% (difference –17.6% points; 95% CI –19.2 to –15.9).

Conclusion: We could identify a low risk for pulmonary embolism during follow-up associated with a combination of a low C-PTP and a D-dimer level of <1,000 ng/mL (Funded by the Canadian Institutes of Health Research and others; PEGeD ClinicalTrials.gov number, NCT02483442.) *Redrafted abstract

"When fear is the disease, faith and confidence is the medicine."

—**Debasish Mridha**

COMMENT

Pulmonary embolism (PE) and deep vein thrombosis (DVT), together known as venous thromboembolism (VTE), are relatively common problems faced by chest specialists on a daily basis. The challenge is to identify patients who require immediate and/or prolonged treatment and avoid unnecessary investigations. Clinical probability scores are available to distinguish patients into groups having low, medium, or high pretest probability of VTE. Some of the common ones include the Wells probability score, the Geneva score, and the Years index.[18,19]

These scores have been combined with use of D-dimer testing to rule out VTE as D-dimer has a good negative predictive value. However, the cut-off levels for D-dimers have not been clearly established and vary from study-to-study and also on the pretest probability. The gold standard for diagnosis of PE is contrast-enhanced pulmonary angiography (CTPA) which entails considerable expense and time, in addition to the risk of radiation exposure and contrast-induced acute kidney injury. Obviously, a strategy that reduces the use of CTPA and allows one to triage patients successfully is required. This would not only reduce the number of unnecessary tests but also allow for clear and precise decision making.

The current study was a prospective trial in which all patients suspected of PE were scored clinically by use of the Wells clinical prediction rule to have low, moderate, or high probability of PE. A D-dimer test was then done in the low and moderate probability groups while the high probability group was evaluated by CTPA. A D-dimer score of <1,000 ng/mL in the low probability group and <500 ng/mL in the moderate probability group was taken as an indication of the absence of PE while any patient who had a score more than mentioned was investigated by CTPA. All patients were followed up for 3 months.

None of the 1,325 patients in the group with low probability and D-dimer score of <1,000 ng/mL and 40 patients in moderate probability group with D-dimer score of <500 ng/mL developed VTE on follow-up. Of all 1,863 patients who did not receive a diagnosis of PE initially and did not receive anticoagulant therapy, one patient had VTE. This diagnostic strategy resulted in a reduction in use of CTPA by –17.6% points as compared to the standard strategy, i.e., PE considered to be ruled out with a low clinical probability score and a D-dimer level of <500 ng/mL.

The strengths of this study include the large sample size, use of CTPA, and use of different D-dimer assays at different sites. Some weaknesses include the short follow-up time and the low prevalence of PE in the target population, limiting the generalizability to other populations where the prevalence of the disease may be higher. Also, almost all of the patients in the study were outpatients which may also be a limiting factor. However, one can also muse that these kinds of prediction rules are meant exactly for this kind of outpatient populations where the chances of PE are low and the interest is mainly in ruling out further investigation!

Overall, this is an interesting study that should be replicated in other populations around the world.

Key Message

⊙ *Combination of a low C-PTP and D-dimer level is useful to identify a group of patients at low risk for pulmonary embolism during follow-up period.*

Interventional Pulmonology

ARTICLE 21

A retrospective study comparing the ultrathin versus conventional bronchoscope for performing radial endobronchial ultrasound in the evaluation of peripheral pulmonary lesions

Sehgal IS, Dhooria S, Bal A, Gupta N, Ram B, Aggarwal AN, et al. A retrospective study comparing the ultrathin versus conventional bronchoscope for performing radial endobronchial ultrasound in the evaluation of peripheral pulmonary lesions.
Lung India. 2019:36:102-7.

Abstract

Background: Few studies have reported on the utility of ultrathin bronchoscopes (UTBs) for performing radial probe endobronchial ultrasound (EBUS). Herein, we describe our experience with UTB and conventional bronchoscope (CB) for performing radial EBUS.

Materials and methods: This was a retrospective study comparing the diagnostic yield of a prototype UTB (external diameter 3 mm, working channel diameter 1.7 mm) versus CBs (external diameter ≥4.9 mm) in performing radial EBUS for the evaluation of peripheral pulmonary lesions (PPLs). Fluoroscopic guidance was not available.

Results: A total of 121 subjects (34, UTB; 87, CB; 69.4% males) with a mean [standard deviation (SD)] age of 55.2 (14.8) years underwent radial EBUS. The mean (SD) size of PPLs on computed tomography of the thorax was 22.2 (13.7) mm. The lesions were significantly smaller in the UTB group (16.4 vs. 24.7 mm, $p = 0.006$). Eight lesions could be visualized within the lumen of the peripheral smaller bronchi with the UTB. The overall yield of radial EBUS was 52.9% and was similar in the two groups (UTB vs. CB, 55.9% vs. 51.7%; $p = 0.7$). The procedure time was significantly shorter in the UTB group. On multivariate logistic regression, the yield was similar in the two groups after adjusting for the size and location of the lesion and position of the radial probe in relation to the lesion.

Conclusion: Despite smaller lesions, radial EBUS performed with the UTB was found to have similar efficacy to that performed with the CB. More lesions could be visualized endobronchially using the UTB making it an attractive alternative for performing radial EBUS.

"Errors like straws upon the surface flow!
He who would search for pearls, must dive below."

COMMENT

The paper describes the experience of the authors with use of ultrathin bronchoscope (UTB) for radial probe endobronchial ultrasound for diagnosis of peripheral lesions. Although the procedure had been used in the Western countries for some years now, there were only a few reports on use of ultrathin bronchoscopes in comparison to conventional bronchoscopy.[20,21] Moreover, this is possibly the first such publication from India. The procedure improves the diagnostic yield for the peripheral nodules. A better diagnostic yield of 70% was observed with improved techniques (such as electromagnetic navigation bronchoscopy, virtual bronchoscopy, radial endobronchial ultrasound, ultrathin bronchoscope, and guide sheath) than with traditional transbronchial biopsy in a meta-analysis of 39 studies.[20] Sehgal and colleagues report a similar efficacy of UTB for significantly smaller lesions of 16.4 mm diameter compared to 24.7 mm diameter lesions for conventional bronchoscopy. Moreover, the procedure-time was significantly shorter. More lesions could be visualized endobronchially with the help of ultrathin bronchoscopy.

Retrospective nature of the study which does not allow a randomized selection and adequate blinding is one major limitation. Nonetheless, there is no doubt that ultrathin bronchoscopy is advantageous for peripheral and small-sized nodules which are often difficult to diagnose with conventional bronchoscopy. Why not straight go for the surgical resection of a small lesion than wasting time and money on a semi-invasive and costly investigation? The issue assumes importance to differentiate between malignant versus nonmalignant infectious or granulomatous nodules. This is especially true in a country such as India where old tubercular granulomas are rather commonly seen on chest roentgenography in adults. Surgical resection of such a benign granulomatous nodule can therefore, be avoided. Percutaneous, image-guided thin-needle aspiration is another alternate technique which is commonly used. UTB has an obvious advantage in view of the greater likelihood of pneumothorax with percutaneous biopsy.

There is a significant learning curve for the procedure. Therefore, the outcome depends upon the experience of the bronchoscopist. But its application is better limited to the specialized centers meant for advanced pulmonary care. Early surgery will be required once a patient is diagnosed with a malignant lesion.

Key Messages

⊙ *Radial EBUS performed with the UTB is better than with conventional bronchoscope.*

⊙ *There is less likelihood of such complications with UTB than percutaneous biopsy.*

REFERENCES (Chest and Critical Care)

1. Dowman L, Hill CJ, Holland AE. Pulmonary rehabilitation for interstitial lung disease. Cochrane Database Syst Rev. 2014;10:CD006322.

2. Richeldi L, Cottin V, du Bois RM, Selman M, Kimura T, Bailes Z, et al. Nintedanib in patients with idiopathic pulmonary fibrosis: Combined evidence from the TOMORROW and INPULSIS® trials. Respir Med. 2016;113:74-9.

3. Cottin V, Wollin L, Fischer A, Quaresma M, Stowasser S, Harari S. Fibrosing interstitial lung diseases: knowns and unknowns. Eur Respir Rev. 2019;28:180100.

4. Distler O, Highland KB, Gahlemann M, Azuma A, Fischer A, Mayes MD, et al. Nintedanib for Systemic Sclerosis-Associated Interstitial Lung Disease. N Engl J Med. 2019;380(26):2518-28.

5. Mortimer K, Gordon SB, Jindal SK, Accinelli RA, Balmes J, Martin WJ II. Household air pollution as a major avoidable risk factor for cardio-pulmonary disease. Chest. 2012;142(5): 1308-15.

6. Dusthackeer A, Sekar G, Chidambaram S, Kumar V, Mehta P, Swaminathan S. Drug resistance among extrapulmonary TB patients: Six years' experience from a supranational reference laboratory. Indian J Med Res. 2015;142(5):568-74.

7. Panda A, Bhalla AS, Goyal A. Bronchial artery embolization in hemoptysis: a systematic review. Diagn Interv Radiol. 2017;23(4):307-17.

8. Ittrich H, Klose H, Adam G. Radiologic management of haemoptysis: diagnostic and interventional bronchial arterial embolisation. Rofo. 2015;187(4):248-59.

9. World Health Organization. (2017). Global tuberculosis report 2017. Geneva: World Health Organization, 2017. [online] Available from https://www.who.int/tb/publications/global_report/gtbr2017_main_text.pdf?ua=1 [Last accessed August, 2020].

10. Van Deun A, Maug AK, Salim MA, Das PK, Sarker MR, Daru P, et al. Short, highly effective, and inexpensive standardized treatment of multidrug-resistant tuberculosis. Am J Respir Crit Care Med. 2010;182:684-92.

11. Liu L, Oza S, Hogan D, Chu Y, Perin J, Zhu J. Global, regional, and national causes of under-5 mortality in 2000–15: an updated systematic analysis with implications for the Sustainable Development Goals. Lancet. 2016;388:3027-35.

12. Semler MW, Kellum JA. Balanced crystalloid solutions. Am J Respir Crit Care Med. 2019;199:952-60.

13. Semler MW, Self WH, Wanderer JP, Ehrenfeld JM, Wang L, Byrne DW, et al. Balanced crystalloids versus saline in critically ill adults. N Engl J Med. 2018;378:829-39.

14. Goyal A, Agarwal N, Pakhre A. Barriers to CPAP Use in India: An Exploratory Study. J Clin Sleep Med. 2017;13(12): 1385-94.

15. Ranjan N, Chaudhary U, Chaudhry D, Ranjan KP. Ventilator-associated pneumonia in a tertiary care intensive care unit: Analysis of incidence, risk factors and mortality. Indian J Crit Care Med. 2014;18(4):200-4.

16. Koulenti D, Parisella FR, Xu E, Lipman J, Rello J. The relationship between ventilator-associated pneumonia and chronic obstructive pulmonary disease: what is the current evidence? Eur J Clin Microbiol Infect Dis. 2019;38: 637-47.

17. Muzaffar SN, Gurjar M, Baronia AK, Azim A, Misra P, Poddar B, et al. Predictors and pattern of weaning and long-term outcome of patients with prolonged mechanical ventilation at an acute intensive care unit in North India. Rev Bras Ter Intensiva. 2017;29(1):23-33.

18. Raja AS, Greenberg JO, Qaseem A, Denberg TD, Fitterman N, Schuur JD. Evaluation of patients with suspected acute pulmonary embolism: best practice advice from the Clinical Guidelines Committee of the American College of Physicians. Ann Intern Med. 2015;163:701-11.

19. van der Hulle T, Cheung WY, Kooij S, Beenen LFM, van Bemmel T, van Es J, et al. Simplified diagnostic management of suspected pulmonary embolism (the YEARS study): a prospective, multicentre, cohort study. Lancet. 2017;390: 289-97.

20. Memoli JS, Nietert PJ, Silvestri GA. Meta-analysis of guided bronchoscopy for the evaluation of the pulmonary nodule. Chest. 2012;142(2):385-93.

21. Shepherd RW. Bronchoscopic pursuit of the peripheral pulmonary lesion: navigational bronchoscopy, radial endobronchial ultrasound, and ultrathin bronchoscopy. Curr Opin Pulm Med. 2016;22(3):257-64.

Section Editor: Siddharth N Shah

Associate Editors: Ragini Maheshwari, Naveen Mittal

ARTICLE 1

Glycaemic durability of an early combination therapy with vildagliptin and metformin versus sequential metformin monotherapy in newly diagnosed type 2 diabetes (VERIFY): a 5-year, multicentre, randomised, double-blind trial

Matthews DR, Paldánius PM, Proot P, Chiang YT, Stumvoll M, Prato SD; VERIFY study group. Glycaemic durability of an early combination therapy with vildagliptin and metformin versus sequential metformin monotherapy in newly diagnosed type 2 diabetes (VERIFY): a 5-year, multicentre, randomised, double-blind trial. *Lancet. 2019;394:1519-29.*

Abstract

Background: Early treatment intensification leading to sustained good glycemic control is essential to delay diabetic complications. Although initial combination therapy has been suggested to offer more opportunities than a traditional stepwise approach, its validity remains to be determined.

Methods: Vildagliptin Efficacy in combination with metfoRmIn For earlY treatment of type 2 diabetes (VERIFY) was a randomised, double-blind, parallel-group study of newly diagnosed patients with type 2 diabetes mellitus (T2DM) conducted in 254 centers across 34 countries. The study consisted of a 2-week screening visit, a 3-week metformin-alone run-in period, and a 5-year treatment period, which was further split into study periods 1, 2, and 3. Patients aged 18–70 years were included if they had T2DM diagnosed within 2 years prior to enrolment, and centrally confirmed glycated hemoglobin (HbA1c) of 48–58 mmol/mol (6.5–7.5%) and a body-mass index of 22–40 kg/m^2. Patients were randomly assigned in a 1:1 ratio either to the early combination treatment group or to the initial metformin monotherapy group, with the help of an interactive response technology system and simple randomization without stratification. Patients, investigators, clinical staff performing the assessments, and data analysts were masked to treatment allocation. In study period 1, patients received either the early combination treatment with metformin (stable daily dose of 1,000 mg, 1,500 mg, or 2,000 mg) and vildagliptin 50 mg twice daily, or standard-of-care initial metformin monotherapy (stable daily dose of 1,000 mg, 1,500 mg, or 2,000 mg) and placebo twice daily. If the initial treatment did not maintain HbA1c below 53 mmol/mol (7.0%), confirmed at two consecutive scheduled visits which were 13 weeks apart, patients in the metformin monotherapy group received vildagliptin 50 mg twice daily in place of the placebo and entered study period 2, during which all patients received the combination therapy. The primary efficacy endpoint was the time from randomization to initial treatment failure, defined as HbA1c measurement of at least 53 mmol/mol (7·0%) at two consecutive scheduled visits, 13 weeks apart from randomization through period 1. The full analysis set included patients who received at least one randomized study medication and had at least one postrandomization efficacy parameter assessed. The safety analysis set included all patients who received at least one dose of randomized study medication. This study is registered with ClinicalTrials.gov, NCT01528254.

Findings: Trial enrolment began on March 30, 2012, and was completed on April 10, 2014. Of the 4,524 participants screened, 2001 eligible participants were randomly assigned to either the early combination treatment group (n = 998) or the initial metformin monotherapy group (n = 1,003). A total of 1,598 (79.9%)

patients completed the 5-year study: 811 (81.3%) in the early combination therapy group and 787 (78.5%) in the monotherapy group. The incidence of initial treatment failure during period 1 was 429 (43.6%) patients in the combination treatment group and 614 (62.1%) patients in the monotherapy group. The median observed time to treatment failure in the monotherapy group was 36.1 [IQR 15.3-not reached (NR)] months, while the median time to treatment failure time for those receiving early combination therapy could only be estimated to be beyond the study duration at 61.9 (29.9-NR) months. A significant reduction in the relative risk for time to initial treatment failure was observed in the early combination treatment group compared with the monotherapy group over the 5-year study duration {hazard ratio 0.51 [95% confidence interval (CI) 0·45–0.58]; p < 0.0001}. Both treatment approaches were safe and well tolerated, with no unexpected or new safety findings, and no deaths related to study treatment.

Interpretation: Early intervention with a combination therapy of vildagliptin plus metformin provides greater and durable long-term benefits compared with the current standard-of-care initial metformin monotherapy for patients with newly diagnosed T2DM.

Funding: Novartis.

"Synergy – the bonus that is achieved when things work together harmoniously."
—**Mark Twain**

COMMENT

Guidelines for the management of hyperglycemia in type 2 diabetes mellitus (T2DM) recommend metformin as first-line pharmacological therapy, with sequential intensification and second-line therapy only when glycemic control (HbA1c ≤53 mmol/mol or ≤7.0%) is not achieved. However, with clinical inertia, treatment intensification is often delayed.

The VERIFY study was therefore designed as a 5-year efficacy and safety study, comparing an early combination therapy of metformin plus dipeptidyl peptidase-4 inhibitor (DPP-4) vildagliptin with standard-of-care metformin monotherapy, defined as a traditional stepwise approach with metformin as initial therapy and vildagliptin added at the time of metformin failure. The choice of exploring the combination of a DDP-4 inhibitor with metformin is supported by glucose-dependent β-cell stimulation by vildagliptin and concomitant insulin sensitization by metformin, and the favorable safety profile of both drugs.

The VERIFY study has shown that early combination treatment improves glycemic durability in patients with T2DM compared with standard-of-care initial metformin monotherapy followed by sequential combination with vildagliptin. Early combination treatment significantly reduced the probability of initial treatment failure, the time to second treatment failure, and the time to treatment failure compared with monotherapy throughout the 5-year study duration (**Fig. 1**).

The early combination treatment was safe and well tolerated and the glycemic control could be achieved with no added hypoglycemia risk and no effect on bodyweight.

As part of safety surveillance, cardiovascular events were monitored and adjudicated. Adjudicated first macrovascular events occurred in 24 (2.4%) patients in the combination treatment group and in 33 (3.3%) patients in the monotherapy group hence favoring the early combination therapy.

The reasons for a potential early cardiovascular benefit beyond glycemia also remain to be determined. Recent meta-analysis and claims database studies[1] have suggested that early use and synergistic effects of DPP-4 inhibitors in combination with metformin could have a potential moderating effect on cardiovascular outcomes.

The findings of VERIFY emphasize the importance of achieving and maintaining early glycemic control which supports the UK Prospective Diabetes Studies, and showed that early treatment intensification was associated with a "legacy effect," and there was a reduction in vascular complications in the intensive group which was maintained or strengthened over 10 years after study completion.[2,3]

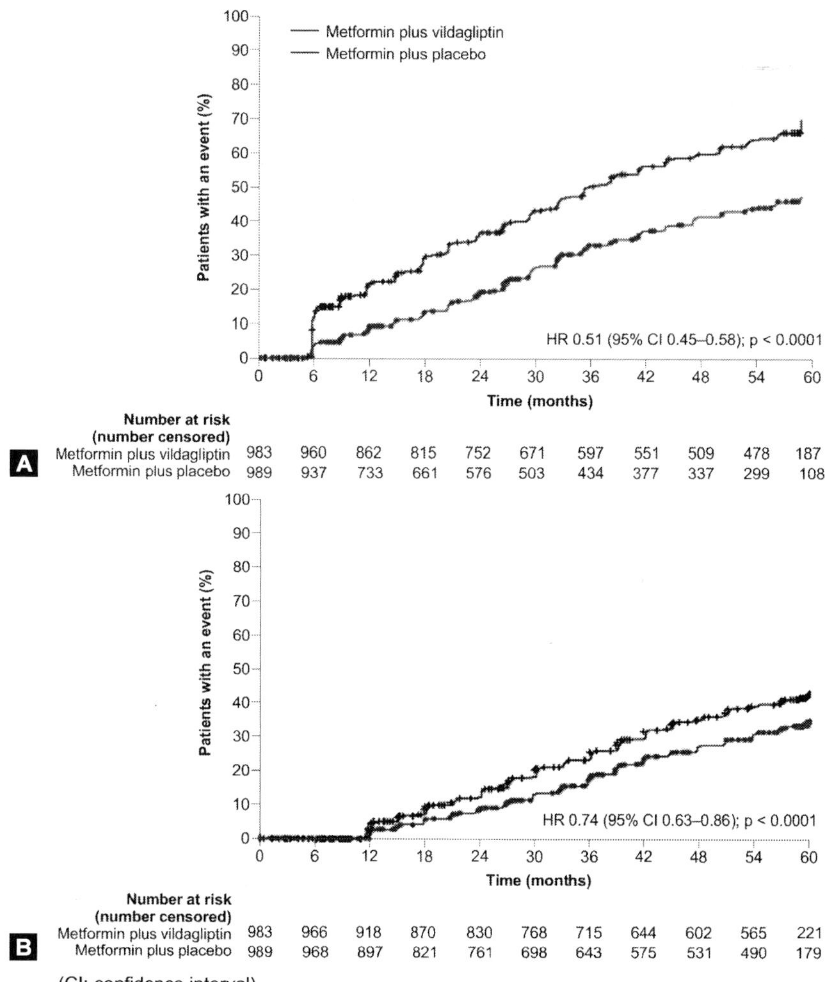

(CI: confidence interval)

FIG. 1: Time to treatment failure. (A) Cumulative probability of initial treatment failure. (B) Cumulative probability of second treatment failure. Hazard ratios (HRs) are based on Cox regression analysis.

Key Message

- *The strategy of early combination treatment approach in VERIFY study significantly and consistently improved long-term glycemic durability as compared with monotherapy. The study also helped to understand the progressive nature and pathophysiological mechanisms of diabetes.*

ARTICLE 2

Management of hypopituitarism

Alexandraki KI, Grossman AB. Management of Hypopituitarism.
J Clin Med. 2019;8:2153.

Abstract

Hypopituitarism includes all clinical conditions that result in partial or complete failure of the anterior and posterior lobe of the pituitary gland's ability to secrete hormones. The aim of management is usually to replace the target-hormone of hypothalamo-pituitary-endocrine gland axis with the exceptions of secondary hypogonadism when fertility is required, and growth hormone deficiency (GHD), and to safely minimize both symptoms and clinical signs. Adrenocorticotropic hormone (ACTH) deficiency replacement is best performed with the immediate-release oral glucocorticoid hydrocortisone (HC) in 2–3 divided doses. However, novel once-daily modified-release HC targets a more physiological exposure of glucocorticoids. GHD is treated currently with daily subcutaneous GH, but current research is focusing on the development of once-weekly administration of recombinant GH. Hypogonadism is targeted with testosterone replacement in men and on estrogen replacement therapy in women; when fertility is wanted, replacement targets secondary or tertiary levels of hormonal settings. Thyroid-stimulating hormone (TSH) replacement therapy follows the rules of primary thyroid gland failure with L-thyroxine replacement. Central diabetes insipidus is nowadays replaced by desmopressin. Certain clinical scenarios may have to be promptly managed to avoid short-term or long-term sequelae such as pregnancy in patients with hypopituitarism, pituitary apoplexy, adrenal crisis, and pituitary metastases.

"A correct diagnosis is three-fourths the remedy."

—Mahatma Gandhi

COMMENT

Hypopituitarism is defined as complete or partial deficiency of hormones secreted by pituitary gland. Defect may be at level of pituitary or hypothalamus. Etiology may be congenital (genetic defect) or acquired (pituitary adenoma, infections, or vascular lesion). Patient may be having single or multiple pituitary hormone deficiencies.

Adrenocorticotropic hormone (ACTH) deficiency: It is managed by oral HC in three divided doses. Total daily dose is 15–20 mg, of which half is given just after waking in morning, other two doses after lunch and late afternoon. To avoid sleep disorder or metabolic side effects, last dose should be taken at least 6 hours before bedtime. Prednisolone may be given as single dose of 5 mg in morning, it being cheaper and has better compliance.

Thyroid-stimulating hormone deficiency: It is diagnosed by low T3 and low T4 levels with inappropriately normal TSH levels. It is treated by giving thyroxin (dose of 1.6 µg/kg daily) in fasting stage early morning, just like primary hypothyroidism. But in monitoring, only free thyroxin (FT4) levels are used and kept at upper half of normal range. TSH cannot be used as monitoring tool. If patient is having central hypothyroidism, first replace cortisol and then only give thyroxin because thyroxin increases catabolism of steroids and hence can precipitate adrenal crisis in undiagnosed secondary adrenal insufficiency.

Central hypogonadism in males: It is diagnosed if serum testosterone is low without elevation of follicle-stimulating hormone (FSH) and luteinizing hormone (LH). Central hypogonadism is treated by giving injection testosterone enanthate 250 mg intramuscularly once in 3 weeks. For monitoring, serum testosterone is measured on 11th day and if level is above 600 ng/dL or below 350 ng/dL, dose needs to be adjusted. If patient wants fertility, testosterone is stopped, gonadotropin therapy is started, in form of human chorionic gonadotropin (hCG) and human menopausal gonadotropin (hMG). Gonadotropins have to be given for 7–10 months.

Central hypogonadism in females: It is confirmed by lower serum estrogen without elevation of FSH and LH levels in previously oligomenorrhic/amenorrhic female (after excluding pregnancy, hyperprolactinemia, polycystic ovarian disease, and thyroid disorders). For treatment, patient is given combined estrogen and progesterone therapy, if no contraindications (breast cancer or thrombosis) are present. Estrogen is given daily with progesterone in last 14 days of 4 weeks cycle. If patient wants to conceive, FSH and LH are given by injections.

Growth hormone deficiency: This deficiency is confirmed by growth hormone stimulation tests. Growth hormone treatment is started with dose of 0.2–0.4 mg/day for patients less than 60 years of age and 0.1–0.2 mg/day if age is more than 60 years.

Central diabetes insipidus: It is diagnosed by measuring serum and urine osmolality in presence of polyuria, i.e., >50 mL/kg body weight per day (3.5 L/day in 70 kg person), in absence of uncontrolled diabetes mellitus, hypercalcemia, or hypokalemia. Treatment of diabetes insipidus is desmopressin 0.1 mg daily orally or 10–20 µg intranasally.

Pituitary apoplexy: Pituitary apoplexy is due to hemorrhage or infarct of pituitary tumor, usually presents as sudden onset of headache, vomiting, visual disturbances, altered sensorium, or cranial nerve palsies. It may be life-threatening. For treatment, after taking blood sample for measuring serum cortisol, give injection HC 100 mg intravenous stat and 200 mg over 24 hours in infusion. Do not wait for report of serum cortisol. Hemodynamics should be monitored and necessary intervention should be done.

In summary, management of pituitary insufficiency involves the appropriate diagnosis and replacement of individual hormone deficiency, simulating physiological rhythm of secretion.

Key Message

⊙ *Management of pituitary insufficiency involves the appropriate diagnosis and replacement of individual hormone deficiency, simulating physiological rhythm of secretion.*

ARTICLE 3

Oral semaglutide and cardiovascular outcomes in patients with type 2 diabetes

Husain M, Birkenfeld AL, Donsmark M, Dungan K, Eliaschewitz FG, Franco DR, et al.; PIONEER 6 Investigators. Oral Semaglutide and Cardiovascular Outcomes in Patients with Type 2 Diabetes.
N Engl J Med. 2019;381:841-51.

Abstract*

Background: The safety of semaglutide, a glucagon-like peptide-1 (GLP-1) receptor agonist in its subcutaneous form, has been well studied for treatment of type 2 diabetes mellitus (T2DM). However, data on its oral form is lacking. Here, we assessed cardiovascular outcomes of once-daily oral semaglutide in high-risk patients.

Methods: An event-driven, randomized, double blind, placebo-controlled trial was conducted enrolling patients at high cardiovascular risk (age of ≥50 years with established cardiovascular or chronic kidney disease, or age of ≥60 years with cardiovascular risk factors only). The first occurrence of a major adverse cardiovascular event (death from cardiovascular causes, nonfatal myocardial infarction, or nonfatal stroke) in a time-to-event analysis was the primary outcome of the study. The trial was designed to rule out 80% excess cardiovascular risk as compared with placebo [noninferiority margin of 1.8 for the upper boundary of the 95% confidence interval (CI) for the hazard ratio for the primary outcome].

Results: Of the 3,183 patients, 2,695 patients (84.7%) were 50 years of age or older and had cardiovascular or chronic kidney disease, with the mean age being 66 years. They were randomly assigned to receive oral semaglutide or placebo. The median time in the trial was 15.9 months. About 61 of 1,591 patients (3.8%) in the oral semaglutide group and 76 of 1,592 (4.8%) in the placebo group had a major adverse cardiovascular event (hazard ratio 0.79; 95% CI 0.57–1.11; p < 0.001 for noninferiority). About 15 of 1,591 patients (0.9%) in the oral semaglutide group and 30 of 1,592 (1.9%) in the placebo group died from cardiovascular causes (hazard ratio 0.49; 95% CI 0.27–0.92); 37 of 1,591 patients (2.3%), and 31 of 1,592 (1.9%), respectively had nonfatal myocardial infarction (hazard ratio 1.18; 95% CI 0.73–1.90); and 12 of 1,591 patients (0.8%) and 16 of 1,592 (1.0%) had nonfatal stroke, respectively (hazard ratio 0.74; 95% CI 0.35–1.57). Death from any cause occurred in 23 of 1,591 patients (1.4%) in the oral semaglutide group and 45 of 1,592 (2.8%) in the placebo group (hazard ratio 0.51; 95% CI 0.31–0.84). Due to gastrointestinal adverse events, discontinuation of oral semaglutide was more common with oral semaglutide.

Conclusion: We concluded that the cardiovascular risk profile of oral semaglutide was not inferior to that of placebo, in patients with T2DM. (Funded by Novo Nordisk; PIONEER 6 ClinicalTrials.gov number, NCT02692716.) *Redrafted abstract

"It is through science that we prove, but through intuition that we discover."

—Henri Poincare

COMMENT

Glucagon-like peptide-1 (GLP-1) receptor agonists used for the treatment of type 2 diabetes mellitus (T2DM) are associated with reductions in body weight and a low risk of hypoglycemia.[4] These agents have shown cardiovascular safety (lixisenatide and exenatide) and benefit (liraglutide, albiglutide, semaglutide,[5] and dulaglutide). In the Trial to Evaluate Cardiovascular and Other Long-term Outcomes with Semaglutide in Subjects with Type 2 Diabetes (SUSTAIN-6), patients who received a once-weekly subcutaneous injection of semaglutide had a 26% lower risk of the primary cardiovascular outcome than those who received placebo.

Oral semaglutide has been developed as a once-daily tablet, which may allay patient's concerns about injections and result in earlier initiation of GLP-1 receptor agonist therapy. As compared with once-weekly subcutaneous semaglutide, oral semaglutide has a different absorption profile.[6] However, the pharmacokinetic properties and effects of semaglutide are similar, regardless of the route of administration.

The present randomized, placebo-controlled, phase 3a trial, Peptide Innovation for Early Diabetes Treatment (PIONEER) 6, is a preapproval cardiovascular outcomes trial specifically designed to rule out an excess in cardiovascular risk with oral semaglutide among patients with T2DM.

This cardiovascular outcomes trial met its primary objective of ruling out an 80% excess cardiovascular risk with oral semaglutide, confirming noninferiority to placebo.

The hazard ratios were similar in the present trial and SUSTAIN-6, which may suggest that the cardiovascular effect of semaglutide is independent of the route of administration.

Oral semaglutide reduced glycated hemoglobin levels and body weight in the present trial, which is consistent with the phase 3a efficacy and safety trial PIONEER 3 and with data for subcutaneous semaglutide in SUSTAIN-6 (**Fig. 1**).

No unexpected adverse events were identified with oral semaglutide. More patients permanently discontinued oral semaglutide than placebo, mostly due to gastrointestinal events.

In SUSTAIN-6, subcutaneous semaglutide was associated with a higher risk of diabetic retinopathy complications than placebo. Most events occurred early in that trial, possibly due to the magnitude and rapidity of the reduction in glycated hemoglobin levels in patients with pre-existing diabetic retinopathy. Given that result, patients with proliferative retinopathy or maculopathy resulting in active treatment were excluded from the current trial.

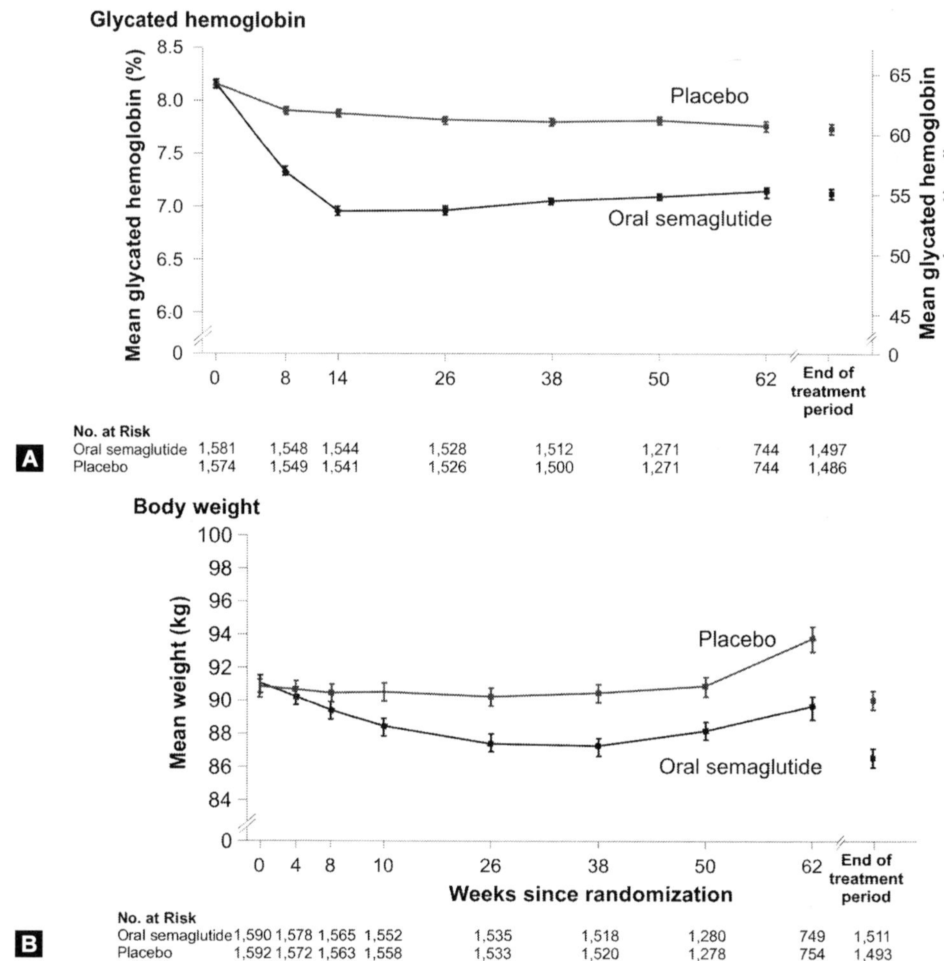

FIG. 1: Efficacy outcomes (In-trial observation period). The curves show the observed change from baseline in the glycated hemoglobin level (A) and body weight (B). Data are for the full analysis set during the in-trial observation period, which was from randomization to the last visit (end of treatment). The end of treatment occurred when the required number of first major adverse cardiovascular events was exceeded. The individual patients' in-trial observation period ranged from 2 to 87 weeks, with a median duration of 69 weeks. I bars indicates standard errors.

Key Message

- *The PIONEER 6 trial showed noninferiority of oral semaglutide to placebo ruling out an 80% of excess cardiovascular risk.*

ARTICLE 4

Adrenal crisis

rushworth RL, Torpy DJ, Falhammar H. Adrenal Crisis.
N Engl J Med. 2019;381:2541-51.

Abstract

In this review article acute adrenal insufficiency also called as Addisonian crisis is discussed in detail. Among patients diagnosed to have adrenal insufficiency 6–8% of them develop adrenal crisis every year. This is despite them being on regular therapy. It is usually precipitated by acute infections and increased demand. Adrenal crisis is more common in primary hypoadrenalism than in secondary adrenal insufficiency. Adrenal crisis can present with hypotension, fever, and gastrointestinal (GI) symptoms of nausea vomiting along with impaired consciousness. Biochemically there will be hyponatremia, hyperkalemia, and hypoglycemia. The condition needs to be recognized early. Treatment involves use of injectable hydrocortisone and plenty of fluids in intravenous (IV) infusion. Adrenal crisis should be diagnosed since it can be life-threatening. In fact it should be anticipated during infection and otherwise increased demands in patients with adrenal insufficiency.

"What remains in diseases after the crisis is apt to produce relapses."
—**Hippocrates, Aphorisms**

COMMENT

It is a review article which tells us about pathophysiology and management of adrenal crisis.

Most severe manifestation of adrenal insufficiency is called adrenal crisis. When will you say that patient is suffering from adrenal crisis: If there is an acute deterioration in clinical status with fall in systolic blood pressure (BP) below 100 mm Hg or relative hypotension (systolic BP >20 mm Hg lower than usual), with resolution of features within 1–2 hours after giving parenteral glucocorticoids.

Associated features are: acute abdominal symptoms (pain, vomiting, or diarrhea), alteration in sensorium, fever, hyponatremia, hyperkalemia, and hypoglycemia. If BP does not improve with steroid administration, presence of other conditions like sepsis should be considered.

At time of crisis, symptoms of mild adrenal insufficiency may also be present, such as fatigue, anorexia, nausea, vomiting, generalized bodyache, postural dizziness, and impaired consciousness.

Why adrenal crisis occurs? It results due to absolute or relative deficiency of cortisol required to maintain homeostasis. Patients with primary adrenal insufficiency are more likely to suffer from adrenal crisis than secondary adrenal insufficiency

due to two reasons: partial preservation of cortisol secretion in secondary adrenal insufficiency and absence of mineralocorticoids in primary hypoadrenalism [as secretion of aldosterone is controlled by renin–angiotensin system independent of adrenocorticotropic hormone (ACTH)].

Adrenal crisis may result in death in 6% of cases.

What are the events which precipitate the crises: Bacterial infections are most common, serious injury and major surgery are other causes. Noncompliance to steroid replacement also leads to adrenal crises. Undiagnosed coexisting thyrotoxicosis or initiating thyroxin therapy in a patient with undiagnosed hypoadrenalism may precipitate adrenal crises (as thyroid hormone increases catabolism of steroids).

When one should suspect adrenal crises in a patient: Unexplained hypotension which is volume nonresponsive, with hyponatremia and hyperkalemia.

How will you treat: Take blood sample for serum cortisol. Without waiting for the report, give hydrocortisone 100 mg intravenously stat followed by 200 mg every 24 hours, administered as a continuous infusion or as frequent IV boluses

(50 mg IV q 6 h) with subsequent doses tailored to clinical response. If hydrocortisone is not available, dexamethasone 4 mg IV once in 24 hours can be given. If serum cortisol taken at time of low BP (<90 mm Hg) is <18 ug/dL, it confirms presence of adrenal insufficiency.

What are fluids you should use: IV normal saline 1,000 mL in first hour. Dextrose normal saline may be given after that if random blood sugar (RBS) is <70 mg/dL. Look for precipitating factors (i.e., infection), investigate and treat.

How one can prevent adrenal crises in a patient with known case of adrenal insufficiency: Patient should be advised to increase the dose of steroids if they have any stress on body (fever, diarrhea, or pneumonia), aim is to replicate normal cortisol stress response of the body. If fever is less than 101°F, double the daily dose of steroids and if it is more than 101°F, dose should be increased to three times, until the illness has resolved. If patient has to undergo surgery, give hydrocortisone 200 mg in 24 hours. If patient is having diarrhea or vomiting, give parenteral hydrocortisone.

Incidence of adrenal crises can be decreased, if patient is educated about use of oral stress dosing and use of parenteral hydrocortisone if required.

Key Messages

- *Adrenal crisis if suspected early, can be treated easily by IV hydrocortisone.*
- *Incidence of adrenal crisis can be decreased, if patient is educated about use of oral stress dosing and use of parenteral hydrocortisone if required.*

ARTICLE 5A

Thyroid function and conception

Chen AX, Leung AM, Tim I M Korevaar. Thyroid Function and Conception.
N Engl J Med. 2019;381:178-81.

Abstract

In this interactive clinical decision-making article a case vignette has been presented. A 30-year-old lady with history of miscarriage who wants to conceive seeks medical advice. She has family history of autoimmune disorders. Her T3, T4, and thyroid-stimulating hormone (TSH) levels are normal. The thyroid peroxidase antibody is positive. It is 78 against upper limit of normal of 35. The case is discussed by two distinguished clinicians, one who feels low dose of levothyroxine will help and the other feels it will not help the lady for getting pregnant. So the other author feels this patient should be kept on close follow-up and monitoring.

The debate shows that there are many grey areas in clinical medicine where we have to use our judgment since the evidence base is borderline. The justification for using low dose levothyroxine is that this therapy is low cost and without any side effects. The author does recognize that a large double blind placebo controlled trial, the TABLET trial, showed that use of levothyroxine in women with normal thyroid functions, who are positive for thyroid per oxidase antibodies, there was no increased live births as compared to placebo. The expert who does not feel levothyroxine will be helpful depends on the literature and feels that if the thyrotropin concentration is more than upper level of normal then it will be helpful. The matter is discussed in detail by the two experts.

ARTICLE 5B

Levothyroxine in women with thyroid peroxidase antibodies before conception

Dhillon-Smith RK, Middleton LJ, Sunner KK, Cheed V, Baker K, Farrell-Carver S, et al. Levothyroxine in Women with Thyroid Peroxidase Antibodies before Conception.
N Engl J Med. 2019;380:1316-25.

Abstract*

Background: There is an increased risk of miscarriage and preterm birth in euthyroid women having thyroid peroxidase antibodies. Levothyroxine, as suggested by small clinical trials, can reduce the incidence of adverse outcomes. Here, we investigate the effect of levothyroxine treatment on incidence of live birth rates among euthyroid women with thyroid peroxidase antibodies and a history of miscarriage or infertility.

Methods: A double blind, placebo-controlled trial was conducted on a total of 19,585 women from 49 hospitals in the United Kingdom who underwent testing for thyroid peroxidase antibodies and thyroid function. About 952 women were randomly assigned to receive either 50 µg once daily of levothyroxine (476 women) or placebo (476 women) before conception through the end of pregnancy. The primary outcome was live birth after at least 34 weeks of gestation.

Results: About 940 of 952 women enrolled in the study followed up for primary outcome. A total of 266 of 470 women in the levothyroxine group (56.6%) and 274 of 470 women in the placebo group (58.3%) became pregnant. Up to 37.4% (176 of 470 women) in the levothyroxine group, and 37.9% (178 of 470 women) in the placebo group, had a live birth ($\geq$34 weeks of gestation) [relative risk 0.97; 95% confidence interval (CI) 0.83–1.14, p = 0.74; absolute difference –0.4 percentage points; 95% CI –6.6–5.8]. No significant difference was found in other pregnancy outcomes, including pregnancy loss or preterm birth, or in neonatal outcomes, across both the groups. Up to 5.9% of women in the levothyroxine group and 3.8% in the placebo group (p = 0.14), had serious adverse events.

Conclusion: Our study could not demonstrate a higher rate of live births in euthyroid women with thyroid peroxidase antibodies as compared to placebo. (Funded by the United Kingdom National Institute for Health Research; TABLET Current Controlled Trials number, ISRCTN15948785.) *Redrafted abstract

"Although the world is full of suffering, it is also full of the overcoming of it."

—Helen Keller

COMMENT

You are sitting in medicine OPD. A female patient comes to you who is trying to conceive for last 2 years. 1 year back she had a miscarriage at 7 weeks of gestation. She has a family history of auto-immune disorders. Her sister is suffering from type 1 diabetes mellitus (T1DM) and her mother is having hypothyroidism. Her gynecologist has got her thyroid function test (TFT) and antithyroid peroxidase antibody (anti-TPOAb) test was also done. Her thyrotropin (TSH) level is 3.1 mIU/L (normal range 0.5–4.0) and her free thyroxin (FT4) level is 15 nmol/L (normal range 12–22). However the test for anti-TPO is positive, i.e., 90 IU/mL (<60).

Now what are you going to do? Are you going to start treatment with thyroxin or not?

The patient is having history of spontaneous loss of pregnancy, her TSH is at upper range of normal, FT4 is normal, and anti-TPOAb is positive.

The latest guidelines from American Thyroid Association (ATA) 2017 state that there is not sufficient evidence that levothyroxine treatment in euthyroid anti-TPO positive decreases pregnancy loss. They recommend that in such cases thyroxin treatment may be considered with minimal risks and potential benefits.

Thyroid autoimmunity does lead to risk of development of hypothyroidism, but it is also an independent risk factor for infertility, abortion, and other poor pregnancy-related outcomes. The mechanisms proposed for these associations are: Cross reactivity between human chorionic gonadotropin (hCG) receptor on oocyte and thyroid antibodies, the effect of other nonspecific autoimmunity, and increased level of endometrial cytokines.

This trial was done in United Kingdom. They took 952 patients and gave them 50 µg of thyroxin (n = 476) or placebo (n = 476), started before conception and continued throughout the pregnancy.

What they found: There was no significant difference in pregnancy outcome, like preterm birth, pregnancy loss, or poor neonatal outcome. One limitation that authors pointed out was that they have used the fixed dose of thyroxin (50 µg) and did not change it according to body weight or TSH concentration.

So in the given case I will not start the treatment before pregnancy, will get her TFT every 3 months till she conceives. Whenever she conceives, if her TSH is more than 2.5 mIU/l at that time, I will start her on treatment.

Key Message

⊚ *If a patient is trying to conceive, thyroid supplementation should be started only if TSH is above the normal range in spite of presence of antithyroid antibodies.*

ARTICLE 6

SGLT2 Inhibitors for primary and secondary prevention of cardiovascular and renal outcomes in type 2 diabetes: a systematic review and meta-analysis of cardiovascular outcome trials

Zelniker TA, Wiviott SD, Raz I, Im K, Goodrich EL, Bonaca MP, et al. SGLT2 Inhibitors for Primary and Secondary Prevention of Cardiovascular and Renal Outcomes in Type 2 Diabetes: A Systematic Review and Meta-analysis of Cardiovascular Outcome Trials.
Lancet. 2019;393:31-9.

Abstract

Background: The magnitude of effect of sodium-glucose cotransporter-2 inhibitors (SGLT2i) on specific cardiovascular and renal outcomes and whether heterogeneity is based on key baseline characteristics remains undefined.

Methods: We did a systematic review and meta-analysis of randomised, placebo-controlled, cardiovascular outcome trials of SGLT2i in patients with type 2 diabetes. We searched PubMed and Embase for trials published up to September 24, 2018. Data search and extraction were completed with a standardized data form and any discrepancies were resolved by consensus. Efficacy outcomes included major adverse cardiovascular events (myocardial infarction, stroke, or cardiovascular death), the composite of cardiovascular death or hospitalization for heart failure, and progression of renal disease. Hazard ratios (HRs) with 95% confidence intervals (CIs) were pooled across trials, and efficacy outcomes were stratified by baseline presence of atherosclerotic cardiovascular disease (ASCVD), heart failure, and degree of renal function.

Findings: We included data from three identified trials and 34,322 patients (60.2% with established ASCVD), with 3,342 major adverse cardiovascular events, 2,028 cardiovascular deaths or hospitalization for heart failure events, and 766 renal composite outcomes. SGLT2i reduced major adverse cardiovascular events by 11% [HR 0.89 (95% CI 0.83–0.96), p = 0.0014], with benefit only seen in patients with ASCVD [0.86

(0.80–0.93)] and not in those without [1.00 (0.87–1.16), p for interaction = 0.0501]. SGLT2i reduced the risk of cardiovascular death or hospitalization for heart failure by 23% [0.77 (0.71–0.84), p < 0.0001], with a similar benefit in patients with and without ASCVD and with and without a history of heart failure. SGLT2i reduced the risk of progression of renal disease by 45% [0.55 (0.48–0.64), p < 0.0001], with a similar benefit in those with and without ASCVD. The magnitude of benefit of SGLT2i varied with baseline renal function, with greater reductions in hospitalizations for heart failure (p for interaction = 0.0073) and lesser reductions in progression of renal disease (p for interaction = 0.0258) in patients with more severe kidney disease at baseline.

Interpretation: SGLT2i have moderate benefits on atherosclerotic major adverse cardiovascular events that seem confined to patients with established ASCVD. However, they have robust benefits on reducing hospitalization for heart failure and progression of renal disease regardless of existing ASCVD or a history of heart failure.

Funding: None.

"Prevention is so much better than healing because it saves the labor of being sick."
—Thomas Adams

COMMENT

Sodium-glucose cotransporter-2 inhibitors (SGLT2i) are the new addition to the list of oral hypoglycemic drugs. Empagliflozin, canagliflozin, and dapagliflozin are the three drugs in this group which have been widely studied. These drugs are beneficial for cardiovascular and renal outcome in patients suffering from diabetes.

Whether these drugs are beneficial for all the patients suffering from diabetes or only in patients who are already diagnosed to be having ASCVD? It means if they are meant for primary prevention or secondary prevention of cardiovascular disease? If any of these drugs is better? These questions have been studied in this meta-analysis.

They have taken three trials: EMPA-REG OUTCOME (involving empagliflozin as active drug), CANVAS Program (canagliflozin), and DECLARE-TIMI 58 (dapagliflozin). In total they have analyzed the data of about 34,000 patients. 60% of patients were known to be suffering from ASCVD and 40% had multiple risk factors but without known ASCVD.

What they found? SGLT2i are very good drugs and they decrease the hospitalization for heart failure (31%) and progression of renal failure (45%). Furthermore the beneficial effects for heart failure and progression of renal failure were observed in all the patients irrespective of whether they were suffering from ASCVD or not. These drugs reduce the major cardiovascular events (myocardial infarction and cardiovascular death) by 11%. But these major cardiovascular events were reduced only in patients who had established ASCVD (i.e., secondary prevention and no effect seen in patients without ASCVD).

While analyzing the individual drugs, it was empagliflozin which was better in reducing cardiovascular death as compared to other two drugs.

For the side effects, genital fungal infections are more common with use of SGLT2i. Rarely, these can be associated with diabetes ketoacidosis. An increased risk of amputation and fractures were seen only with canagliflozin. Overall no increase incidence of stroke was seen.

This meta-analysis suggests that SGLT2i reduce the risk of hospitalization for heart failure and progression of renal failure and should be used in all patients suffering from diabetes. In addition they also reduce myocardial infarction and cardiovascular deaths in patients with pre-existing ASCVD.

Key Messages

- Sodium-glucose cotransporter-2 inhibitors reduce the risk of hospitalization for heart failure and progression of renal failure and should be used in all patients suffering from diabetes.
- Sodium-glucose cotransporter-2 inhibitors also reduce myocardial infarction and cardiovascular deaths in patients with pre-existing ASCVD.

ARTICLE 7

Intensive glucose control in patients with type 2 diabetes—15-year follow-up

Reaven PD, Emanuele NV, Wiitala WL, Bahn GD, Reda DJ, McCarren M, et al.; for the VADT Investigators. Intensive Glucose Control in Patients with Type 2 Diabetes—15-Year Follow-up.
N Engl J Med. 2019;380:2215-24.

Abstract*

Background: As reported in our previous study that a median of 5.6 years of intensive glucose lowering in type 2 diabetes resulted in lowered risk of major cardiovascular events after a total of 10 years of combined intervention and observational follow-up. We now report the full 15-year follow-up.

Methods: We observationally followed enrolled participants (complete cohort) after the conclusion of the original clinical trial by using central databases to identify cardiovascular events, hospitalizations, and deaths. Participants were asked whether they would be willing to provide additional data by means of surveys and chart reviews (survey cohort). The prespecified primary outcome was a composite of major cardiovascular events, including nonfatal myocardial infarction, nonfatal stroke, new or worsening congestive heart failure, amputation for ischemic gangrene, and death from cardiovascular causes. Death from any cause was a prespecified secondary outcome.

Results: There were 1,655 participants in the complete cohort and 1,391 in the survey cohort. During the trial (which originally enrolled 1,791 participants), the separation of the glycated hemoglobin curves between the intensive-therapy group (892 participants) and the standard-therapy group (899 participants) averaged 1.5 percentage points, and this difference declined to 0.2–0.3 percentage points by 3 years after the trial ended. Over a period of 15 years of follow-up (active treatment plus post-trial observation), the risks of major cardiovascular events or death were not lower in the intensive-therapy group than in the standard-therapy group [hazard ratio for primary outcome 0.91; 95% confidence interval (CI) 0.78–1.06; p = 0.23; hazard ratio for death 1.02; 95% CI 0.88–1.18]. The risk of major cardiovascular disease outcomes was reduced, however, during an extended interval of separation of the glycated hemoglobin curves (hazard ratio 0.83; 95% CI 0.70–0.99), but this benefit did not continue after equalization of the glycated hemoglobin levels (hazard ratio 1.26; 95% CI 0.90–1.75).

Conclusion: Participants with type 2 diabetes mellitus who had intensive glucose control for 5.6 years had a lower risk of cardiovascular events than those who received standard therapy only. However, there was no evidence of a legacy effect or a mortality benefit with intensive glucose control. (Funded by the VA Cooperative Studies Program; VADT ClinicalTrials.gov number, NCT00032487.) *Redrafted abstract

"Try to learn something about everything and everything about something."
—**Thomas Huxley**

COMMENT

The VADT–F (Veterans Affairs Diabetes Trial Follow-up Study group) was designed to examine long-term consequences of intensive glycemic control on cardiovascular disease outcomes, quality of life and mortality, and for assessing the legacy effects.

In the 5-year period after the glycated hemoglobin levels equalized in the treatment groups, the intensive-therapy group had a modestly higher risk of major cardiovascular events than the standard-therapy group.

The results show that during the approximate 10-year period of separation of the glycated hemoglobin curves (median duration, approximately 7.1 years), there was a significant reduction of 17% in the risk of the primary cardiovascular disease outcome. These latter results suggest that there are modest long-term cardiovascular benefits of intensive glucose-lowering therapy in patients with more advanced diabetes.

In fact, there was a decline in benefit with regard to the risk of cardiovascular disease that coincided with equalization of glucose control within treatment groups and this continued during the 5 (or more) years of equal glycemic control that followed.

In this 15-year follow-up study, we found that 5.6 years of intensive glucose lowering that led to a median separation of 1.5 percentage points in the glycated hemoglobin curves did not result in a significantly lower risk of major cardiovascular events than standard therapy.

There is a reduced benefit from glucose lowering in older patients with long-standing type 2 diabetes such as the participants in the ACCORD (Action to Control Cardiovascular Risk in Diabetes) and ADVANCE (Action in Diabetes and Vascular Disease: Preterax and Diamicron MR Controlled Evaluation) trials and in this trial[7,8] it is possible that underlying atherosclerosis and cardiovascular injury were too advanced in these participants to be effectively altered by glucose lowering.

The DCCT (Diabetes Control and Complications Trial) and UKPDS (United Kingdom Prospective Diabetes Study) were also conducted at a time before widespread statin use and tight blood pressure control, whereas participants in the VADT and other recent trials have had aggressive treatment of all cardiovascular disease risk factors.

In conclusion In this group of participants who were at high risk for cardiovascular disease 5.6 years of intensive glucose lowering to a glycated hemoglobin level of 6.9% did not reduce the incidence of major cardiovascular events over a follow-up of 13.6 years or reduce total mortality or improve quality of life over a follow-up of 15 years. However, there was a significantly lower risk of major cardiovascular events during 7.1 years of separation of the glycated hemoglobin curves (**Fig. 1**).

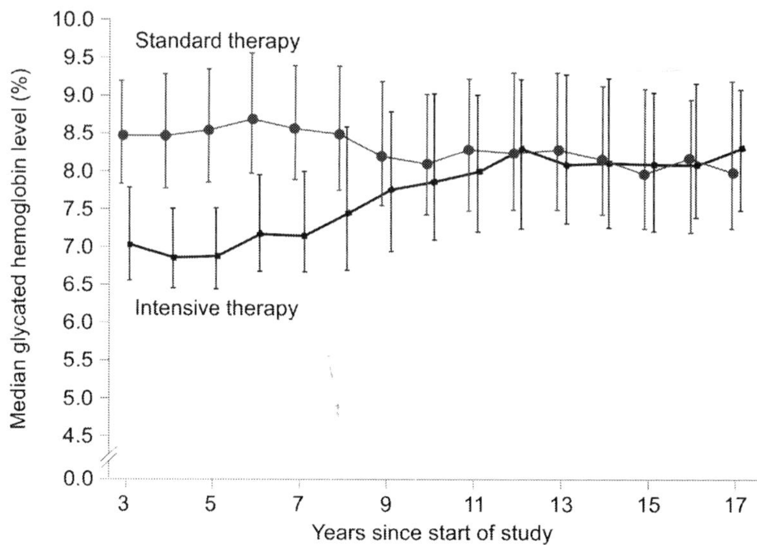

FIG. 1: Median glycated hemoglobin levels according to year since start of the trial, starting at year 3. Year 3 was a point at which all the participant had been enrolled and had been receiving treatment per protocol for at least 3 months. The I bars (slightly offset for better visibility) represent interquartile ranges. The dotted line represents the end of the interventional component of the trial and the beginning of the follow-up period. To convert values for glycated hemoglobin to millimoles per moles, multiply by 10.93 and then subtract 23.50.

Key Message

- *There is no evidence of a legacy effect or a mortality benefit with intensive glucose control hence treatment should be individualized according to the patient profile.*

ARTICLE 8

Hypoparathyroidism

Gafni RI, Collins MT. Hypoparathyroidism.
N Engl J Med. 2019;380:1738-47.

Abstract

A case presenting with hypocalcemia and features of tetany with family history of autoimmune disorders is presented in this article. This is a patient with hypoparathyroidism. These patients present with neuropsychiatric manifestations like paresthesias, muscle spasms specially carpopedal spasm. Diagnosis is suggested by low calcium and high phosphate levels with normal for mildly decreased parathyroid hormone (PTH) levels. Hypoparathyroidism is most commonly due to a complication of surgical thyroidectomy. It is seen in 2–8% patients. In two-thirds it is transient and in one-third it is persistent. Besides postsurgical it can be due to genetic or autoimmune causes. These patients are treated with life-long calcium and vitamin D (calcitriol) supplementation. Some intractable cases need to be given injectable recombinant parathormone hormone. These patients need magnesium supplementation also. On treatment, calcium levels should be kept in low normal range. During treatment they can have basal ganglia calcification and nephrocalcinosis.

Those patients who present with acute tetany including laryngospasm with breathing difficulty need slow intravenous (IV) infusion of calcium gluconate to tide over the acute phase. The diagnosis of this condition can be made with high index of suspicion and looking at calcium and phosphorus levels in patients presenting with above mentioned symptoms. This patient was also put on long-term calcium and vitamin D supplementation. The patient responded well.

"Continuous improvement is better than delayed perfection."

—Mark Twain

COMMENT

This article discusses about clinical features and treatment of hypoparathyroidism.

Parathyroid hormone is responsible for keeping serum calcium in the normal range by acting on bone, kidney, and intestine. Serum calcium regulates secretion of PTH hormone by acting on calcium-sensing receptor (CaSR) present on cells of parathyroid glands.

Clinical features of hypoparathyroidism: Paresthesia, muscle cramps, are seen in mild cases, but may lead to cardiac arrhythmia (due to prolonged QTc interval), laryngospasm or convulsions in severe cases. Bone mass increases because of low bone turnover. Basal ganglion calcification, cataract, hypodontia, and enamel hypoplasia are observed in long-standing cases. Nonspecific features like lethargy, depression, and lack of focus (brain fog) may also be present.

Etiology: Most common cause for hypoparathyroidism is anterior neck surgery (2% of postoperative patients in experienced hands). Patients who are at high risk to develop hypoparathyroidism after surgery are: bilateral neck exploration, repeat neck surgery, extensive neck dissection, parathyroid glands not visualized during surgery and re-exploration for postoperative bleeding. It may be autoimmune in etiology if other autoimmune diseases are also present especially in young patient.

Diagnostic evaluation: If patient is having hypocalcemia, hyperphosphatemia, and PTH level is normal (not increased), diagnosis of hypoparathyroidism is confirmed.

Treatment: If patient is having tetany or seizures, give one ampule 10% calcium gluconate slowly over 10 minutes followed by continuous infusion. It can be given by injecting 5 ampules of calcium gluconate in 500 mL of Dextrose 5% and given over 5 hours.

Oral treatment should be started simultaneously. Parenteral calcium should be continued for 2–3 days till oral treatment has started acting.

As PTH activates 1-alpha hydroxylation of 25-hydroxy vitamin D, we have to give activated vitamin D analogs which have already undergone 1-alpha hydroxylation (calcitriol and alphacalcidol). These have short half-lives and so should be given twice daily.

Patient should receive oral calcium as well: calcium carbonate 0.5–2 g of elemental calcium divided into 2–4 doses daily.

If economy is the issue, plain vitamin D can also be given in high doses (Cholecalciferol 10,000–100,000 units daily).

Patient on calcium and vitamin D can develop nephrocalcinosis, so one should keep calcium in lower range of normal. Oral phosphate binders (Sevelamer) may be given to treat hyperphosphatemia.

Parathyroid hormone therapy: This is the new development in treatment of hypoparathyroidism. Hypocalcemia can be adequately treated with once or twice daily subcutaneous injections of tripartite (PTH 1-34 fragment) or intact PTH (PTH 1-84).

Monitoring: Blood calcium, phosphate, serum creatinine, and 24-hour urine calcium should be measured once in 3–6 months. Ultrasonography of abdomen should be done once a year to look for nephrocalcinosis and nephrolithiasis.

With these measures we can manage the problem of hypoparathyroidism adequately.

Key Messages

- *If patient is having hypocalcemia, hyperphosphatemia, and PTH level is normal (not increased), diagnosis of hypoparathyroidism is confirmed.*
- *Activated vitamin D (calcitriol and alphacalcidol) plays a key role in the management of hypoparathyroidism.*

ARTICLE 9

Drug effects on the thyroid

burch HB. Drug Effects on the Thyroid.
N Engl J Med. 2019;381:749-61.

Abstract*

Thyroid function can be adversely affected by a wide range of drugs ranging from over-the-counter supplements to advanced medical therapy, and include antiarrhythmic agents, antineoplastic agents, and glucocorticoids, and also has an effect on interpretation of the results of standard thyroid laboratory testing. From artifactual laboratory effects to severe thyroid dysfunction, the consequences of drug therapy on the thyroid vary in importance. This review provides a systematic approach to drug-induced thyroid dysfunction, with an emphasis on clinically relevant interactions and on artifacts on laboratory assays.
*Redrafted abstract

"Decisions are the frequent fabric of our daily design."

—Don Yaeger

COMMENT

This review article discusses the effect of commonly used drugs on thyroid dysfunction, with stress on relevant interactions.

Proton pump inhibitors and H2 blockers: These decrease the acid milieu in stomach, which is required for dissolution of thyroxin and hence its absorption. So in patient with exogenous thyroid replacement, dose of thyroxin has to be increased by 25% if taking proton pump inhibitors or H2 blockers.

Ferrous sulfate, calcium carbonate, aluminum hydroxide, sucralfate, bile acid sequestrant, and raloxifene: These drugs interfere with intestinal absorption of thyroxin. So there should be a gap of minimum 4 hours between thyroxin intake and the consumption of these drugs. Patient is advised to consume thyroxin in empty stomach because milk, coffee, or soya formulae impair its absorption.

There are the drugs which increase catabolism of thyroxin by inducing glucronization enzyme. These drugs are phenobarbitone, phenytoin, carbamazepine, and rifampicin. So if hypothyroid patient is put on these drugs, dose of thyroxin has to be increased.

Estrogen-containing drugs (oral contraceptives): These drugs increase the protein binding of thyroxin. Hence patient on exogenous thyroxin replacement has to increase the dose of thyroxin after the starting of oral estrogen treatment. But if estrogens are given as local application on skin or vagina, it has minimal effect on protein binding globulins because this route circumvents the first pass effect on the liver.

A patient can get excess of *iodine* if he is given iodinated contrast agents, for computed tomography (CT scan), and if he is receiving amiodarone or topical povidone iodine. Excess iodine in thyroid inhibits synthesis of thyroid hormone, called Wolff–Chaikoff effect. It is thought to be due to inhibition of thyroid peroxidase enzyme involved in thyroid hormone synthesis. If thyroid is normal, person will escape this effect in 1–2 weeks, but patient having lymphocytic thyroiditis, or has received radioiodine ablation or has undergone partial thyroidectomy, this effect persists and patient develops hypothyroidism. Iodine excess can also lead to thyrotoxicosis (Jod-Basedow phenomenon), especially in patients with autonomous thyroid nodule (single or multiple).

Amiodarone, and antiarrhythmic drug, has 33% iodine by weight, releases 7 mg of iodine per 200 mg tablet (approximately 45 times the daily recommended intake of 150 μg). It leads to hypothyroidism in patients with autoimmune thyroid disease (Wolff–Chaikoff). If patient is having autonomous nodular goiter, it leads to hyperthyroidism (Jod-Basedow), known as type 1 amiodarone-induced thyrotoxicosis. Amiodarone also has direct cytotoxic effect on thyroid cells leading to destructive thyroiditis—known as type 2 amiodarone induce thyrotoxicosis. Treatment of type 1 thyrotoxicosis is antithyroid drugs, but type 2 disease is managed with glucocorticoids.

Lithium can lead to hypothyroidism and goiter by inhibiting pinocytosis of colloid and hence decreases release of thyroid hormone. Lithium use increases chances of developing hypothyroidism by 6 times.

Interferon alfa used in treatment of hepatitis C results in thyroid dysfunction 16% of patients with painless thyroiditis resulting in thyrotoxicosis followed by hypothyroidism. Risk factors for thyroid dysfunction are female gender, presence of thyroid antibodies, and marginally normal thyrotropin [thyroid-stimulating hormone (TSH)] levels.

Biotin interferes with laboratory measurement of T4 and TSH, resulting in false high T4, false low TSH, and false positive anti-TPO antibody, thus simulating picture of Graves' disease. This effect lasts for 48 hours after the last dose of biotin. Patient should be asked to stop biotin 5–7 days before giving blood sample for thyroid function test.

One has to be aware about the interaction of drugs with thyroid gland and exogenous thyroid hormone administration, so as to monitor the patient more efficiently.

Key Messages

- *Many of commonly used drugs like oral iron, calcium, antacids, and oral contraceptives interfere with thyroid physiology.*
- *One has to be aware about the interaction of drugs with thyroid gland and exogenous thyroid hormone administration, so as to monitor the patient more efficiently.*

ARTICLE 10

Efficacy and safety of alirocumab and evolocumab: a systematic review and meta-analysis of randomized controlled trials

Guedeney P, Giustino G, Sorrentino S, Claessen BE, Camaj A, Kalkman DN, et al. Efficacy and Safety of Alirocumab and Evolocumab: A Systematic Review and Meta-Analysis of Randomized Controlled Trials.
Eur Heart J. 2019;ehz430.

Abstract*

Aim: Proprotein convertase subtilisin-kexin type 9 (PCSK9) inhibitors, alirocumab or evolocumab, have been approved by the US Food and Drug Administration (FDA) in 2015, for treatment of hypercholesterolemia and mixed dyslipidemia. Here, we aim to evaluate the efficacy and safety of alirocumab and evolocumab in patients with dyslipidemia or atherosclerotic cardiovascular disease (ASCVD).

Methods and results: A systematic review of randomized controlled trials (RCTs) comparing treatment with alirocumab or evolocumab vs. placebo or other lipid-lowering therapies up to March 2018, was conducted. All-cause death, cardiovascular death, myocardial infarction (MI), and stroke were the primary efficacy endpoints. Risk ratios (RRs) and 95% confidence intervals (CIs) were estimated using random effect models. A total of 39 RCTs comprising 66,478 patients of whom 35,896 were treated with PCSK9 inhibitors (14,639 with alirocumab and 21,257 with evolocumab) and 30,582 with controls, were included in the study. Mean weighted follow-up time across trials was 2.3 years with an exposure time of 150,617 patient-years. Overall, no statistically significant association was found between the effects of PCSK9 inhibition and all-cause death and cardiovascular death ($p = 0.15$ and $p = 0.34$, respectively). However, PCSK9 inhibitors were associated with lower risk of MI (1.49 vs. 1.93 per 100 patient-year; RR 0.80; 95% CI 0.74–0.86; I2 = 0%; $p < 0.0001$), ischemic stroke (0.44 vs. 0.58 per 100 patient-year; RR 0.78; 95% CI 0.67–0.89; I2 = 0%; $p = 0.0005$), and coronary revascularization (2.16 vs. 2.64 per 100 patient-year; RR 0.83; 95% CI 0.78–0.89; I2 = 0%; $p < 0.0001$), when compared with the control group. Use of these PCSK9 inhibitors was not associated with increased risk of neurocognitive adverse events ($p = 0.91$), liver enzymes elevations ($p = 0.34$), rhabdomyolysis ($p = 0.58$), or new-onset diabetes mellitus ($p = 0.97$).

Conclusion: PCSK9 inhibitors like alirocumab or evolocumab were associated with lower risk of MI, stroke, and coronary revascularization, and had a favorable safety profile. *Redrafted abstract

"Opportunity dances with those on the dance floor."

—**Anonymous**

COMMENT

If a patient suffering from ASCVD, is having high cholesterol in spite of receiving high-intensity statins or is intolerant to statins, what to do?

We have to use PCSK9 inhibitors. Two monoclonal antibodies that have been approved by FDA are—alirocumab and evolocumab.

This meta-analysis has told us about beneficial and harmful effects of PCSK9 inhibitors. They have taken 39 RCTs involving about 66,000 patients out of which about 50% received one of these antibodies. Mean follow-up was 2.3 years.

What they found: Use of PCSK9 inhibitors was associated with lower risk of ischemic stroke (22%), MI (20%), coronary revascularization (17%) compared with controls. But mortality was not decreased with use of these drugs. Among the side effects, like neurocognitive adverse events, liver enzyme elevation, rhabdomyolysis, allergic reactions, or diabetes mellitus were not increased with use of these antibodies. Local reaction at injection site was the only side-effect which was more common with use of these antibodies.

What is the mechanism of action of PCSK9 inhibitors? PCSK9 inhibitors reduce the level of circulation of low-density lipoprotein (LDL) concentration by increasing the extracellular membrane density of LDL receptors. These antibodies when used over and above the maximum dose of statins, reduce LDL level by 75 mg/dL from baseline as compared with controls.

Overall use of PCSK9 inhibitors was not associated with significant decrease in mortality except in one trial using alirocumab (ODYSSEY-OUTCOME). I feel that to found mortality benefits with any drug, observation period has to be 5–6 years as was seen with statins. But in PCSK9 inhibitors trial, mean follow-up was only 2.3 years.

So we conclude that use of PCSK9 inhibitors reduces the risk of ischemic stroke, MI, and coronary revascularization. But they do not have a mortality benefit. Not many side-effects were observed.

This meta-analysis supports the use of PCSK9 inhibitors to further decrease ASCVD in patients already on maximum doses of statins or who are intolerant to statins.

Key Messages

- *Proprotein convertase subtilisin-kexin type 9 inhibitors reduce the risk of ischemic stroke, MI, and coronary revascularization.*
- *Proprotein convertase subtilisin-kexin type 9 inhibitors are not having mortality benefit.*
- *These drugs are not associated with many side effects.*

ARTICLE 11

A prospective study of thyroid function test in geriatric population and its clinical correlation

Natasha, Badiger R. A prospective study of thyroid function test in geriatric population and its clinical correlation. *J Assoc Physicians India. 2019;67:33-6.*

Abstract

Background and Objectives: Thyroid disorders in elderly population are of prime importance as it has emphasis on various metabolic activity and disease states. There is limited data regarding the prevalence of thyroid disorders in elderly from India. This study was an attempt to assess the thyroid function tests in elderly population and to correlate them with clinical symptoms.

Methodology: This 1-year hospital based prospective cross sectional study was done in outpatient Department, Department of General Medicine and Geriatric Medicine, KLES Dr Prabhakar Kore Hospital and Medical Research Centre, Belagavi on a total of 100 elderly patients who presented for regular check-ups with clinical suspicion of thyroid disorders from January 2017 to December 2017. The selected patients were investigated for T3, T4, thyroid stimulating hormone (TSH) and thyroid antibodies.

Results: Majority of the patients were females (67%), the male to female ratio was 1:2.03. The mean age was 67.69 ± 7.21 years. The mean T3 levels were 1.32 ± 0.88 ng/mL, the mean T4 levels were 7.69 ± 4.13 µg/mL and mean TSH levels were 12.31 ± 22.82 mIU/mL. The mean TPO antibodies were noted as 95.97 ± 211.82 IU/mL. Thyroid abnormalities were diagnosed in 28% of the patients and hypothyroidism was the most common thyroid abnormality noted in 12% of the patients. No association was found between thyroid abnormalities and sex (p = 0.349) as well as age (p = 0.946). Easy fatigability (94%) and generalized weakness (93%) were the common clinical complaints and mild pallor was the common clinical sign noted in 26% of the patients followed by dry/coarse skin in 25% of the patients. Thyroid abnormalities were significantly associated with easy fatigability, generalized weakness, swelling of limb/face, weight gain, constipation, and with clinical signs of pallor, dry/coarse skin, hoarseness, ankle jerk and edema. Family history of thyroid disorders was reported by 47% of the patients and it was significantly associated with of thyroid disorders (p = 0.001).

Conclusion and Interpretation: There is higher incidence of thyroid abnormalities among elderly population in the study area and overt hypothyroidism is the common thyroid abnormality.

"It's not how old you are, it's how you are old."

—**Jules Renard**

COMMENT

Many changes that occur during healthy aging mimic those of hypothyroidism, e.g., fatigue, dry skin, cold intolerance and constipation. The evaluation of thyroid function test (TFT) becomes complicated due to many chronic diseases and use of medications, both of which can affect the concentration of thyroid hormone.

Thyroid dysfunction is difficult to diagnose clinically in elderly because symptoms and signs seen in young people may not occur in older population. Levothyroxine treatment deserves special attention in older people because of significant incidence of iatrogenic hyperthyroidism and its associated risks of atrial fibrillation and bone loss. Furthermore studies have shown that thyrotropin (TSH) concentration increases as age advances from 70 years to 100 years.

If an elderly person comes to you with clinical features suggestive of hypothyroidism, you order TFT, what are the chances of having abnormal TFT? Are these clinical features just because of old age or is it because of thyroid disorder? This is what this article has tried to find out.

They have taken 100 elderly patients (age >60 years) who came to OPD, and in whom thyroid disorders were suspected clinically. Who were already known case of thyroid disorder or on drugs which alter TFT, were excluded. Their clinical features were recorded and TFT were done.

What they found? Thyroid abnormalities were found in 28% of patients. Hypothyroidism was the most common disorder, present in 43% of thyroid disorders, followed by subclinical hypothyroidism in 36% of patients. Subclinical hyperthyroidism was seen in 14% of patients whereas hyperthyroidism was seen in 7% of patients.

If the patient presents with generalized weakness, easy fatigue, weight gain, swelling of face/feet, constipation, there was higher chances of having thyroid abnormality. On the other hand if patient presents with anorexia, sweating, weight loss, palpitation, diarrhea, increased appetite, tremors, these features were not associated with increased probability of finding thyroid abnormality. Among the clinical signs pallor, hoarseness of voice, dry skin, edema feet and delayed ankle reflex were more common in dysthyroid patients. However body mass index was not associated with thyroid disorder.

Keeping this data in mind, you should be vigilant about presence of thyroid abnormalities in elderly patients and investigate accordingly.

Key Messages

⊙ *Thyroid dysfunction is difficult to diagnose clinically in elderly.*

⊙ *If the patient presents with generalized weakness, weight gain, swelling of face/feet, constipation, or is having hoarseness of voice, dry skin, delayed ankle reflex, there is higher chances of having thyroid abnormality.*

ARTICLE 12

A prospective, open-label, randomized study comparing efficacy and safety of teneligliptin versus sitagliptin in Indian patients with inadequately controlled type 2 diabetes mellitus: INSITES study

Mohan V, Ramu M, Poongothai S, Kasthuri S. A Prospective, OpeN-Label, Randomized Study Comparing Efficacy and Safety of Teneligliptin versus Sitagliptin in Indian patients with inadequately controlled type 2 diabetes mellitus: INSITES Study. *J Assoc Physicians India. 2019;67:14-9.*

Abstract

Background: Teneligliptin is widely prescribed dipeptidyl peptidase-4 inhibitor (DPP-4i) in India because of its economical pricing. However, there is no head-to-head trial comparing teneligliptin with any other

DPP-4i in Indian setting. We evaluated the efficacy and safety of teneligliptin versus sitagliptin as add-on to metformin and/or sulfonylureas in patients with type 2 diabetes mellitus (T2DM).

Methods: This prospective, open-label, randomized, active-controlled study enrolled 76 patients (1:1) at 2 centers. Patients received teneligliptin 20 mg or sitagliptin 100 mg orally once daily for 12 weeks as add-on to ongoing metformin or sulfonylurea therapy. Primary endpoint was mean change in glycosylated hemoglobin (HbA1c) from baseline at week 12 **(Fig. 1)**.

Results: Both arms were comparable (p > 0.05) at baseline in terms of age, gender, metformin daily dose, sulfonylurea use, HbA1c, fasting and postprandial blood glucose (FBG and PPBG). At the end of 12 weeks, statistically significant reductions were observed in both teneligliptin and sitagliptin arms in HbA1c (–1.19 ± 1.16% p < 0.0001 and –0.92 ± 0.95%, p < 0.0001), in FBG (-28.3 ± 63.0 mg/dL, p = 0.01 and –22.9 ± 47.4 mg/dL, p = 0.006) and PPBG (–41.3 ± 85.4 mg/dL, p = 0.006 and –54.7 ± 85.6 mg/dL, p = 0.0005). The reductions in all glycemic parameters were similar between the arms. Both gliptins were well-tolerated with no difference in the number of adverse events. There was no change in QT/QTc intervals or other ECG parameters at week 12 in both arms. In post-hoc comparison, percentage of patients achieving target HbA1c <7% (as per American Diabetes Association guidelines) at week 12 favored teneligliptin arm over sitagliptin arm (33.3% vs. 19.4% patients).

Conclusion: Teneligliptin provided similar glycemic control as compared to sitagliptin and reduced HbA1c, FBG and PPBG values significantly within 12 weeks of treatment. Both gliptins were found to be safe and well-tolerated in Indian patients with T2DM.

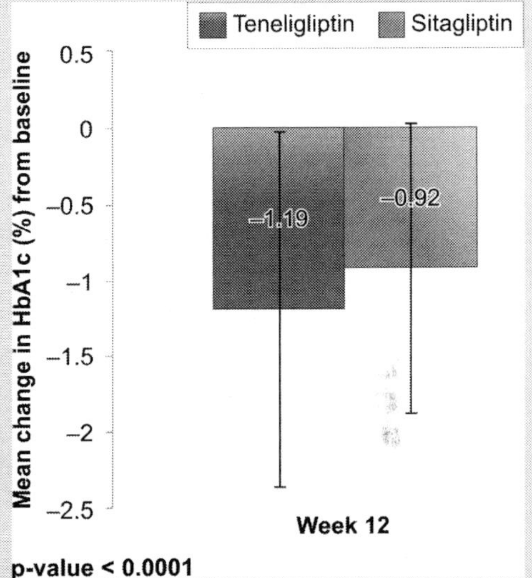

FIG. 1: Mean (SD) change HbA1c from baseline to week 12.

"Knowing is not enough; we must apply. Willing is not enough; we must do."
—**Johann Wolfgang von Goethe**

COMMENT

The pharmacokinetic properties, and the elimination route differs among DPP-4i and these differences are related to the need for dose adjustments in patients with renal or hepatic dysfunctions.

Teneligliptin was extensively evaluated for efficacy, safety and tolerability in Japanese and Korean patients with T2DM. A pooled analysis of two phase III trials has shown that teneligliptin as monotherapy or combination therapy has similar adverse event (AE) profile with lesser risk of hypoglycemia as compared to sulfonylurea for as long as 52 weeks. Teneligliptin monotherapy significantly reduced HbA1c by –0.94% in a 24-week placebo-controlled trial in Korea. Teneligliptin improved first phase of insulin secretion thus decreasing post meal glucose excursions in a 12-week study in drug-naïve Japanese patients.

There is long-term safety of teneligliptin in T2DM patients with any stage of renal impairment[9] and in hepatic impairment.

In a real world study, addition of sitagliptin was effective in lowering HbA1c by about 1% in patients who failed on sulfonylurea/metformin.[10]

Teneligliptin can reduce the average pharmacotherapy cost by about 80% in India when compared to other DPP-4i.

This study demonstrated that 3-month treatment with either teneligliptin or sitagliptin reduced HbA1c significantly by about 1% and there was a significant decrease in the fasting and postprandial glucose levels at week 12 with both DPP-4i. The mean ± SD HbA1c level achieved after 12 weeks of teneligliptin and sitagliptin treatment was 7.6 ± 1.1% and 7.7 ± 0.8%, respectively. The mean reduction in HbA1c at week 12 was statistically significant and comparable between the treatment arms. Similarly, mean reductions in FBG and PPBG at week 6 and 12 were comparable between teneligliptin and sitagliptin.

The long-term 52-week pooled analysis of Japanese studies also demonstrated that the reductions in HbA1c were dependent on the baseline values: −1.0 ± 0.9% for HbA1c >8.0% at baseline.

There were no significant changes in any of the lipid parameters with either teneligliptin or sitagliptinin line with the finding reported by Kim et al.

Both teneligliptin and sitagliptin were well-tolerated with no difference in the number of adverse effects and no hypoglycemia events. The QT interval did not increase significantly from baseline to week 12 with either of the two gliptins.

Key Message

- *Teneligliptin and Sitagliptin both are safe and well-tolerated gliptins and all international guidelines advocate use of DPP4 inhibitors as first- and second-line agents in the treatment of type 2 diabetes, however teneligliptin is more cost-friendly.*

ARTICLE 13

Management of diabetes during fasting and feasting in India

Saboo B, Joshi S, Shah SN, Tiwaskar M, Vishwanathan V, Bhandari S, et al. Management of diabetes during fasting and feasting in India.
J Assoc Physicians India. 2019;67:70-7.

Abstract

Fasting and feasting are integral part of many religions and cultures. As the amount of food and fluid intake are markedly altered during these phases, patients with diabetes are prone to higher risk of complications (**Table 1**). Even though several guidelines for fasting and feasting are available; Indian specific recommendations are the need of the hour, because of the distinct dietary habits and the diet content (high carbohydrate) of Indians. To fill this void, the current guidelines have been developed by experts from India who extensively reviewed the literature, shared their practical knowledge and ultimately arrived at a consensus.

TABLE 1: Risk stratification of patients with diabetes during fasting.

Very high risk	High risk	Moderate risk	Low risk
• Severe hypoglycemia/ketoacidosis/hyperosmolar hyperglycemic coma within last 3 months prior to Ramadan • History of recurrent hypoglycemia • Hypoglycemia unawareness • Sustained poor glycemic control • Patients on dialysis • Patients who perform intense physical labor • Acute illness • Gestational diabetes mellitus treated with insulin • Pregnancy • Type 1 diabetes mellitus	• Moderate hypoglycemia (Average blood glucose 150–300 mg/dL) • Renal insufficiency • People living alone that are treated with multiple insulin injections • Old age with ill health • Patiets with macro and microvascular complications that present additional risk factors	• Well controlled patients (HbA1c <7%) treated with short-acting insulin secretagogues and modern sulfonylureas	• Well controlled patients (HbA1c <7%) treated with diet alone, metformin, or a thiazolidinedione who are otherwise healthy

Patients with the following conditions should refrain from fasting: Pregnant and lactating women; Type 1 diabetes; Acute peptic ulcer; Cancer; Severe bronchial asthma, pulmonary tuberculosis; Overt cardiovascular diseases recent MI, sustained angina; Hepatic dysfunction

Adapted from: South Asian Consensus Guideline, ADA 2005, IDF 2016, and IGDR 2015.

"The best of all medicines is resting and fasting."

—**Benjamin Franklin**

COMMENT

Fasting and feasting are common practices observe by people for traditional or cultural reasons.
- *Hindu fasts and feasts:*
  - "Nirahara": No food
  - "Phalahara": Fruit and milk allowed
  - "Alpahara": Broken rice
- *Islamic fasts and feasts:* Fast known as *Sawn*, is avoiding eating and drinking during day. In Ramadan, high calorie food at *Iftar*; evening meal after fast and at *Suhoor* (meal consumed early in the morning).
- *Jain fasts and feasts:* "Paryushan" is the most observed, which lasts 8 days in Svetambara Jains and 10 days in Digambar Jains.
- *Buddhist fasts and feasts:* Vassa or Buddhist Lent is the fast and feast observed for 3 lunar months every year in the rainy season.

■ MANAGEMENT

The **Table 2** suggests the management of diabetes complications.

Management of T1DM

The evidence suggests that fasting for 25 hours is safe and can be observed by patients with T1DM.[11]

The South Asian Consensus Guideline on insulin use during Ramadan; advocates that once- or twice daily injections of intermediate or long-acting insulin along with pre-meal rapid-acting insulin can be safely used in patients during fasting.

Management of T2DM (Table 3)

- **Nonpharmacological management**
  - Physical activity and yoga can be performed however excessive and aggressive activity should be avoided during prolonged fasting periods.
  - Nutrition: The pre-fast meal should be composed of complex carbohydrates with low glycemic index and proteins. The post-fast meal should have simple carbohydrates such as bread, rice, etc. Adequate fluids to be taken.
- **Pharmacological management**
  - Metformin can be safely used during fasting periods due to minimal chances of hypoglycemia.
  - Gliclazide due to its efficacy in glycemic control, lower risk of hypoglycemia, less CV complications and death and lower

TABLE 2: Management of diabetes complications (hypoglycemia, hyperglycemia, diabetic ketoacidosis, and dehydration) during fasting and feasting period.

Lifestyle modification	• Attend pre-fast counseling and learn the warning symptoms of hyperglycemia and hypoglycemia • Strict adherence to the diabetic diet • Take medication regularly as per instruction • Do not overeat after fast is broken and minimize eating sweet or fatty foods • Record weight daily and inform doctor for gain or loss of more than 2 kg • If a complication occurs, break the fast immediately and seek medical help • Patients/family should be aware of potential problems and alert doctor immediately • Serving of meal supplements may be added to pre-fast meals or intra fast liquids, to prevent hypoglycemia
Frequent blood glucose monitoring	• Test blood glucose regularly especially for patients on insulin therapy during prolonged fasting such as Ramadan, *Navaratri*, Vassa, etc. • Test blood glucose before and 2 h after *Iftar*, before *Suhoor* and at mid-day • Frequent SMBGs testing should be done
Exercise	• Normal levels of physical activity may be maintained. However, excessive physical activity may lead to higher risk of hypoglycemia and should be avoided • Less fluid intake for prolonged time may attribute to dehydration, and this may become severe for individuals who perform hard physical labor
Breaking the fast	• If the blood sugar level is <70 mg/dL (3.9 mmol/L) or >300 mg/dL (16.7 mmol/L) and/or development of diabetes complication, the fast should be broken • After breaking the fast due to hypoglycemia, patients should consume a little amount of a fast-acting carbohydrate diet
Medication	• Patients taking insulin and sulfonylurea should be closely monitored for hypoglycemia • SGLT2 inhibitors should not be used in elderly and frail patients and those residing at hot and humid conditions • Dose modification should be done as per individual patients risk and the preference

(SMBG: self-monitoring of blood glucose; SGLT2: sodium-glucose cotransporter-2)

cost can be a suitable alternative and safely used during fasting periods in Indian patients.[12]

- ○ DPP-4 inhibitors can be safely used during fasting due to reduced risk of hypoglycemia as they work by increasing insulin secretion in a dose dependent manner.
- ○ The STEADFAST study compared vildagliptin and gliclazide during Ramadan and did not find any significant difference between two treatments in terms of hypoglycemic episodes.
- ○ SGLT2 inhibitors can be used during fasting due to low risk of hypoglycemia, however the fasting for long period without fluids may aggravate risk of hypotension and dehydration.
- ○ Pioglitazone: There is low risk of hypoglycemia, however weight gain is a concern.
- ○ Alpha–glucosidase inhibitors: Acarbose, voglibose, miglitol can be safely used, however their ineffectiveness as monotherapy and GI side effects reduce their usage.
- ○ GLP-1 receptor agonists are associated with weight loss and low risk of hypoglycemia, hence chosen in overweight and obese patients during the fasting period. Trials such as Treat 4 Ramadan and Lira-Ramadan trial did not find any significant difference between liraglutide and sulfonylurea and can be safely used.
- ○ Insulin analogs are recommended over regular human insulin due to lower hypoglycemia.

TABLE 3: Approach to adjustment or modification of continued antidiabetic medications in patients with diabetes during fasting period (IDF 2016, Sadikot S 2017, Kalra S 2015, Jhulka S 2017, and Latt TS and Kalra S 2012).

Anti-diabetic agents	Muslim fast prolonged	Hindu fast infrequent but brief	Infrequent but prolonged	Frequent	Jain fast High-risk	Low-risk	Buddhist fast
	Ramadan	Karva chauth	Navratri	Somvaar, Mangalvaar	Tiwihar upavas, Upavas, Bela (Chhath), Tela (Asththam)	Byasana, Ekasana, Ratri Bhojan Tyag	Vaasa
Metformin	• One daily: Take at Iftar • Twice daily: Take at Iftar and Suhoor • Thrice daily: Take 2/3rd of the total daily dose at the Iftar and 1/3rd at the Suhoor	• Once daily: Take at night • Twice daily: Take at morning and night • Thrice daily: Omit the lunch dose and follow above	• Once daily: Take at night • Twice daily: Take at morning and night • Thrice daily: Take 2/3 of the total daily dose at night and 1/3 at the morning	• Once daily: Take at night • Twice daily: Take at morning and night • Thrice daily: Omit the lunch dose and follow above	Omit the therapy on the day of fast	No change required	No change required
Sulfonyl-ureas*	• Once daily: Take at Iftar • Twice daily: Take 1/2 of usual evening dose with the Suhoor and the usual morning dose with the Iftar	• Once daily: Take at dinner • Twice daily: Omit he morning dose in absence of breakfast	• Once daily: Take at dinner • Twice daily: Omit the morning dose	• Omit the therapy on the day of fast	Avoided, or taken in half dose at night	Full dose at morning and half dose at night	• Once daily: Take at morning • Twice daily: Take 2/3rd at morning
DPP-4 inhibitors	• No dose adjustments is required	• No change, take at dinner	• No change, take at dinner	• No change	Omit the therapy on the day of fast	Taken at night	• No change
SGLT2 inhibitors†	• No dose adjustment is required and the dose be taken with Iftar	• No change, take at dinner	• No change, take at dinner	• No change	Omit the therapy on the day of fast	Evening dose avoided, or taken in half dose	• No change
Pioglitazone	• No dose adjustment is required	• No change	• No change, or 2/3rd take at dinner	• No change	No change	No change required	• No change
AGIs	• No dose adjustment is required	• No change	• No change	• No change	Omit the therapy on the day of fast	No change required	• No change
GLP-1 analogues	• The dose should be titrated 6 weeks prior to Ramadan and no dose adjustment is required	• Reduce the dose to 1/2 and take at dinner	• The dose should be titrated prior to Navratri	• No change or reduce the dose to 1/2	Once weekly dose: No change (postpone due doses till the completion of fasting)	No change required	

Continued

Continued

Anti-diabetic agents	Muslim fast prolonged	Hindu fast infrequent but brief	Infrequent but prolonged	Frequent	Jain fast High-risk	Low-risk	Buddhist fast
	Ramadan	Karva chauth	Navratri	Somvaar, Mangalvaar	Tiwihar upavas, Upavas, Bela (Chhath), Tela (Asththam)	Byasana, Ekasana, Ratri Bhojan Tyag	Vaasa
Long-acting insulin	• Once-daily: ↓ dose by 15–30% and take at *Iftar* • Twice daily: Take usual morning dose at *Iftar* and ↓ evening dose by 50% and take at *Suhoor*	• Need no change or may reduce the dose to 2/3rd	• Need no change or may reduce the dose to 2/3rd	Reduce the dose to 2/3rd	25% reduction in dose	10–20% reduction in dose	Once dialy: before the main meal of 24 h period
Short-acting insulin	• Take normal dose at *Iftar* and lunch dose at dinner • ↓ *Suhoor* dose by 50%	Reduce the dose to 1/2th	Reduce the dose to 1/2	Reduce the dose to 1/2	1 bolus	2 bolus	Reduce the dose to 1/2
Premixed insulin	• Once daily: Take normal dose at *Iftar* • Twice daily: Take 1/2 of evening dose with *Suhoor* and the usual moring dose with the *Iftar* • Thrice Daily: Omit afternoon dose and adjust *Iftar* and *Suhoor* doses	• 30:70 or 25:75: reduce the dose to 2/3rd • 50:50: reduce the dose to 1/2	• 30:70 or 25:75: Reduce the dose to 2/3rd • 50:50: Reduce the dose to 1/2	Reduce the dose to 2/3rd and prefer 30:70 or 25:75	30:70 at night or 50:50 at day	50:50 once daily	Can be given once daily, before the main meal of the 24 h period

(AGIs: alpha-glucosidase inhibitors; DPP-4: dipeptidyl peptidase-4; SGLT2: sodium-glucose co-transporter-2)

*Gliclazide and glimepiride should be preferred among all other sulfonylureas

† Elderly patients, patients with renal impairment, hypotensive individuals, those at risk of dehydration or those taking diuretics should not be treated with SGLT2 inhibitors.

Key Message

⊙ *Structured diabetes education plan along with proper treatment dose adjustment or modification are important to ensure a safe fasting or feasting period.*

ARTICLE 14

IMPACT India: insights for insulin therapy in routine clinical practice

Mohan V, Das AK, Unnikrishnan AG, Shah SN, Kumar A, Zargar AH, et al. IMPACT India: Insights for insulin therapy in routine clinical practice.
J Assoc Physicians India. 2019;67:34-8.

Abstract

Objective: Widely used in the management of diabetes, insulin therapy is influenced by several patient preferences and physician choices. This article reports the findings of the IMPACT survey, designed to assess insights on various factors which influence the choice of insulin therapy in India.

Methods: We administered a questionnaire which focused on the practice and patient profiles and the preferred regimens in specific clinical situations using a case scenario. Respondents were asked about preferred insulin regimens for various phases of life, comorbid conditions, dietary choices and psychological factors.

Results: Overall, 314 doctors participated in the survey. Majority were general physicians (51%) and diabetologists (37%). In clinical practice, the most preferred regimens included premix insulin BD in adults (59%) and elderly (53%), and basal bolus therapy in pregnant women (>47%) and in acute illness (62%). Both regimens were equally preferred for symptomatic patients (41% basal bolus and 38% premix insulin) and those with renal or hepatic failure (36% each). Premix insulin was preferred for patients with high carbohydrate intake (73%) while basal bolus was preferred for patients with variable meal timings (39%) and in pronounced postprandial glucose excursions (45%). Insulin coformulation and high-mix insulins were not a part of the survey questionnaire.

Summary: Indian physicians exercise logic in the choice of insulin regimens. Preference is based on patient characteristics including glucophenotype, dietary patterns, psychosocial needs, clinical situations, and comorbid conditions.

"There is only one cardinal rule: One must always listen to the patient."
—Oliver Sacks

COMMENT

The American Association of Clinical Endocrinologists (AACE) and American Diabetes Association (ADA) recommend basal insulin while the Indian National Consensus Group (INCG)[13] recommends premix insulin for the initiation of therapy in diabetes.

The adoption of insulin in routine practice is guided by the duration and severity of diabetes, patient preferences, overall health, cost and accessibility. Delayed initiation of insulin is common in India.

In IMPACT INDIA Survey

Total 12 questions included key factors which determined therapeutic choices, i.e., patient characteristics, presenting symptoms, diversity in meal patterns and patient preferences, severity and patterns of hyperglycemia, and diversity in meal patterns (**Fig. 1**).

The INCG recommends premixed insulins, preferably analog formulations, for the management of all stages of diabetes as these offer a simple and safe option for the initiation of treatment.[14]

According to the survey, Indian physicians prefer to use twice daily dosing of premix insulin in adults, elderly with no limitations of activities of daily living, and the frail elderly. Physicians prefer premix insulin twice daily dosing for patients with high carbohydrate intake which matches the INCG guidelines for the high glycemic responses to high carbohydrate meals.

In India the basal bolus therapy is the most preferred therapy for pregnant women. In the survey, 28% of respondents used premixed insulins during pregnancy with good results (**Fig. 2**).

Basal bolus regimens are reported to be efficacious and safe for use in patients of diabetes with medical and surgical complications.

The Indian Council of Medical Research (ICMR) guidelines also recommend the use of premix insulin twice a day as an alternative to multiple insulin injection regimen.

Insulin coformulations make a logical choice in several scenarios with advantages of similar efficacy to basal bolus or basal plus regimens along with proven reduction in hypoglycemia events as well as reducing burden of injections. Unfortunately, insulin coformulations were not part of the survey questionnaires.

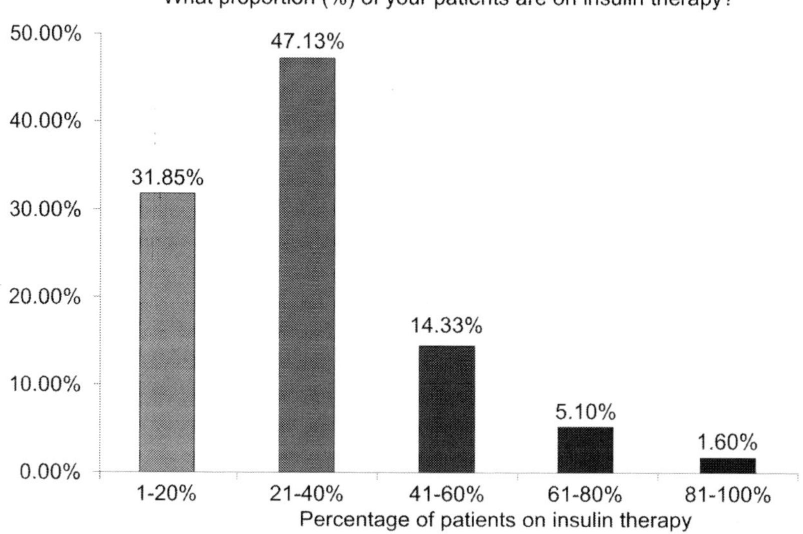

FIG. 1: Proportion of patients on insulin therapy.

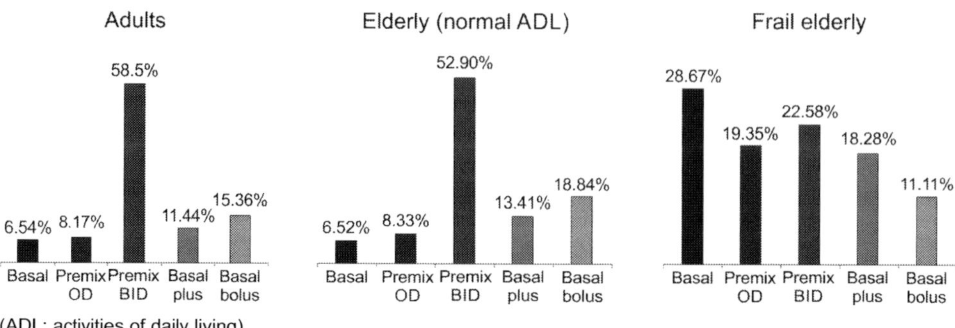

FIG. 2: Preferred insulin therapy in adults and elderly patients with diabetes.

> **Key Message**
>
> ⊚ *By assessing stage of life, clinical situation, diet, cost, accessibility and psychosocial factors individualization and customization of insulin regime and dosage should be done. Premix insulins are the preferred option by most physicians in India.*

ARTICLE 15

Anti-diabetic agent and cancer

Pareek KK, Mathur G, Ramchandani GD. Anti-diabetic agent and cancer.
J Assoc Physicians India. 2019;67:66-9.

Abstract

In this update article Dr KK Pareek et al. have looked at association and chances of cancer occurrence in patients of diabetes. There have been some reports of increase in the chances of liver, pancreas, colorectal and breast cancer in patients of diabetes. Patients of cancer when they have associated diabetes have a 40% higher mortality than cancer patients without diabetes. The association of diabetes with cancer is more through the antidiabetic drugs rather than the disease itself. Insulin is the drug of choice in type 1 diabetes mellitus (T1DM) and is used in many patients of long standing type 2 diabetes mellitus (T2DM). Insulin has structural and functional similarity to insulin like growth factor 1 (IGF-1). The IGF-1 stimulates cell proliferation which could be related to cancer occurrence. There is some data that higher doses of insulin may be related to increased risk of cancer.

Insulin secretagogues especially sulfonylurea agents increase the insulin secretion can thus also be related to oncogenesis. This may happen indirectly due to increase in IGF-1 activity. Many trials have shown patients of diabetes who are taking metformin have lesser cancer mortality than diabetic patients who are on insulin or sulfonylureas. The cancer protective effect of metformin may be due to PPARg pathway. Although there are studies correlating antidiabetic drugs with cancer occurrence there has been no large randomized trial which has associated a link between cancer and antidiabetic drugs.

"Diseases can rarely be eliminated through early diagnosis or good treatment, but prevention can eliminate disease."

—Denis Parsons Burkitt

COMMENT

Coexistence of cancer and diabetes is related to the elevated risk of all-cause mortality by 41%, compared to the presence of cancer without diabetes (**Flowchart 1, Table 1**).[15]

■ INSULIN

According to Gu et al., the overall risk of cancer in patients with type 2 diabetes mellitus (T2DM) treated with human insulin was not elevated compared to patients without insulin treatment. However, the site-specific analysis showed a significantly higher risk of liver cancer in this group, higher risks of overall mortality and cancer mortality.

The study conducted by Hemkens et al. involved more than 127,000 cancer naïve patients with T1DM or T2DM, were treated with human insulin or short-acting (lispro and aspart) or long-acting (glargine) insulin analogs with average follow-up 1.63 years. For each type of insulin a positive relationship between the dose and the risk of cancer development was demonstrated.

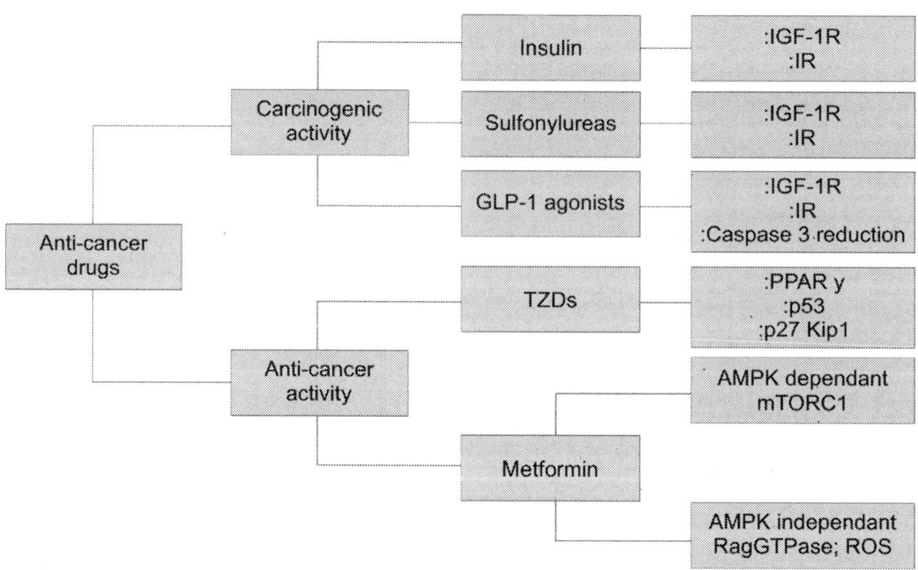

(GLP: glucagon-like peptide; TZD: thiazolidinediones; IGF-1R: insulin-like growth factor type 1 receptor; PPAR: peroxisome proliferated activated receptor; AMPK: adenosine monophosphate-activated protein kinase; ROS: reactive oxygen species)

FLOWCHART 1: Anti-diabetic drugs and role in cancer disease.

TABLE 1: Possible risks to develop cancer by anti-diabetic agents

Drug		Drug	Risk of cancer	Cancer site
Insulin	Human insulin	Insulin	Not elevated	Overall
			Increased	Liver, colorectum, pancreas
	Fast acting insulin analogs	Lispro	Not elevated vs. insulin	-
		As part	Not elevated vs. insulin	-
		Glulisine*	Not elevated vs. insulin	Breast
	Long acting insulin analogs	Glargine	Increase	Breast
			Not elevated	Breast
Insulin secretagogues	Sulfonylureas	In general	Increased	Overall, pancreas
		Glibenclamide	Increase	-
			Reduced	-
		Glipizide	Not reduced	-
		Gliclazide	Reduced	-
	Meglitinides	**Repaglinide**	**Reduced (in vitro)**	**Breast, hepatic, cervical carcinoma cells**
	GLP-1 agonists	Exenatide	Not elevated	Intestine
		Liraglutide	Not elevated	Intestine, pancreas
	DPP-4 inhibitors	**Sitagliptin**	Not elevated	Intestine

Continued

Continued

Drug		Drug	Risk of cancer	Cancer site
Insulin sensitizers	Biguanides	Metformin	Reduced	Pancreas, **breast, lung, prostate,** colorectum, liver
	TZDs	In general	Reduced	Lung
			Not elevated	Lung, bladder, breast, colon, prostate
		Pioglitazone	Reduced	Liver
			Increased	Bladder
		Rosiglitazone	Reduced	Liver, colorectum
		Troglitazone	Reduced	Stomach, liver
Others	Alpha-glucosidase inhibitors	Acarbose	Decreased	Lung
			Not elevated	Thyroid
	SGLT2 inhibitors	Canagliflozin	Not elevated	Kidney, bladder, breast
		Dapagliflozin	**Not elevated**	**Bladder**

*Bold letters are showing animal or preclinical studies.

Insulin degludec does not increase any type cancer as per recent meta-analysis, while detemir reduces risk of cancer incidences in type 1 and 2 diabetic patients compared to human insulin.

■ INSULIN SECRETAGOGUES

The latest meta-analysis of 18 sulfonylurea studies showed that sulfonylurea use in T2DM was linked with an increase in overall cancer risk in cohort studies, though, the results from randomized control trials and case–control studies proved no statistically significant effect.[16]

■ INCRETIN MIMETICS

No excess risk of pancreatic cancer was observed with Liraglutide. To date there is no sufficient evidence to show significant coexistence between incretin mimetics and cancer.

■ INSULIN SENSITIZERS

Diabetic patients taking metformin have lower mortality rate from cancer than in those treated with insulin and sulfonylurea.

Mutations of loss-of-function type of PPARγ have been found in numerous cancer types, e.g., lung, breast, colon, liver, prostate and thyroid cancer. Due to inhibitory role of PPARγ Thiazolidinediones (TZDS) can be a new agent in hepatocellular carcinoma (HCC) treatment.

Increased risk of bladder cancer was noted among patients with the highest cumulative dose and the longest exposure to pioglitazone, which may be minimized by the appropriate patient selection and exclusion criteria. Using these medicines in patients with current bladder cancer history or macroscopic hematuria of unknown origin should be avoided. TZDS have not been found to increase cancer risk in meta-analyses, however currently association is under assessment.[17]

Canagliflozin, Dapagliflozin therapy did not increase the risk of renal, bladder, or breast cancer compared to placebo.

Currently there is no any strong evidence to prove acarbose or voglibose adverse effect on oncological disease.

Key Message

⊙ *Insulin and insulin secretagogues can possibly increase risk of breast, pancreas, liver and colorectal cancer, whereas insulin sensitizers seem to exert a cancer protective effect on the above cancers along with lung and stomach cancers.*

ARTICLE 16

Application of non-HDL cholesterol for population-based cardiovascular risk stratification: results from the multinational cardiovascular risk consortium

Brunner FJ, Waldeyer C, Ojeda F, Salomaa V, Kee F, Sans S, et al. Application of non-HDL cholesterol for population-based cardiovascular risk stratification: results from the Multinational Cardiovascular Risk Consortium. *Lancet. 2019;394:2173-83.*

Abstract

Background: The relevance of blood lipid concentrations to long-term incidence of cardiovascular disease (CVD) and the relevance of lipid-lowering therapy for CVD outcomes is unclear. We investigated the CVD risk associated with the full spectrum of bloodstream non-HDL cholesterol concentrations. We also created an easy-to-use tool to estimate the long-term probabilities for a CVD event associated with non-HDL cholesterol and modeled its risk reduction by lipid-lowering treatment.

Methods: In this risk-evaluation and risk-modeling study, we used Multinational Cardiovascular Risk Consortium data from 19 countries across Europe, Australia, and North America. Individuals without prevalent cardiovascular disease at baseline and with robust available data on cardiovascular disease outcomes were included. The primary composite endpoint of atherosclerotic CVD was defined as the occurrence of the coronary heart disease event or ischemic stroke. Sex-specific multivariable analyses were computed using non-HDL cholesterol categories according to the European guideline thresholds, adjusted for age, sex, cohort, and classical modifiable cardiovascular risk factors. In a derivation and validation design, we created a tool to estimate the probabilities of a CVD event by the age of 75 years, dependent on age, sex, and risk factors, and the associated modeled risk reduction, assuming a 50% reduction of non-HDL cholesterol.

Findings: Of the 524,444 individuals in the 44 cohorts in the Consortium database, we identified 398,846 individuals belonging to 38 cohorts [184,055 (48.7%) women; median age 51.0 years (IQR 40.7–59.7)]. 199,415 individuals were included in the derivation cohort [91,786 (48.4%) women] and 199,431 [92,269 (49.1%) women] in the validation cohort. During a maximum follow-up of 43.6 years (median 13.5 years, IQR 7.0–20.1), 54,542 cardiovascular endpoints occurred. Incidence curve analyses showed progressively higher 30-year cardiovascular disease event-rates for increasing non-HDL cholesterol categories (from 7.7% for non-HDL cholesterol <2.6 mmol/L to 33.7% for ≥5.7 mmol/L in women and from 12.8% to 43.6% in men; p < 0.0001). Multivariable adjusted Cox models with non-HDL cholesterol lower than 2.6 mmol/L as reference showed an increase in the association between non-HDL cholesterol concentration and CVD for both sexes (from hazard ratio 1.1, 95% CI 1.0–1.3 for non-HDL cholesterol 2.6 to <3.7 mmol/L to 1.9, 1.6–2.2 for ≥5.7 mmol/L in women and from 1.1, 1.0–1.3 to 2.3, 2.0–2.5 in men). The derived tool allowed the estimation of CVD event probabilities specific for non-HDL cholesterol with high comparability between the derivation and validation cohorts as reflected by smooth calibration curves analyses and a root mean square error lower than 1% for the estimated probabilities of CVD. A 50% reduction of non-HDL cholesterol concentrations was associated with reduced risk of a CVD event by the age of 75 years, and this risk reduction was greater the earlier cholesterol concentrations were reduced.

Interpretation: Non-HDL cholesterol concentrations in blood are strongly associated with long-term risk of atherosclerotic CVD. We provide a simple tool for individual long-term risk assessment and the potential benefit of early lipid-lowering intervention. These data could be useful for physician-patient communication about primary prevention strategies.

Funding: EU Framework Programme, UK Medical Research Council, and German Centre for Cardiovascular Research.

"Only the inquiring mind solves problems."

—Edward Hodnett

COMMENT

A 45-year-old patient comes to you with no cardiovascular risk factor, having non-HDL cholesterol of 150 mg/dL. What are chances of this patient having cardiovascular events in next 30 years? Would you prescribe him lipid-lowering drugs?

These are the questions which are taken up by this article.

Non-HDL cholesterol represents all the atherogenic lipoproteins, including LDL cholesterol. It is calculated by subtracting HDL cholesterol from total cholesterol. The concentration of non-HDL cholesterol is usually 30 mg/dL (0.76 mmol/L) higher than LDL cholesterol.

Till now we have firm evidence for beneficial effects of statins for preventing cardiovascular events in high-risk groups as primary prevention and patients with known cardiovascular disease as secondary prevention. But there is not much data about relationship of high cholesterol in young individuals and incidence of cardiovascular events in next 30 years. Most of guidelines take person's 10 year cardiovascular risk into consideration. There is evidence that 30 year risk of cardiovascular events is ten times higher than 10 year risk especially in young persons.

In this study, total of about 400,000 individuals were taken for analysis. Maximum follow-up was 43.6 years (median 13.5 years). A total of 55,000 cardiovascular events were reported. There was direct correlation between increased non-HDL concentration and incidence of CVD events. The 30 year CVD event rate was 3–4 times more in higher non-HDL category (>220 mg/dL) as compared to lowest category (<100 mg/dL). If the hyperlipidemia is present before age of 45 years, it is more harmful than if it is present after the age of 45 years. If non-HDL is between 100 and 145 mg/dL before the age of 45 years, it increases the chance of CVD by 10–20% more than when it is present after the age of 45 years.

In this article, they have also given a risk prediction tool that takes into consideration age, sex, cardiovascular risk factors to estimate the long term probability of CVD events linked to non-HDL cholesterol level. They also predicted that if you lower the cholesterol with interventions, incidence of CVD events decreases over next 30 years.

This data tells us impact of non-HDL cholesterol on very long term CVD outcome. This information can be used for primary prevention in young individuals.

So based on this knowledge, if a 45-year-old person comes with non-HDL cholesterol of 150 mg/dL, he should be treated with lipid lowering drugs throughout his life.

Key Message

⊙ *Elevated non-HDL cholesterol is associated with long term increased risk of atherosclerotic cardiovascular disease. This information should be used for primary prevention in young individuals.*

ARTICLE 17

Sodium-glucose cotransporter-2 inhibitors and the risk for severe urinary tract infections: a population-based cohort study

Dave CV, Schneeweiss S, Kim D, Fralick M, Tong A, Patorno E. Sodium–glucose cotransporter-2 inhibitors and the risk for severe urinary tract infections: a population-based cohort study.
Ann Intern Med. 2019;171:248-56.

Abstract*

Background: The US Food and Drug Administration (FDA) warned about the risk for severe urinary tract infections (UTIs) with sodium-glucose cotransporter-2 (SGLT2) inhibitors, in 2015. However, few studies evaluating this could not find any association.

Objective: We aim to assess the risk of severe UTI events in patients initiating use of SGLT2 inhibitors and compare them with those initiating use of dipeptidyl peptidase-4 (DPP-4) inhibitors or glucagon-like peptide-1 receptor (GLP-1) agonists.

Design: Population-based cohort study.

Setting: Two large, US-based databases of commercial claims (March 2013 to September 2015).

Participants: Within each database, 2 cohorts were created and matched 1:1 on propensity score. Patients included in the cohort were ≥18 years of age, had type 2 diabetes mellitus, and were initiating use of SGLT-2 inhibitors versus DPP-4 inhibitors (cohort 1) or GLP-1 agonists (cohort 2).

Measurements: Occurrence of a severe UTI event, defined as a hospitalization for primary UTI, sepsis with UTI, or pyelonephritis was the primary outcome. An outpatient UTI treated with antibiotics was the secondary outcome. Hazard ratios (HRs) were estimated in each propensity score-matched cohort, with adjustment for more than 90 baseline characteristics.

Results: A total of 123,752 patients were identified in cohort 1 and 111,978 in cohort 2 in the 2 databases, after 1:1 matching on propensity score. In cohort 1, 61 and 57 events of severe UTI were reported with use of SGLT2 inhibitors [incidence rate (IR) per 1,000 person-years, 1.76] and DPP-4 inhibitors (IR, 1.77) [HR, 0.98 (95% CI 0.68–1.41)], respectively. In cohort 2, those receiving SGLT2 inhibitors had 73 events (IR, 2.15), compared with 87 events in the GLP-1 agonist group (IR, 2.96) [HR 0.72 (CI 0.53–0.99)]. Findings were robust across sensitivity analyses; within several subgroups of age, sex, and frailty; and for canagliflozin and dapagliflozin individually. There was no significant association between SGLT2 inhibitors and outpatient UTIs [cohort 1: HR, 0.96 (CI 0.89–1.04); cohort 2: HR, 0.91 (CI 0.84–0.99)] (**Fig. 1**).

Limitation: Generalizability of the study findings may be limited to patients with commercial insurance.

Conclusion: No increased risk for severe and nonsevere UTI events was observed among patients initiating SGLT-2 inhibitor therapy compared to those initiating treatment with other second-line antidiabetic medications.

Primary funding source: Brigham and Women's Hospital, Division of Pharmacoepidemiology and Pharmacoeconomics. *Redrafted abstract

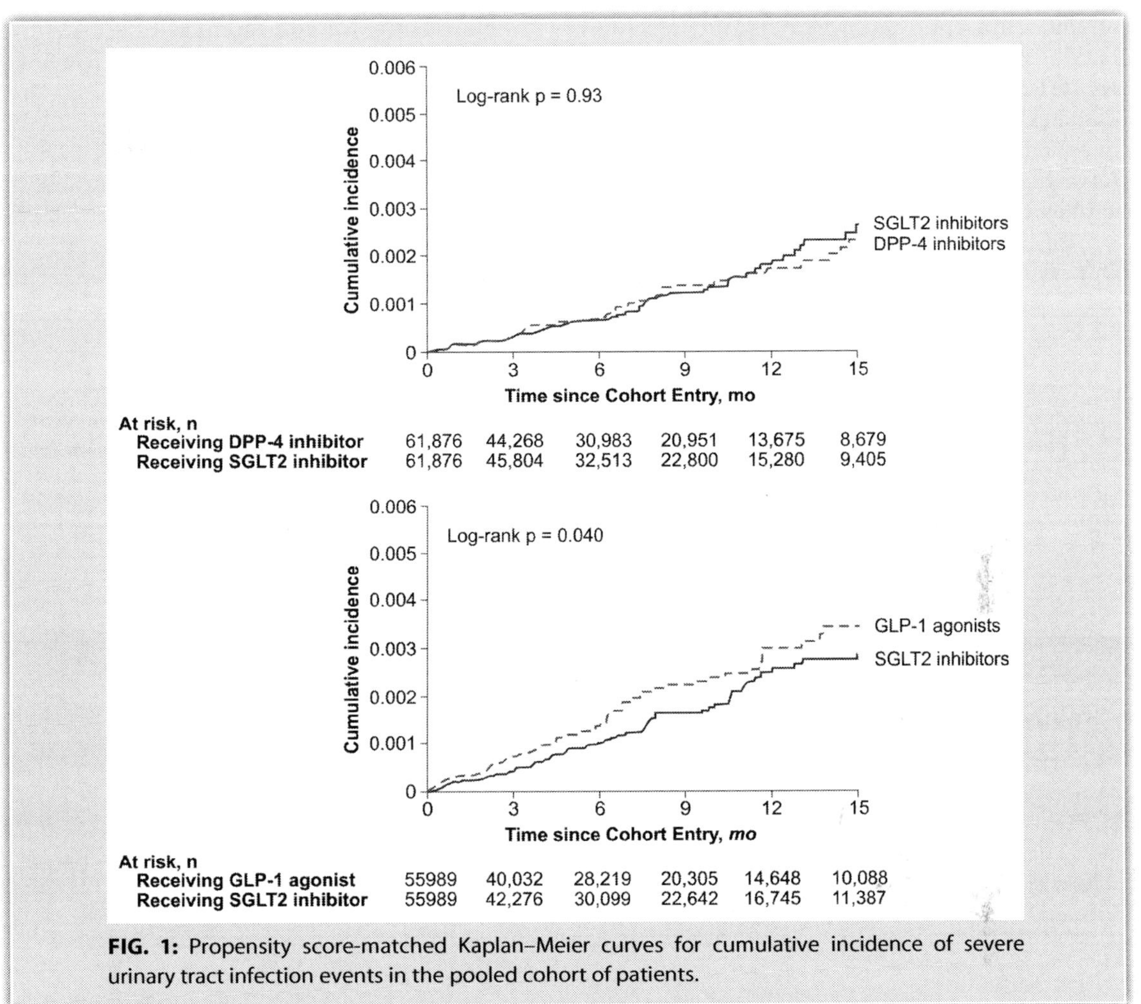

FIG. 1: Propensity score-matched Kaplan–Meier curves for cumulative incidence of severe urinary tract infection events in the pooled cohort of patients.

"Somewhere, something incredible is waiting to be known."

— **Carl Sagan**

COMMENT

Sodium-glucose cotransporter-2 (SGLT2) inhibitors reduce the serum glucose by inhibiting its resorption in the proximal tubule thus increasing the availability of glucose in the urinary tract which provides substrate for bacteria to grow. Although SGLT-2 inhibitors have consistently been shown to increase risk for genital infections, their association with urinary tract infections (UTIs) is less clear, and prior meta-analyses have reported conflicting findings.[18] Most UTIs caused by SGLT2 inhibitors are of mild to moderate severity.

This study examined data from two large commercial claims databases and found that compared with patients initiating use of a DPP-4 inhibitor or GLP-1 agonist, those initiating use of an SGLT2 inhibitor for type 2 diabetes had a similar rate of severe or nonsevere UTI events. Study findings were consistent across a range of predefined sensitivity analyses; within several subgroups of age, sex, and frailty; and for individual SGLT2 agents.

Patients with diabetes have a higher frequency and severity of UTIs;[19-21] hence antidiabetic agents that increase risk of UTIs may decrease quality of life, predisposing patients to therapy discontinuation and poor glycemic control. In addition, uroseptic and pyelonephritic infections have been found to contribute to patient mortality. As UTIs are highly prevalent in patients with diabetes, this could exclude a substantial number of patients from receiving SGLT2 inhibitors which have been shown to decrease risk for major cardiovascular events and death.

This study did not find an increase in risk for UTI events among new users of SGLT2 inhibitors.

The results are consistent with a recent a recent meta-analysis of 72 clinical trials which found only 17 cases of sepsis with UTI in the SGLT2 inhibitor group (0.67 events per 1,000 patients). A network meta-analysis by Li and colleagues examined individual SGLT2 inhibitors and similarly did not find an elevated risk for UTI (with a possible exception of dapagliflozin at higher doses).

Key Message

⊙ *Sodium-glucose cotransporter-2 inhibitor was not associated with an increase in risk for serious or nonserious UTIs; hence the additional beneficial effect on blood pressure, reduced cardiovascular events and mortality, kidney disease progression should be evaluated and SGLT2 therapy should be prescribed for patients with diabetes.*

ARTICLE 18

Prevalence and predictors of "new-onset diabetes after transplantation" (NODAT) in renal transplant recipients: an observational study

Choudhury PS, Mukhopadhyay P, Roychowdhary A, Chowdhury S, Ghosh S. Prevalence and predictors of "new-onset diabetes after transplantation" (NODAT) in renal transplant recipients: an observational study.
Indian J Endocr Metab. 2019;23:273-7.

Abstract

Objective: New-onset diabetes after transplantation (NODAT) develops frequently after renal transplant. The study aims at the prevalence of NODAT, predictors for developing it and therapeutic glycemic responses in NODAT.

Materials and methods: Consecutive renal transplant recipients excluding diabetic kidney disease (DKD) or pretransplant diabetes were evaluated. Forty-three out of 250 persons were found to have NODAT. Ninety age-matched transplant recipients from the rest were recruited as control. Fasting blood sugar (FBS), HbA1c, lipid profile, and trough tacrolimus level (T_0) were examined in all. HOMA IR C-peptide and HOMA-beta C-peptide were calculated.

Results: Prevalence of NODAT in renal transplant recipients was 17.2% (43/250). Twenty-four (55.8%) developed early NODAT (<1 year) and 19 (44.2%) developed late NODAT (>1 year). Significantly higher pretransplant body mass index (BMI) (kg/m^2) (p < 0.001), waist circumference (WC) (cm) (p < 0.001), pretransplant cholesterol (mg%) (p = 0.04), triglyceride (mg%) (p < 0.001), and FBS (mg%) (p < 0.001) were found in NODAT compared with non-NODAT. Trough tacrolimus (ng/mL) was found to be higher in NODAT (10.2 vs. 5.37, p < 0.001). Though HOMA IR was not found to be different between groups, HOMA-beta C-peptide was low in NODAT compared with non-NODAT (p = 0.03). Predictors of NODAT were WC [odds ratio (OR) = 01.15] and trough tacrolimus level (OR = 1.316). Best cut-off of WC for predicting NODAT was 87.5 cm for male and 83.5 cm for female. Best cut-off of T_0 was 8.5 ng/mL. In NODAT, 9.3%

were treated by lifestyle modification, 67.4% by oral hypoglycemic agents, 11.6% by insulin, and 11.6% by combined insulin and oral antidiabetic agents with HbA1c <7% (**Table 1**).

Conclusion: NODAT in renal transplant recipients is more common in those with higher pretransplant BMI, WC, pretransplant total cholesterol, triglyceride, and FBS. Beta-cell secretory defect is more relevant as etiological factor rather than insulin resistance. Higher WC and trough tacrolimus level above 8.5 ng/mL may be important factors for predicting NODAT.

TABLE 1: Demographic, clinical, and biochemical characteristics of NODAT and non-NODAT patients

Characteristics	NODAT (n = 43)	Non-NODAT (n = 90)	P
Age (years)	37.4 ± 10.4	35.87 ± 9.1	0.381
Sex (male:female)	33.10	68:22	0.881
Pretransplant BMI (kg/m^2)	22.4 ± 2.8	20.3 ± 2.01	<0.001
Waist circumference (cm)	91.77 ± 7.47	82.58 ± 6.37	<0.001
Pretransplant FBS (mg/dL)	109 ± 18	85 ± 11.5	<0.001
Hypertension (%)	76.7	63.3	0.175
Family h/o diabetes mellitus (%)	27.9	18.9	0.239
Family h/o hypertension (%)	39.5	27.8	0.172
Smoking (%)	18.6	17.8	0.908
Alcoholism (%)	4.7	3.3	0.709
Total cholesterol (mg/dL)	244.8 ± 46	230 ± 34.1	0.04
Triglyceride (mg/dL)	209 ± 62.5	168.9 ± 32.8	<0.001
T_0 (ng/mL)	10.2 ± 2.28	5.37 ± 1.19	<0.001
HOMA IR C-peptide	1.02 ± 0.70	1.06 ± 0.80	0.817
HOMA-beta C-peptide	0.62 ± 0.89	1.29 ± 1.44	0.03

(BMI: body mass index; FBS: fasting blood sugar; NODAT: new-onset diabetes mellitus after transplantation)

Note: Comparison of mean was done by Student's unpaired t-test for continuous variables and comparison of proportions (expressed as percentage) was done by Chi-square test.

"If we knew what it was we were doing, it would not be called research, would it?"

—Albert Einstein

COMMENT

New-onset diabetes after transplantation is defined as development of diabetes for the first time after transplantation in previously nondiabetic transplant recipients. Prevalence of NODAT may vary from 2 to 53%. An Indian study showed prevalence of NODAT to be 26.7%.[22]

Immunosuppression with Tacrolimus (FK-506), mycophenolate mofetil and prednisolone may play a role as risk factors of NODAT. Higher trough levels of FK-506 during the first month, acute rejections, and higher body mass index (BMI) are the most obvious risk factors for development of post-transplant diabetes in a study done by Maes et al.[23]

In this study, diagnosis of NODAT was done by "International consensus guidelines of NODAT (2003)" by the criteria of the American Diabetes Association.

Early NODAT and late NODAT are defined as occurrence of NODAT less than 1 year and more than 1 year after renal transplantation, respectively.

In this study, among 43 patients with NODAT, 24 (55.8%) had early NODAT and the rest 19 patients (44.2%) had late NODAT. Moreover, among those having early NODAT, most of the patients 46.5% (20/24) developed NODAT within 6 months after renal transplantation.

Bonato et al. showed that overweight or obese patients were more prone to develop NODAT.

In this study, the mean pretransplant BMI was more in NODAT subjects compared with non-NODAT subjects. Waist circumference (WC), pretransplant total cholesterol, triglyceride, and FBS were other notable variables which were significantly worse in NODAT subjects. Among the several variables examined in this study, independent predictors of NODAT were WC (best cut-off in male was 87.5 cm and in female was 83.5 cm).

A study by Sinangil et al. also found pretransplant triglyceride as a risk factor of NODAT as was shown by Porrini et al. also.

In a study by Maes et al., high trough tacrolimus level more than 15 ng/mL in the first month after transplantation was also shown as an important risk factor for NODAT.

Most of the subjects in this study (67.4%) were managed by OAD (metformin, gliclazide, glimepiride, voglibose) whereas only 9.3% were treated solely by lifestyle modification. About 11.6% of subjects received insulin therapy and the rest 11.7% were treated by combined insulin and OAD. Almost all patients were maintaining HbA1c less than 7%.

Key Message

⊙ *New-onset diabetes after transplantation is considered to be a major determinant of loss of renal allograft, development of infections and increased morbidity and mortality. Higher pretransplant BMI, WC, pretransplant total cholesterol, triglyceride, FBS and trough tacrolimus level (above 8.5 ng/mL) appears to be important factors for predicting NODAT.*

ARTICLE 19

Vitamin D toxicity: a prospective study from a tertiary care centre in Kashmir valley

Misgar RA, Sahu D, Bhat MH, Wani AI, Bashir MI. Vitamin D toxicity: a prospective study from a tertiary care centre in Kashmir valley.
Indian J Endocr Metab. 2019;23:363-6.

Abstract

Background: Vitamin D toxicity (VDT), a "not uncommon" cause of hypercalcemia, can be life-threatening and cause substantial morbidity, if not treated promptly.

Aims: To describe presentation, management, and outcome in 32 patients with VDT diagnosed over 3 years.

Materials and methods: Patients presenting with VDT at a tertiary care center in Srinagar Kashmir India were included. Evaluation included detailed history and biochemical tests including serum calcium, phosphate, creatinine, intact parathyroid hormone (iPTH), 25-hydroxy Vitamin D (25-OHD), and 24-hour urinary calcium.

Results: The clinical manifestations of the 32 patients (median age 65; range 3–77 years) included gastrointestinal symptoms (constipation and vomiting), polyuria/polydipsia, altered sensorium, pancreatitis, acute kidney injury, and nephrocalcinosis. The median total serum calcium level was 13.95 (range 11.10–17.20) mg/dL and median 25-OHD level was 306 (range 105–2,800) ng/mL. All patients had suppressed or low normal iPTH and hypercalciuria and 78% had azotemia. All patients had received multiple intramuscular injections of vitamin D3. The median cumulative dose was 4,200,000 (range, 1,800,000–30,000,000) IU. The median time to resolution of hypercalcemia was 7 months (range 4–18 months).

Conclusion: We conclude that VDT is an increasingly common cause of symptomatic hypercalcemia. VDT needs prolonged follow-up as it takes months to abate its toxicity. Enhancing awareness among general practitioners regarding the toxicity resulting from high doses of vitamin D is the key to prevent VDT. We suggest that VDT be considered in patients, especially the elderly, presenting with polyuria, polydipsia, vomiting, azotemia, or encephalopathy.

"The art of clinical diagnosis lies in the ability to ask the right questions."
—**Harriet B. Braiker**

COMMENT

Vitamin D toxicity is an important cause of hypercalcemia in India. I feel that after ruling out hyperparathyroidism, one should look for hypervitaminosis D as the potential cause for increased calcium.

There is increased awareness about vitamin D deficiency in general public and doctors. Vitamin D is being used by people without prescription and by doctors in therapeutic doses just to treat symptoms presumably associated with hypovitaminosis D without monitoring vitamin D levels.

What is mechanism of hypercalcemia with vitamin D intoxication: 25 (OH) vitamin D acts directly on 1,25 (OH) vitamin D receptor and also 25 (OH) vitamin D displaces 1,25 (OH) vitamin D form its binding proteins, leading to increased concentration of active free calcitriol levels.

In this study from Kashmir they have taken 32 patients of vitamin D intoxication, presenting with hypercalcemia in the hospital. They have described clinical features, etiology, management and time taken for resolution of hypercalcemia in these patients.

It is almost always iatrogenic to have vitamin D toxicity. Patients are usually given vitamin D for nonspecific aches, fatigue, knee osteoarthritis and back pain. Dose of vitamin D given is always more than the recommended pharmacological dose.

What doses of vitamin D lead to intoxication: Usually patients have received intramuscular injections of vitamin D (300,000–600,000 IU) daily or weekly without monitoring of blood levels. According to literature, toxicity occurs if patient has received 50,000 IU/day for several weeks, whereas doses below 10,000 IU/day are not associated with toxicity.

How the patient is going to present: Gastrointestinal symptoms (nausea, vomiting, constipation), anorexia, fatigue, polyurea, dehydration and neurological symptoms (irritability, altered sensorium or coma). Hypercalcemia leads to nephrogenic diabetes insipidus, and hence polyuria and dehydration. Pancreatitis can occur rarely. Nephrocalcinosis is due to ectopic calcification.

How will you confirm the diagnosis: High serum calcium with normal or suppressed parathyroid levels. But serum 25 (OH) Vitamin D levels are always above 100 ng/mL. In this article mean vitamin D levels were 306 (105–2,800) ng/mL.

Treatment: First line of treatment is intravenous normal saline. After adequate hydration, loop diuretics can be given. Glucocorticoids have an important role in the management as it prevents the activation of 25 (OH) vitamin D by the kidneys. Additionally, you can use calcitonin and Zoledronic acid.

With this treatment, patient usually comes out of hypercalcemia crisis and can be discharged in 7–10 days. But next question is for how long patient needs to be treated on OPD basis. As vitamin D is fat soluble vitamin, it gets deposited in adipose tissue from where is gradually released. Average body half-life of vitamin D is 62 days. In this study, time of resolution varies from 4 to 18 months, with a median of 7 months. It is the first study which has documented time for resolution of high calcium in vitamin D toxicity. Furthermore, in older patients it took a longer time to resolve hypercalcemia.

With these measures, we can diagnose and treat hypervitaminosis D leading to hypercalcemia.

Key Messages

- ◉ *Vitamin D toxicity is important cause of hypercalcemia.*
- ◉ *It takes months (median time 7 months) for resolution of hypercalcemia caused by vitamin D toxicity.*

ARTICLE 20

Continuation of metformin till night before surgery and lactate levels in patients undergoing coronary artery bypass graft surgery

Bano T, Mishra SK, Kuchay MS, Mehta Y, Trehan N, Sharma P, et al. Continuation of metformin till night before surgery and lactate levels in patients undergoing coronary artery bypass graft surgery.
Indian J Endocr Metab. 2019;23:416-21.

Abstract

Background: Lactic acidosis is a rare but serious complication associated with metformin therapy in certain high-risk patients. NICE guidelines and the British National Formulary advise the discontinuation of metformin before surgery. The drug manufacturer's datasheet advises the withdrawal of metformin 48 hour before surgery. However, the data regarding perioperative use of metformin is scarce.

Aims: To evaluate the effect of continuation of metformin till night before surgery on lactate levels in patients undergoing coronary artery bypass graft (CABG) surgery.

Materials and methods: In this prospective cohort study, 1,800 consecutive patients who underwent CABG between November 1st 2015 and October 31st 2016 were enrolled. Following exclusion criteria, a total of 790 subjects were included for final analysis. Three-hundred and eight seven (48.9%) patients with diabetes received metformin till night before surgery (Met group), 239 (30.3%) patients with diabetes were non-metformin users (Non-Met group), and 164 (20.8%) patients were having no diabetes (Non-Diab group) (**Fig. 1**). Lactate levels and arterial pH were measured using arterial blood gas machine. Postoperative morbidity outcome data were obtained by collecting clinical data, routine biochemistry, and chest imaging.

Results: The mean metformin dose was 1,124.6 mg/day (SD 509.3; range: 500–2,500 mg/day). Mean postoperative lactate levels were 1.91 ± 0.7 in Met group, 2.04 ± 0.79 in Non-Met group, and 2.07 ± 0.78 in Non-Diab group. Lactic acidosis occurred in 41 patients and there was no difference among the groups [Met group = 18 (4.7%); Non-Met group = 14 (5.9%)]. Among secondary outcome measures, acute renal failure occurred more frequently in diabetic patients [Met group = 46 (11.9%) and Non-Met group = 32 (13.4%)] as compared with non-diabetic patients. There were no differences with regard to pneumonia, length of ICU stay, and duration of ventilatory support among the three groups.

Conclusions: Continuation of metformin till night before surgery is not associated with significant changes in lactate levels in patients undergoing CABG.

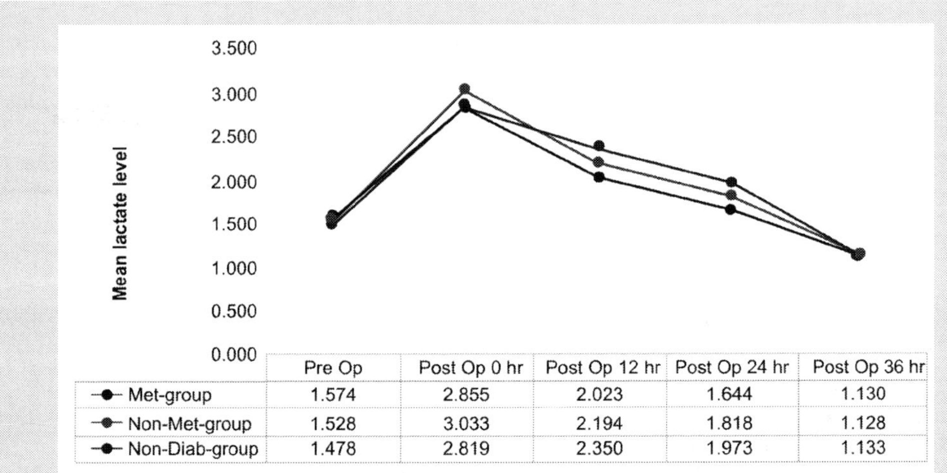

	Pre Op	Post Op 0 hr	Post Op 12 hr	Post Op 24 hr	Post Op 36 hr
Met-group	1.574	2.855	2.023	1.644	1.130
Non-Met-group	1.528	3.033	2.194	1.818	1.128
Non-Diab-group	1.478	2.819	2.350	1.973	1.133

FIG. 1: Changes in lactate levels (mmol/L) in the three groups. Met group, patients receiving metformin till night before surgery; non-Met group, patients who have diabetes but not receiving metformin; non-Diab group, patients who have no diabetes and underwent CABG surgery.

"To simplify complications is the first essential of success."

—George Earle Buckle

COMMENT

Metformin-associated lactic acidosis (MALA) is more likely in patients with underlying predisposing conditions, such as renal impairment, hepatic disease, congestive heart failure, or severe sepsis. NICE guidelines and the British National Formulary advise the discontinuation of metformin before surgery.

The current large study demonstrated that continuation of metformin till night before CABG surgery in patients with type 2 diabetes was not associated with increase in blood lactate levels or lactic acidosis. The study also revealed that there was rise in serum lactate levels in all the three groups postoperatively but was more common in patients without diabetes and non-metformin users.

In a systematic review by Salpeter et al., pooled data from 347 comparative trials (no cardiac surgery) compared the incidence of lactic acidosis in patients with diabetes using metformin versus those not using metformin. Similar to our study, a lower incidence of lactic acidosis was found in the metformin group (0.0043% vs. 0.0054%).[24]

In a retrospective study by Duncan et al., postoperative outcomes were compared between metformin users and nonusers. They evaluated 1,284 diabetic patients who had received metformin within 8–24 hours before cardiac surgery. There were no significant differences in overall mortality and immediate postoperative morbidity. There was no case of lactic acidosis during early postoperative period.

Manlapaz et al. analyzed the data of 4,528 diabetic patients who underwent cardiac surgical procedures. The patients received metformin within 8–24 hours before surgery. Mortality and morbidity were lower in these patients as compared with patients treated with other hypoglycemic agents. This suggests beneficial effect of metformin use.[25] In the study by Nazer et al., there were no differences in clinical outcomes between groups; and higher lactate levels in non-metformin users did not result in adverse postoperative outcome measures.

> ## Key Message
>
> ⊙ *This study does not support the guidance that metformin be discontinued 24–48 hours before a major surgery as metformin is not associated with significant changes in lactate levels or adverse immediate postoperative complications.*

REFERENCES (Diabetes and Metabolic Disorders)

1. Evans M, Kozlovski P, Paldánius PM, Foley JE, Bhosekar V, Serban C, et al. Factors that may account for cardiovascular risk reduction with a dipeptidylpeptidase-4 inhibitor, vildagliptin, in young patients with type 2 diabetes mellitus. Diabetes Ther. 2018;9:27-36.

2. Crowley MJ, Williams JW Jr, Kosinski AS, D'Alessio DA, Buse JB. Metformin use may moderate the effect of DPP-4 inhibitors on cardiovascular outcomes. Diabetes Care. 2017;40:1787-9.

3. Crowley MJ, Gokhale M, Pate V, Sturmer T, Buse JB. Impact of metformin use on the cardiovascular effects of the use of dipeptidyl peptidase-4 inhibitors: an analysis of Medicare claim data from 2007 to 2015. Diabetes Obes Metab. 2019;21:854-65.

4. Aroda VR, Ahmann A, Cariou B, Chow F, Davies MJ, Jódar E, et al. Comparative efficacy, safety, and cardiovascular outcomes with once-weekly subcutaneous semaglutide in the treatment of type 2 diabetes: Insights from the SUSTAIN 1-7 trials. Diabetes Metab. 2019;45:409-18.

5. Marso SP, Bain SC, Consoli A, Eliaschewitz FG, Jódar E, Leiter LA, et al. Semaglutide and cardiovascular outcomes in patients with type 2 diabetes. N Engl J Med. 2016;375:1834-44.

6. Davies M, Pieber TR, Hartoft-Nielsen ML, Hansen OKH, Jabbour S, Rosenstock J. Effect of oral semaglutide compared with placebo and subcutaneous semaglutide on glycemic control in patients with type 2 diabetes: a randomized clinical trial. JAMAN. 2017;318:1460-70.

7. Mazzone T. Intensive glucose lowering and cardiovascular disease prevention in diabetes: reconciling the recent clinical trial data. Circulation. 2010;122:2201-11.

8. Bianchi C, Miccoli R, Del Prato S. Hyperglycemia and vascular metabolic memory: truth or fiction? Curr Diab Rep. 2013;13:403-10.

9. Haneda M, Kadowaki T, Ito H, Sasaki K, Hiraide S, Ishii M, et al. Safety and efficacy of teneligliptin in patients with type 2 diabetes mellitus and impaired renal function: interim report from post-marketing surveillance. Diabetes Ther. 2018;9:1083.

10. Sudhakaran C, Kishore U, Anjana RM, Unnikrishnan R, Mohan V. Effectiveness of sitagliptin in Asian Indian patients with type 2 diabetes-an Indian tertiary diabetes care center experience. Diabetes Technol Ther 2011;13:27-32.

11. Sadikot S, Jothydev K, Zargar AH, Ahmad J, Arvind SR, Saboo B. Clinical practice points for diabetes management during RAMADAN fast. Diabetes Metab Syndr. 2017;11:S811-9.

12. Kalra S, Aamir AH, Raza A, Das AK, Azad Khan AK, Shrestha D, et al. Place of sulfonylureas in the management of type 2 diabetes mellitus in South Asia: a consensus statement. Indian J Endocrinol Metab. 2015;19:577-96.

13. Indian National Consensus Group. Premix insulin: initiation and continuation guidelines for management of diabetes in primary care. J Assoc Physicians India. 2009;57:42-6.

14. Das AK, Sahay BK, Seshiah V, Mohan V, Muruganathan A, Kumar A, et al. Indian National Consensus Group: National Guidelines on Initiation and Intensification of Insulin Therapy with Premixed Insulin Analogs. In: Medicine Update. Mumbai: API India; 2013. pp. 227-36.

15. Barone BB, Yeh HC, Snyder CF, Peair KS, Stein KB, Derr RL, et al. Long-term all-cause mortality in cancer patients with preexisting diabetes mellitus: a systematic review and meta-analysis. JAMA. 2008;300:2754-64.

16. Thakkar B, Aronis KN, Vamvini MT, Shields K, Mantzoros CS. Metformin and sulfonylureas in relation to cancer risk in type II diabetes patients: a meta-analysis using primary data of published studies. Metabolism. 2013;62:922-34.

17. Mamtani R, Haynes K, Wilker WB, Vaughn DJ, Strom BL, Glanz K, et al. Association between longer therapy with thiazolidinediones and risk of bladder cancer: a cohort study. J Natl Cancer Inst. 2012:1411-4.

18. Puckrin R, Saltiel MP, Reynier P, Azoulay L, Yu OHY, Filion KB. SGLT-2 inhibitors and the risk of infections: a systematic review and meta-analysis of randomized controlled trials. Acta Diabetol. 2018;55:503-14.

19. Zhanel GG, Nicolle LE, Harding GK, Manitoba Diabetic Urinary Infection Study Group. Prevalence of asymptomatic bacteriuria and associated host factors in women with diabetes mellitus. Clin Infect Dis. 1995;21:316-22.

20. Ronald A, Ludwig E. Urinary tract infections in adults with diabetes. Int J Antimicrob Agents. 2001;17:287-92.

21. Gadzhanova S, Pratt N, Roughead E. Use of SGLT2 inhibitors for diabetes and risk of infection: analysis using general practice records from the NPS MedicineWise MedicineInsight program. Diabetes Res Clin Pract. 2017;130:180-5.

22. Memon SS, Tandon N, Mahajan S, Bansal VK, Krishna A, Subbiah A. The prevalence of new onset diabetes mellitusafter renal transplantation in patients with immediate post transplantation with immediate hyperglycemia in a tertiary care centre. Indian J Endocr Metab. 2017;21:871-5.

23. Maes BD, Kuypers D, Messiaen T, Evenepoel P, Mathieu C, Coosemans W, et al. Post-transplantation diabetes mellitus in FK-506-treated renal transplant recipients: analysis of incidence and risk factors. Transplantation. 2001;72:1655-61.

24. Salpeter SR, Greyber E, Pasternak GA, Salpeter EE. Risk of fatal and nonfatal lactic acidosis with metformin use in type 2 diabetes mellitus. Cochrane Database Syst Rev. 2010;CD002967.

25. Manlapaz MR, Duncan AI, Koch CG, Xu M, Starr NJ. Diabetic patients treated with metformin have decreased pulmonary morbidity following cardiac surgery. Anesthesiology. 2005;103:A32.

Section Editor: Ajay Kumar

Associate Editors: Sandeep Lakhtakia, Manav Wadhawan, Vineet Ahuja

ARTICLE 1

Endoscopic ultrasound-guided transmural approach versus ERCP-guided transpapillary approach for primary decompression of malignant biliary obstruction: a meta-analysis

Bishay K, Boyne D, Yaghoobi M, Khashab MA, Shorr R, Ichkhanian Y, et al. Endoscopic ultrasound-guided transmural approach versus ERCP-guided transpapillary approach for primary decompression of malignant biliary obstruction: a meta-analysis. *Endoscopy. 2019;51:950-60.*

Abstract*

Background: In the patients who have malignant biliary obstruction, primary decompression can be achieved through endoscopic retrograde cholangiopancreatography (ERCP) along with transpapillary stenting or, recently, through transmural endoscopic ultrasound-guided biliary drainage (EUS-BD). It is still not clear whether, in the primary setting, either approach is superior with respect to clinical success or adverse events.

Methods: This study included a comprehensive systematic electronic search for studies that compared EUS-BD and ERCP as the primary approach in terms of clinical success as well as any other outcome(s). By using Laird and DerSimonian random effects models, the pooled relative risks (RRs) and weighted mean differences were calculated as appropriate. Sensitivity analyses were also done.

Results: Out of total 776 studies, five studies enrolling total 396 patients were included. There was no significant difference in overall clinical between EUS-BD and ERCP [RR 0.98; 95% confidence interval (CI) 0.93–1.03]. Overall adverse events were comparable (RR 0.84; 95% CI 0.35–2.01), although results indicated an association between EUS-BD and decreased risk of pancreatitis (RR 0.22; 95% CI 0.05–1.02). EUS-BD and ERCP were similar with respect to the risk of stent occlusion or procedure time.

Conclusion: Findings of meta-analysis, which included a modest number of patients, showed that in the primary decompression of malignant biliary obstruction, there was no significant difference in the clinical success rates and occlusion rates between EUS-BD and ERCP. In such patients, EUS-BD may be a practical option to the ERCP-guided approach. More well-designed prospective studies that include greater numbers of patients are needed to more clearly define potential differences in adverse events as well as cost.
*Redrafted abstract

"Transmural or transpapillary biliary drainage? Not yet ready for prime time—need more data."

COMMENT

Endoscopic retrograde cholangiopancreatography (ERCP) is considered as standard of care for biliary drainage from benign as well as malignant biliary obstruction. However, ERCP failure remains an area of concern either due to failed cannulation or failure to access the papilla. Percutaneous biliary drainage or surgical bypass was the standard fallback option. However, endoscopic ultrasound (EUS) is increasingly being used for biliary access and drainage in such instances. Therapeutic EUS has gained momentum recently and is establishing itself into the mainstream practice.

In this meta-analysis, ERCP and EUS were compared in patients with malignant biliary obstruction for biliary drainage. The analysis of five studies including 396 patients, EUS or ERCP biliary drainage was comparable. There was no difference in technical or clinical success, duration of stent patency, and overall adverse events. There was trend toward increased post-ERCP pancreatitis with transpapillary approach when compared with EUS biliary drainage (EUS-BD). Stent occlusion rates were higher with EUS-BD compared to ERCP. EUS-BD approach is a recent endoscopic intervention and decision to use is based upon operator expertise and availability of dedicated equipment or accessories.

The EUS-BD is comparable to ERCP for safety and efficacy in expert hands (all the studies analyzed here were from single and high-volume centers). Also, there was heterogeneity in types of stents used. However, cost-effective analyses and multicenter studies should be performed to determine optimal primary approach.

Key Message

⊙ *Primary EUS-guided biliary drainage is an emerging option for biliary decompression of malignant biliary obstruction with similar safety and efficacy. It needs to be evaluated in multicenter randomized trials in future.*

ARTICLE 2

Non-superiority of lumen-apposing metal stents over plastic stents for drainage of walled-off necrosis in a randomised trial

Bang JY, Navaneethan U, Hasan MK, Sutton B, Hawes R, Varadarajulu S. Non-superiority of lumen-apposing metal stents over plastic stents for drainage of walled-off necrosis in a randomised trial.
Gut. 2019;68:1200-9.

Abstract*

Objective: There is an increase in the use of lumen-apposing metal stents (LAMS) walled-off necrosis (WON) drainage; however, their advantage above plastic stents is still not clear. This study aimed to compare the efficacy of LAMS and plastic stents for drainage of WON.

Design: Randomization of patients with WON was done to endoscopic ultrasound-guided drainage by using plastic stents or LAMS. Primary outcome in the study was to compare total number of procedures for achieving treatment success, which was defined as relief in symptom in combination with resolution of WON on computed tomography (CT) at 6 months. The secondary outcomes included duration of procedure, treatment success, clinical or stent-related adverse events, length of hospital stay (LOS) and costs, and readmissions.

Results: Out of total 60 patients, 31 underwent LAMS and 29 patients plastic stent placement. No significant difference was observed between cohorts in terms of total number of procedures performed [median 2 (range 2–7) LAMS vs. 3 (range 2–7) plastic, p = 0.192], clinical adverse events, treatment success, readmissions, LOS, and overall treatment costs. In patients in LAMS group, duration of procedure was shorter (15 vs. 40 min, p < 0.001), and stent-related adverse events (32.3% vs. 6.9%, p = 0.01) and procedure costs (US $12,155 vs. US $6609, p < 0.001) were higher. In LAMS cohort, significant stent-related adverse events were noted 3 weeks or more postintervention. Interim audit led to protocol amendment where CT scan was performed at 3 weeks postintervention followed by removal of LAMS, if WON resolved. No significant difference was observed in adverse events between cohorts after protocol amendment.

Conclusion: No significant difference was found between LAMS and plastic stents in treatment outcomes; only procedure duration was shorter with LAMS. For minimizing adverse events associated with LAMS, follow-up imaging and stent removal should be performed in patients at 3 weeks, if WON has resolved. *Redrafted abstract

"Walled off necrosis drainage: LAMS versus plastic stent—What is primary aim?"

COMMENT

For drainage of walled off necrosis (WON), lumen-opposing metal stents (LAMS) are increasingly being used. However, there are limited studies that compare efficacy of LAMS versus plastic stents for endoscopic ultrasound (EUS)-guided drainage of WON. In this randomized controlled trial (RCT), the total number of procedures to achieve "treatment success" defined as symptom relief with WON resolution at 6 months was compared.

Total 60 patients of WON were randomized to EUS-guided drainage using either LAMS (31) or plastic stent (29). There was no significant difference between two groups in the median total number of interventions/procedures performed [LAMS 2 (range 2–7), plastic stent 3 (median 2–7)], treatment success, clinical adverse events, and readmission rates. LAMS had shorter procedure duration, more stent-related adverse events, and procedure costs. There were more stent-related adverse events in LAMS group, if kept in place for >3 weeks.

However, in LAMS cohort 8 of 31 (25.8%) patients and in plastic stent cohort 16 of 29 (55.2%), patients required additional intervention within 72 hours of drainage due to suboptimal treatment response. This finding indicates that approximately 75% of LAMS group (compared to 45% in plastic stent) improve with single procedure drainage procedure. This is similar to Lakhtakia et al. study (GI Endoscopy, 2017) that showed efficacy of endoscopic ultrasound guided of WON using step-up approach. Adverse events related to prolonged duration of metal stent can be mitigated by its removal early, preferably within 3 or 4 weeks. (Vinay Dhir, et al. Endoscopy)

We suggest use of LAMS in majority patients and plastic stent in patients with small WONs with <30% debris in whom reinterventions may not be required.

Key Message

⊛ *In majority of patients with walled-off pancreatic necrosis (WON), LAMS achieve clinical improvement with fewer number of reinterventions. After WON resolution, early endoscopic removal of LAMS reduces adverse events related to it.*

ARTICLE 3

Superiority of step-up approach vs open necrosectomy in long-term follow-up of patients with necrotizing pancreatitis

Hollemans RA, Bakker OJ, Boermeester MA, Bollen TL, Bosscha K, Bruno MJ, et al. Superiority of step-up approach vs open necrosectomy in long-term follow-up of patients with necrotizing pancreatitis.
Gastroenterology. 2019;156:1016-26.

Abstract

Background and aims: In a 2010 randomized trial (the PANTER trial), a surgical step-up approach for infected necrotizing pancreatitis was found to reduce the composite endpoint of death or major complications compared with open necrosectomy; 35% of patients were successfully treated with simple catheter drainage only. There is concern, however, that minimally invasive treatment increases the need for reinterventions for residual peripancreatic necrotic collections and other complications during the long term. We, therefore, performed a long-term follow-up study.

Methods: We re-evaluated all the 73 patients (of the 88 patients randomly assigned to groups) who were still alive after the index admission, at a mean 86 months (±11 months) of follow-up. We collected data on all clinical and healthcare resource utilization endpoints through this follow-up period. The primary endpoint was death or major complications (the same as for the PANTER trial). We also measured exocrine insufficiency, quality of life (using the Short Form-36 and EuroQol 5 dimensions forms), and Izbicki pain scores.

Results: From index admission to long-term follow-up, 19 patients (44%) died or had major complications in the step-up group compared with 33 patients (73%) in the open-necrosectomy group (p = 0.005). Significantly lower proportions of patients in the step-up group had incisional hernias (23% vs. 53%; p = 0.004), pancreatic exocrine insufficiency (29% vs. 56%; p = 0.03), or endocrine insufficiency (40% vs. 64%; p = 0.05). There were no significant differences between groups in proportions of patients requiring additional drainage procedures (11% vs. 13%; p = 0.99) or pancreatic surgery (11% vs. 5%; p = 0.43), or in recurrent acute pancreatitis, chronic pancreatitis, Izbicki pain scores, or medical costs. Quality of life increased during follow-up without a significant difference between groups.

Conclusion: In an analysis of long-term outcomes of trial participants, we found the step-up approach for necrotizing pancreatitis to be superior to open necrosectomy, without increased risk of reinterventions.

"Infected pancreatic necrosis—team-work counts."

COMMENT

The 2010 randomized PANTER trial in (infected) necrotizing pancreatitis found a minimally invasive step-up approach to be superior to primary open necrosectomy for the primary combined endpoint of mortality and major complications. Surgery could be avoided in up to one-third of patients by using step-up approach. But, long-term results are unknown. There was always a concern that minimal invasive approach will increase the rate of reinterventions. This study is a post-hoc analyses of PANTER trial at mean 86 months of follow-up analyzed death or major complication as primary endpoint. This study also evaluated exocrine insufficiency, quality of life, and pain.

With extended follow-up, the primary endpoint was reached in 19 (44%) in step-up group and 33 (73%) in open necrosectomy—a significant difference. Also, in the minimally invasive step-up group, patients had fewer incisional hernias, less exocrine insufficiency, and a trend toward less endocrine insufficiency. There were no significant differences between two groups for recurrent or chronic pancreatitis, pancreatic endoscopic or surgical interventions, quality of life, or costs.

Follow-up to the PANTER trial, there was TENSION trial looking at step-up endoscopic approach versus step-up surgical approach and found no major difference in complications or death. Thus, in infected pancreatic necrosis patients requiring intervention, step-up approach starting either with endoscopic drainage or percutaneous drainage should be considered. Further surgical intervention should be considered depending on local expertise and location of collections. In patients with collections unsuitable for endoscopic drainage, percutaneous approach should be preferred, with surgical options whenever required. As infected pancreatic necrosis is a heterogeneous condition, a single rigid protocol cannot be followed everywhere. The minimally invasive approaches result in better long-term outcomes. A careful consideration by multidisciplinary team should improve outcomes. Considering both the short- and long-term results, the step-up approach is superior to open necrosectomy for the treatment of infected necrotizing pancreatitis.

Key Message

- *Infected necrotizing pancreatitis is heterogeneous disease that requires a personalized approach for management as a standard of care. A multidisciplinary team comprising of gastroenterologist, surgeon, intervention radiologist, and critical care physician should discuss and together decide the management of the individual.*

ARTICLE 4

Meta-analysis of randomized clinical trials of early versus delayed cholecystectomy for mild gallstone pancreatitis

Moody N, Adiamah A, Yanni F, Gomez D. Meta-analysis of randomized clinical trials of early versus delayed cholecystectomy for mild gallstone pancreatitis.
Br J Surg. 2019;106:1442-51.

Abstract

Background: Gallstones account for 30–50% of all presentations of acute pancreatitis. While the management of acute pancreatitis is usually supportive, definitive treatment of gallstone pancreatitis is cholecystectomy. Guidelines from the British Society of Gastroenterology suggest definitive treatment on index admission or within 2 weeks of discharge; whereas, joint recommendations from the International Association of Pancreatology and the American Pancreatic Association recommend definitive treatment on index admission. Evidence suggests that uptake of these guidelines is low.

Methods: Embase, MEDLINE, and Cochrane databases were searched for randomized controlled trials (RCTs) investigating early versus delayed cholecystectomy in patients with a confirmed diagnosis of mild gallstone pancreatitis. The pooled synthesis was undertaken using a random effect meta-analysis of the primary outcome of recurrent biliary complications causing hospital readmission. Secondary outcomes included intraoperative and postoperative complications, and total length of hospital stay (LOS). All analyses were performed using RevMan5 software.

Results: Five RCTs were identified, which included 629 patients [318 in the early cholecystectomy (EC) group and 311 in the delayed cholecystectomy (DC) group]. Recurrent biliary events that required readmission were reduced in patients undergoing EC compared with the number in patients having DC [odds ratio (OR) 0.17; 95% CI 0.09–0.33]. There was no difference in the rate of intraoperative (OR 0.58, 0.17–1.92) or postoperative (OR 0.78, 0.38–1.62) complications.

Conclusion: EC following mild gallstone pancreatitis does not increase the risk of intraoperative or postoperative complications, but reduces the readmission rate for recurrent biliary complications.

"Cholecystectomy for mild gallstone pancreatitis: Just do it now!"

COMMENT

Gallstones account for 30–50% of acute pancreatitis. For patients developing acute pancreatitis due to gallstones, cholecystectomy is a definitive treatment. There has been a debate on early (during index hospital admission) or delayed as an elective procedure. Issues that matter are increased incidence of recurrent pancreatitis in delayed group versus difficult dissection due to inflammation, and more conversions to open group or infection of the pancreatic necrosis in early group. In presence of difference of opinion among various scientific societies (BSG, IAP, and APA), this meta-analysis provides valuable information. Also, in spite of guidelines, in practice, most of the centers do not seem to be following these guidelines and there is a trend toward delaying surgery thereby increasing the risk of readmissions due to recurrent pancreatitis.

This meta-analysis of five randomized controlled trials (RCTs) with 629 patients found that recurrent biliary events requiring readmission were reduced in patients undergoing early cholecystectomy with no difference in rate of intraoperative or postoperative complications. Also, there was no significant difference in the rate of conversion to the open cholecystectomy. There is significant increase in recurrent biliary events not requiring admission in delayed cholecystectomy group.

Though there is some heterogeneity in the various studies, this meta-analysis reinforces that early cholecystectomy, preferably during index hospital admission, is safe and effective approach in patients with mild gallstone pancreatitis.

Key Message

⊙ *Patients with mild gallstone pancreatitis should undergo cholecystectomy in the same admission to reduce re-admissions or further complications.*

ARTICLE 5

Laparoscopic versus open pancreatoduodenectomy for pancreatic or periampullary tumours (LEOPARD-2): a multicentre, patient-blinded, randomised controlled phase 2/3 trial

van Hilst J, de Rooij T, Bosscha K, Brinkman DJ, van Dieren S, Dijkgraaf MG, et al. Laparoscopic versus open pancreatoduodenectomy for pancreatic or periampullary tumours (LEOPARD-2): a multicentre, patient-blinded, randomised controlled phase 2/3 trial.
Lancet Gastroenterol Hepatol. 2019;4:199-207.

Abstract

Background: Laparoscopic pancreatoduodenectomy may improve postoperative recovery compared with open pancreatoduodenectomy. However, there are concerns that the extensive learning curve of this complex procedure could increase the risk of complications. We aimed to assess whether laparoscopic pancreatoduodenectomy could reduce time to functional recovery compared with open pancreatoduodenectomy.

Methods: This multicenter, patient-blinded, parallel-group, randomized controlled phase 2/3 trial was performed in four centers in the Netherlands that each do 20 or more pancreatoduodenectomies annually; surgeons had to have completed a dedicated training program for laparoscopic pancreatoduodenectomy and have done 20 or more laparoscopic pancreatoduodenectomies before trial participation. Patients with a benign, premalignant, or malignant indication for pancreatoduodenectomy, without signs of vascular involvement, were randomly assigned (1:1) to undergo either laparoscopic or open pancreatoduodenectomy using a central web-based system. Randomization was stratified for annual case volume and preoperative estimated risk of pancreatic fistula. Patients were blinded to treatment allocation. Analysis was done according to the intention-to-treat principle. The main objective of the phase 2 part of the trial was to assess the safety of laparoscopic pancreatoduodenectomy (complications and mortality), and the primary outcome of phase 3 was time to functional recovery in days, defined as all of the following: Adequate pain control with only oral analgesia, independent mobility, ability to maintain >50% of the daily required caloric intake, no need for intravenous fluid administration, and no signs of infection (temperature <38.5°C). This trial is registered with Trialregister.nl, number NTR5689.

Findings: Between May 13 and December 20, 2016, 42 patients were randomized in the phase 2 part of the trial. Two patients did not receive surgery and were excluded from analyses in accordance with the study protocol. Three (15%) of 20 patients died within 90 days after laparoscopic pancreatoduodenectomy, compared with none of 20 patients after open pancreatoduodenectomy. Based on safety data from the phase 2 part of the trial, the data and safety monitoring board and protocol committee agreed to proceed with phase 3. Between January 31 and November 14, 2017, 63 additional patients were randomized in phase 3 of the trial. Four patients did not receive surgery and were excluded from analyses in accordance with the study protocol. After randomization of 105 patients (combining patients from both phase 2 and phase 3), of whom 99 underwent surgery, the trial was prematurely terminated by the data and safety monitoring board because of a difference in 90-day complication-related mortality [five (10%) of 50 patients in the laparoscopic pancreatoduodenectomy group vs. one (2%) of 49 in the open pancreatoduodenectomy group; risk ratio (RR) 4.90; (95% CI 0.59–40.44); p = 0.20]. Median time to functional recovery was 10 days (95% CI 5–15) after laparoscopic pancreatoduodenectomy versus 8 days (95% CI 7–9) after open pancreatoduodenectomy (log-rank p = 0.80). Clavien–Dindo grade III or higher complications [25 (50%) of 50 patients after laparoscopic pancreatoduodenectomy vs. 19 (39%) of 49 after open pancreatoduodenectomy; RR 1.29 (95% CI 0.82–2.02); p = 0.26] and grade B/C postoperative pancreatic fistulas [14 (28%) vs. 12 (24%); RR 1.14 (95% CI 0.59–2.22); p = 0.69] were comparable between groups.

Interpretation: Although not statistically significant, laparoscopic pancreatoduodenectomy was associated with more complication-related deaths than was open pancreatoduodenectomy, and there was no difference between groups in time to functional recovery. These safety concerns were unexpected and worrisome, especially in the setting of trained surgeons working in centers performing 20 or more pancreatoduodenectomies annually. Experience, learning curve, and annual volume might have influenced the outcomes; future research should focus on these issues.

"Major surgeries—making a way for laparoscopy."

COMMENT

The previous two randomized controlled trials (RCTs) (PLOT and PADULET) comparing laparoscopic and open pancreatoduodenectomy (Whipple's surgery) showed that laparoscopic pancreatoduodenectomy can reduce postoperative recovery time, though there is concern for increased complications due to steep learning curve. PADULOP trial also showed decrease in postoperative complications.

This phase 2/3 RCT (LEOPARD-2) trial is the first and largest multicenter, patient-blinded trial in setting of experienced surgeons. In phase 2, safety (complications and mortality) of laparoscopic approach was studied. In phase 3, time to functional recovery in days was studied.

In phase 2, there was 15% (3/20) mortality in laparoscopic arm compared to none (0/20) in open arm. Phase 3 trial was prematurely terminated because 90-day complication-related mortality 10% (5/50) in laparoscopic arm compared to 2% (1/50) in open arm, higher severe complication in laparoscopic arm (50% vs. 39%), and comparable grade 2/3 postoperative pancreatic fistula and recovery time.

As there were worrisome safety concerns in laparoscopic pancreatoduodenectomy arm, the trial was terminated prematurely, even though difference was nonsignificant statistically. In spite of including experienced surgeons, higher mortality in laparoscopic arm appeared to be related to "relative inexperience" associated with intraoperative vascular injury and post-operative morbidity. This study included surgeons who had performed 20 laparoscopic pancreatoduodenectomy before participating, which may not be adequate to overcome learning curve. A meta-analysis comparing laparoscopic and open pancreatoduodenectomy (six studies; 282 laparoscopic and 982 open) showed that two groups were similar in number of lymph nodes and R0 resection, time of start of adjuvant chemotherapy after surgery and similar survival rate up to 2 years. Interestingly, the survival rates were higher in laparoscopic group at 3–5 years.

In short, laparoscopic pancreatoduodenectomy does not reduce the time to patient recovery in hands of surgeons having experience of 20 surgeries annually. Experience (learning curve) and annual volume may influence the results of this trial. This needs more evaluation in future studies.

Key Message

⊙ *Not all surgeons are same. A steep learning curve needs to be overcome before adopting laparoscopic pancreatoduodenectomy in standard practice for Whipple's procedure. Till then, open pancreato-duodenectomy is as good.*

ARTICLE 6

Prognostic role of ammonia in patients with cirrhosis

Shalimar, Sheikh MF, Mookerjee RP, Agarwal B, Acharya SK, Jalan R. Prognostic role of ammonia in patients with cirrhosis. *Hepatology. 2019;70:982-94.*

Abstract

Ammonia is thought to be central to the pathogenesis of hepatic encephalopathy (HE), but its prognostic role in patients with cirrhosis and acute decompensation is unknown. The aims of this study were to determine the relationship between ammonia levels and severity of HE and its association with organ dysfunction and short-term mortality. We identified 498 patients from two institutions as part of prospective observational studies in patients with cirrhosis. Plasma ammonia levels were measured on admission and Chronic Liver Failure-Sequential Organ Failure Assessment criteria were used to determine the presence of organ failures. The 28-day patient survival was determined. Receiver operating characteristic analysis was used to identify the cutoff points for ammonia values, and multivariable analysis was performed using the Cox proportional hazard regression model. The 28-day mortality was 43.4%. Plasma ammonia correlated with severity of HE ($p < 0.001$), was significantly higher in nonsurvivors [93 (73–121) vs. 67 (55–89) µmol/L; $p < 0.001$], and was an independent predictor of 28-day mortality (hazard ratio: 1.009; $p < 0.001$). An ammonia level of 79.5 µmol/L had sensitivity of 68.1% and specificity of 67.4% for predicting 28-day mortality. An ammonia level of ≥79.5 µmol/L was associated with a higher frequency of organ failures [liver ($p = 0.004$), coagulation ($p < 0.001$), kidney ($p = 0.004$), and respiratory ($p < 0.001$)]. Lack of improvement in baseline ammonia at day 5 was associated with high mortality (70.6%).

Conclusion: Ammonia level correlates with not only the severity of HE but also the failure of other organs and is an independent risk factor for mortality; lack of improvement in ammonia level is associated with high risk of death, making it an important biomarker and a therapeutic target.

"Ammonia levels revisited—should we measure in all cirrhotics?"

COMMENT

Ammonia is an important prognostic marker in patients with acute liver failure (ALF). Higher ammonia denotes higher incidence of cerebral edema and mortality in ALF. However, in cirrhosis, the role of ammonia measurements is poorly defined. We understand that patients with HE have high ammonia levels, normal ammonia levels virtually rule out hepatic cause of encephalopathy. On the other hand, patients without encephalopathy may have high serum ammonia levels. There is no data on correlation the level of ammonia with severity of liver disease in cirrhotic population. This paper from AIIMS, India gives us a long-awaited evidence in this regard.

This is a retroprospective study that analyzes three cohorts of patients (prospective cohorts from AIIMS, India and UCL, London and a retrospective cohort from UCL, London). A total of 498 patients of cirrhosis admitted in hospital with acute decompensation (AD) were included. All patients had arterial ammonia level measured at the time of admission. The authors found that ammonia levels correlated with the grade of HE. Levels were significantly higher in patients with

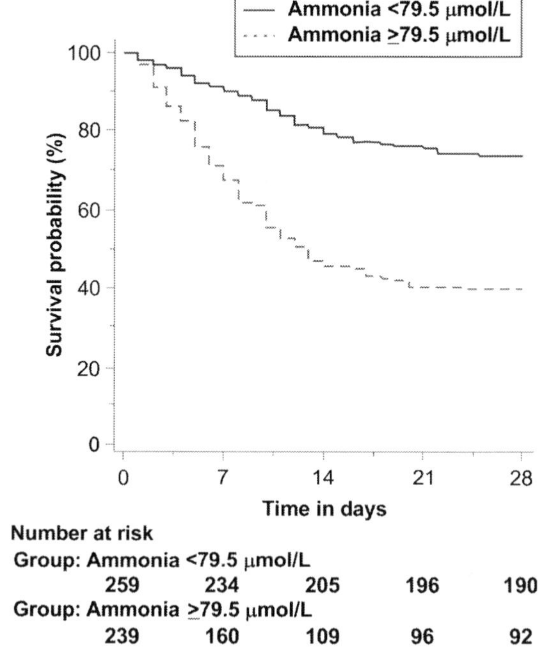

FIG. 1: Cumulative survival at 28 days in patients with ammonia above and below 79.5 µmol/L.

grade 3/4 HE (97 µmol/L) compared to grade 2 (77 µmol/L) and grade 0/1 HE (73 µmol/L). Also, they arrived at an arterial ammonia cut-off of 79.5 µmol/L to predict organ failures (coagulation, renal dysfunction, as well respiratory dysfunction). The proportion of patients with acute-on-chronic liver failure (ACLF) was also higher in the group with ammonia >79.5 compared to lower ammonia group (75.3% vs. 49.4%; p < 0.001). On a multivariate analysis, ammonia was independently predictive of mortality. Those with an ammonia level of ≥79.5 µmol/L had higher mortality compared to lower ammonia (61.5% vs. 26.6%; p < 0.001). Also, the authors reported that failure to lower ammonia at 5 days was associated with a poor survival at 28 days [70.6% vs. 35.7% mortality in those with an improvement in baseline ammonia (p = 0.007)].

This paper gives us an important message that high arterial ammonia (>79.5 µmol/L) in patients with cirrhosis admitted due to AD is predictive of complications and mortality. Ammonia-lowering therapies may help in reducing mortality in this group of patients over and above the improvement in HE (**Fig. 1**).

Key Messages

- *Ammonia levels have a prognostic significance in patients of cirrhosis admitted with acute decompensation.*
- *Measures to lower ammonia may be indicated in all admitted cirrhotics irrespective of the presence of hepatic encephalopathy.*

ARTICLE 7A

Daily aspirin use associated with reduced risk for fibrosis progression in patients with nonalcoholic fatty liver disease

Simon TG, Henson J, Osganian S, Masia R, Chan AT, Chung RT, et al. Daily aspirin use associated with reduced risk for fibrosis progression in patients with nonalcoholic fatty liver disease.
Clin Gastroenterol Hepatol. 2019;17:2776-84.e4.

Abstract

Background and aims: There are few data from prospective studies on the effects of aspirin on fibrosis in patients with nonalcoholic fatty liver disease (NAFLD).

Methods: We performed a prospective cohort study of 361 adults with biopsy-confirmed NAFLD; from 2006 through 2015, examined every 3–12 months for incident advanced fibrosis defined using serial measurements of validated indices (the Fibrosis-4, NAFLD fibrosis score, and aspartate aminotransferase to platelet ratio indices). Histological analyses of liver biopsies collected at baseline were performed by a blinded pathologist. Information collected at baseline and, at each examination, included frequency and duration of aspirin and nonsteroidal anti-inflammatory drug (NSAID) use. Using multivariable-adjusted logistic regression, we estimated the association of aspirin use with prevalent nonalcoholic steatohepatitis (NASH) and fibrosis. Using multivariable-adjusted Cox proportional hazards modeling, we estimated the association between aspirin use and risk for fibrosis progression.

Results: At enrollment, 151 subjects used aspirin daily. Compared with nonregular use, daily aspirin use was associated with significantly lower odds of NASH [adjusted odds ratio (OR) 0.68; 95% confidence interval (CI) 0.37–0.89] and fibrosis (adjusted OR 0.54; 95% CI 0.31–0.82). Among individuals with baseline F0-2 fibrosis (n = 317), 86 developed advanced fibrosis over 3,692 person-years. Daily aspirin users had significantly lower risk for developing incident advanced fibrosis versus nonregular users [adjusted hazard ratio (aHR) 0.63; 95% CI 0.43–0.85]. This relationship appeared to be duration dependent (adjusted p trend = 0.026), with the greatest benefit found with at least 4 years or more of aspirin use (aHR 0.50; 95% CI 0.35–0.73). Conversely, use of nonaspirin NSAIDs was not associated with risk for advanced fibrosis (aHR 0.93; 95% CI 0.81–1.05).

Conclusion: In a prospective study of patients with biopsy-proven NAFLD, daily aspirin use was associated with less severe histologic features of NAFLD and NASH, and lower risk for progression to advanced fibrosis with time.

ARTICLE 7B

Association of daily aspirin therapy with risk of hepatocellular carcinoma in patients with chronic hepatitis B

Lee TY, Hsu YC, Tseng HC, Yu SH, Lin JT, Wu MS, et al. Association of daily aspirin therapy with risk of hepatocellular carcinoma in patients with chronic hepatitis B.
JAMA Intern Med. 2019;179:633-40.

Abstract*

Background and objective: In patients with chronic hepatitis B, risk of hepatocellular carcinoma (HCC) cannot be erased by the antiviral therapy; it is not indicated for most of the carriers of hepatitis B virus (HBV). There is a need to develop an effective way to decrease HCC risk. Use of aspirin may prevent development of cancer; however, clinical evidence in patients having HBV-related HCC is still limited. This study aimed to evaluate the association of daily aspirin therapy with HBV-related HCC risk.

Material and methods: This was a Taiwan nationwide cohort study in which total 204,507 patients were screened for chronic hepatitis B for the duration from January 1, 1997 to December 31, 2012. After exclusion of patients who had confounding conditions, total 2,123 patients who continuously received daily aspirin for ≥90 days (i.e., treated group) were randomly matched 1:4 with 8,492 patients who never received antiplatelet therapy (i.e., untreated group) through propensity scores, comprising baseline characteristics, follow-up index date, and use of potentially chemopreventive drug during follow-up. From August 1 to November 30, 2018, analysis of data was done. During the study period, patients were given daily aspirin therapy. Cumulative incidence of and hazard ratios (HRs) for development of HCC were assessed after adjusting patient mortality as a competing risk event.

Results: Out of total 10,615 patients, 72.4% (n = 7,690) were males; mean (±SD) age of the patients was 58.8 (±11.8) years. In 5 years, the cumulative incidence of HCC in the treated group was found to be significantly lower as compared to that of untreated group [5.20%; 95% confidence interval (CI) 4.11–6.29% vs. 7.87%; 95% CI 7.15–8.60%; p < 0.001]. Multivariable regression analysis showed aspirin therapy to be independently associated with a decreased HCC risk (HR 0.71; 95% CI 0.58–0.86; p < 0.001). This association was also verified by the sensitivity subgroup analyses (all HRs <1.0). Also, old age (HR 1.01 per year; 95% CI 1.00–1.02); male sex (HR 1.75; 95% CI 1.43–2.14), and cirrhosis (HR 2.89; 95% CI 2.45–3.40) were found to be independently associated with an enhanced HCC risk; however, nucleos(t)ide analog (HR 0.54; 95% CI 0.41–0.71) or statin (HR 0.62; 95% CI 0.42–0.90) use was observed to be correlated with a reduced HCC risk.

Conclusion: Use of daily aspirin therapy may be associated with a decreased risk of HBV-related HCC.
*Redrafted abstract

"Aspirin, a panacea for all your medical problems?"

COMMENT

Aspirin is the most commonly used anti-inflammatory drug in the world. Lately a lot of data has emerged on the efficacy of aspirin in reducing inflammatory markers in a variety of diseases. Also, evidence is emerging on the preventive effect of aspirin on the tumors that are related to chronic inflammation. These articles discuss the two diverse effects of aspirin in decreasing inflammation and hence fibrosis in nonalcoholic fatty liver disease (NAFLD) patients, and also reducing the risk of hepatocellular carcinoma (HCC) in chronic hepatitis B patients.

The first study explores the possible benefit of aspirin in reducing the risk of fibrosis in NAFLD patients. Around 361 patients with biopsy-proven NAFLD (with F0-2 fibrosis) were prospectively followed over 9 years and monitored 3–12 monthly for development of advanced fibrosis (F3-4). The use of aspirin was dictated by established indications (cardiovascular and others). Simply stated, aspirin was not used to look at prevention of fibrosis, but the patients already on aspirin were followed to observe for incident fibrosis. Development of fibrosis on follow-up was assessed by noninvasive indices [Fibrosis-4 (FIB-4), NAFLD fibrosis score, and aspartate aminotransferase to platelet ratio indices (APRI)]. These are simple scores that can be calculated using free apps available online/offline. Each one of these indices uses simple parameters detailed below, and picks up advanced fibrosis with a very high accuracy.

- *FIB-4*: Age, aspartate aminotransferase (AST), alanine aminotransferase (ALT), and platelet count
- *NAFLD fibrosis score*: Age, AST, ALT, platelet count, body mass index (BMI), albumin, and impaired glucose tolerance
- *APRI*: AST to platelet ratio.

Of 361 patients with NAFLD and F0-2 fibrosis, 151 were using aspirin daily. The biopsies at baseline were compared according to aspirin use.

Interestingly, daily aspirin use was associated with 36% lower odds of inflammation and 46% lower odds of fibrosis at baseline. Out of 361 patients included, 317 had F0-2 fibrosis at baseline; these were then followed up as described earlier. A total 86 patients (of 317) developed advanced fibrosis over 3,692 person-years. The risk of new onset advanced fibrosis was 37% lower in daily aspirin users compared to nonregular users. Also, longer the use of aspirin, higher the benefit. The greatest benefit was found with at least 4 years or more of aspirin use. The use of nonaspirin nonsteroidal anti-inflammatory drugs (NSAIDs) did not provide risk reduction in fibrosis.

The second study investigates, if aspirin can prevent HCC in chronic hepatitis B patients. It uses national database of chronic hepatitis B patients in Taiwan. More than 2 lakh hepatitis B patients were screened (between 1997 and 2012) and 2,123 patients with daily aspirin use were identified after all exclusions. These 2,123 patients were then randomly matched in 1:4 ratio with aspirin nonusers (n = 8,492). These patients were followed up till HCC diagnosis, death, or the end of the study period (up to December, 2012). At the end of follow-up, the incidence of HCC in daily aspirin users was significantly lower than in nonusers in 5 years (5.20% vs. 7.87%; p < 0.001). The authors also did a multivariate analysis to identify the predictors of HCC. While older age, male sex, and cirrhosis were associated with higher risk of HCC, use of nucleoside analogs or statins decreased the HCC risk. Daily aspirin therapy was an independent factor decreasing the HCC risk by 29% [hazard ratio (HR) 0.71; p < 0.001).

These two studies add more evidence to the emerging fact that aspirin use may decrease inflammation and fibrosis as well as cancers associated with inflammation in a variety of disorders (**Figs. 1** and **2**).

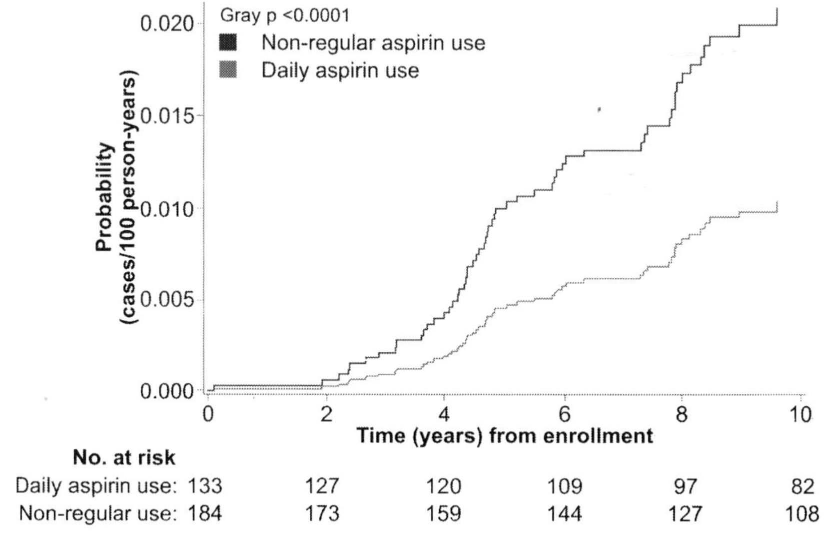

No. at risk

Daily aspirin use: 133	127	120	109	97	82
Non-regular use: 184	173	159	144	127	108

FIG. 1: Incidence of advanced fibrosis in aspirin users versus aspirin nonusers in patients with early stage nonalcoholic fatty liver disease (NAFLD) at baseline.

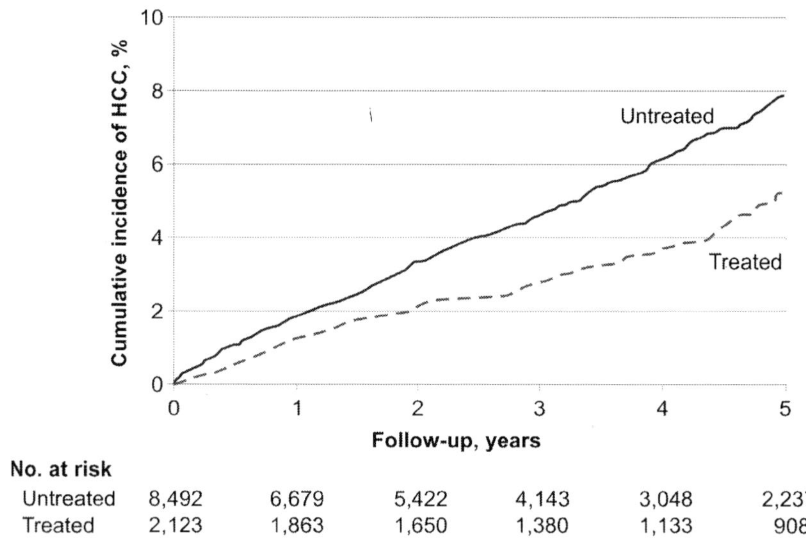

No. at risk

Untreated	8,492	6,679	5,422	4,143	3,048	2,237
Treated	2,123	1,863	1,650	1,380	1,133	908

Key Messages

- *Aspirin usage has been shown to decrease development of new onset fibrosis in NAFLD patients.*
- *Aspirin also has been associated with lower risk of incident HCC in chronic hepatitis B population.*
- *Important fact to understand is that association may or may not mean benefit. Prospective RCTs are needed before aspirin can be used primarily for these indications.*

ARTICLE 8

β blockers to prevent decompensation of cirrhosis in patients with clinically significant portal hypertension (PREDESCI): a randomised, double-blind, placebo-controlled, multicentre trial

Villanueva C, Albillos A, Genescà J, Garcia-Pagan JC, Calleja JL, Aracil C, et al. β blockers to prevent decompensation of cirrhosis in patients with clinically significant portal hypertension (PREDESCI): a randomised, double-blind, placebo-controlled, multicentre trial.
Lancet. 2019;393:1597-608.

Abstract

Background: Clinical decompensation of cirrhosis is associated with poor prognosis. Clinically significant portal hypertension (CSPH), defined by a hepatic venous pressure gradient (HVPG) ≥10 mm Hg, is the strongest predictor of decompensation. This study aimed at assessing whether lowering hepatic venous pressure gradient (HVPG) with β-blockers could decrease the risk of decompensation or death in compensated cirrhosis with CSPH.

Methods: This study on β-blockers to prevent decompensation of cirrhosis with portal hypertension (PREDESCI) was an investigator-initiated, double-blind, randomized controlled trial done in eight hospitals in Spain. We enrolled patients with compensated cirrhosis and CSPH without high-risk varices. All participants had HVPG measurements with assessment of acute HVPG-response to intravenous propranolol. Responders (HVPG-decrease ≥10%) were randomly assigned to propranolol (up to 160 mg twice a day) versus placebo and nonresponders to carvedilol (≤25 mg/day) versus placebo. Doses were individually determined during an open-label titration period after which randomization was done with 1:1 allocation by a centralized web-based system. The primary endpoint was incidence of cirrhosis decompensation (defined as development of ascites, bleeding, or overt encephalopathy) or death. Since death in compensated cirrhosis is usually unrelated to the liver, an intention-to-treat analysis considering deaths unrelated to the liver as competing events was done. This study is registered with ClinicalTrials.gov, number NCT01059396. The trial is now completed.

Findings: Between January 18, 2010 and July 31, 2013, 631 patients were evaluated and 201 were randomly assigned. Around 101 patients received placebo and 100 received active treatment (67 propranolol and 33 carvedilol). The primary endpoint occurred in 16 (16%) of 100 patients in the β-blockers group versus 27 (27%) of 101 in the placebo group [hazard ratio (HR) 0.51; 95% confidence interval (CI) 0.26–0.97; p = 0.041]. The difference was due to a reduced incidence of ascites (HR 0.44; 95% CI 0.20–0.97; p = 0.0297). The overall incidence of adverse events was similar in both groups. Six patients (four in the β-blockers group) had severe adverse events.

Interpretation: Long-term treatment with β-blockers could increase decompensation-free survival in patients with compensated cirrhosis and CSPH, mainly by reducing the incidence of ascites.

"Beta blockers—a uniform prescription for all patients with cirrhosis."

COMMENT

Beta-blockers are one of the most commonly prescribed drugs in cirrhosis. The role of β-blockers is well defined in patients with large high-risk varices. Their use in this group is recommended to prevent variceal bleeding and also prevents decompensation. However, in patients with low-risk varices, β-blockers are currently not recommended to prevent variceal bleeding. Conceptually speaking, the portal pressure is high in patients with varices (small or large, high risk or low risk). Portal pressure contributes to liver injury in cirrhosis. Hence, lowering portal pressure may ameliorate liver injury and prevent decompensation of liver disease. The proof to this concept is provided in this elegant randomized controlled trial (RCT) published from Spain.

This is a multicenter, double blind, RCT done to assess the role of β-blockers in altering natural history of cirrhotics. Patients with clinically significant portal hypertension [(CSPH), defined as hepatic venous pressure gradient (HVPG) ≥10 mm Hg] with low-risk varices were included in the trial. High-risk varices were excluded, as β-blockers are indicated in these patients anyway. All patients underwent HVPG measurement at recruitment, and response to IV propranolol was assessed. Those with HVPG ≥10 mm Hg were included, patients who decreased HVPG after propranolol were randomized to propranolol versus placebo, patients who had no decrease after propranolol were randomized to carvedilol versus placebo. The clinical endpoints were decompensation events (ascites, variceal bleeding, or encephalopathy) or death. A total of 631 patients were evaluated, 201 were randomized [101 patients in placebo arm and 100 to treatment arm (67 propranolol and 33 carvedilol)].

Decompensation or death occurred in 27 patients out of 101 in the placebo group and in 16 out of 100 in the β-blockers group. β-blockers decreased the risk of decompensation or death by 49% (HR 0.51; p = 0.041). The reduction in decompensation was primarily due to reduction in development of ascites (20 in placebo developed ascites compared to 9 in treatment arm). If endpoints were compared individually between treatment and placebo arm, the incidence of high-risk varices, encephalopathy, and death from any cause did not differ between the two groups (only ascites was different as described) (**Fig. 1**).

This is the first RCT addressing this important issue. This clearly changes our clinical practice, as β-blockers can now be recommended for all patients with cirrhosis and low-risk varices also.

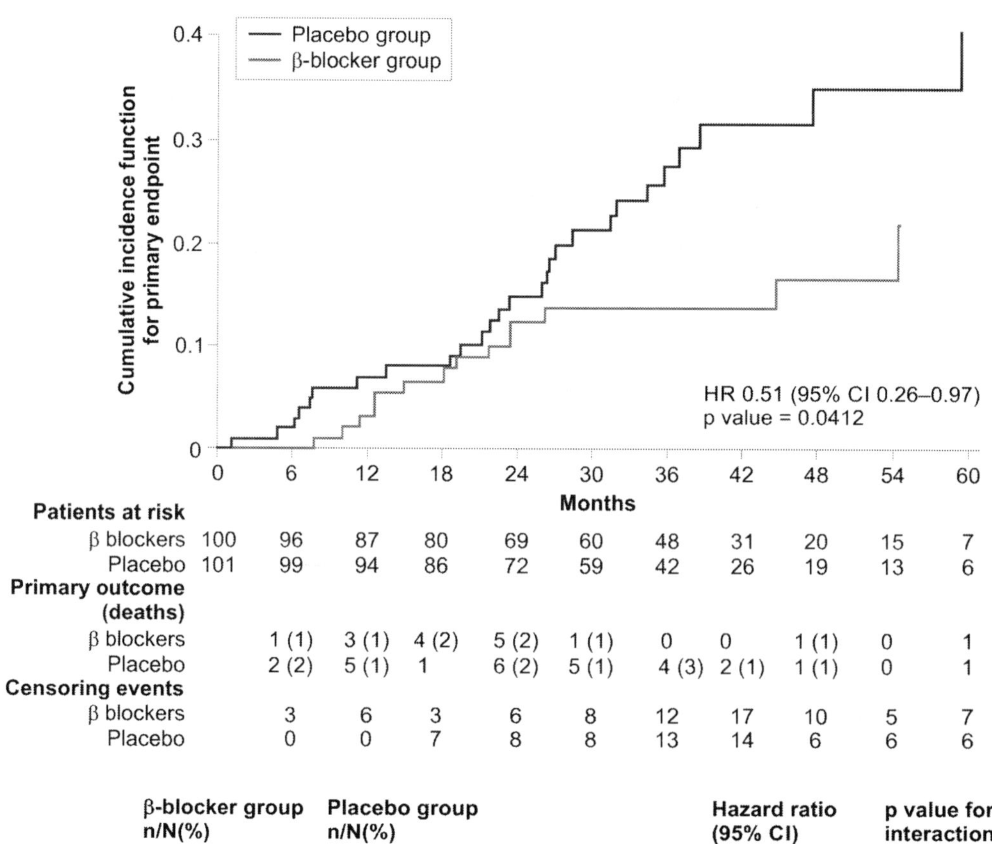

Patients at risk	0	6	12	18	24	30	36	42	48	54	60
β blockers	100	96	87	80	69	60	48	31	20	15	7
Placebo	101	99	94	86	72	59	42	26	19	13	6
Primary outcome (deaths)											
β blockers		1 (1)	3 (1)	4 (2)	5 (2)	1 (1)	0	0	1 (1)	0	1
Placebo		2 (2)	5 (1)	1	6 (2)	5 (1)	4 (3)	2 (1)	1 (1)	0	1
Censoring events											
β blockers		3	6	3	6	8	12	17	10	5	7
Placebo		0	0	7	8	8	13	14	6	6	6

β-blocker group n/N(%)	Placebo group n/N(%)	Hazard ratio (95% CI)	p value for interaction

FIG. 1: Incidence of decompensation or death in placebo versus β-blocker group.

Key Messages

- *Beta-blockers should be used in all patients of early cirrhosis, if portal pressures are high (documented by presence of varices, or low platelet counts or HVPG, if available).*
- *Even patients with low-risk varices may benefit from use of β-blockers.*

ARTICLE 9

Effects of intermittent fasting on health, aging, and disease

de Cabo R, Mattson MP. Effects of intermittent fasting on health, aging, and disease.
N Engl J Med. 2019;381:2541-51.

Abstract

In this review article, authors discuss the benefits of intermittent fasting on health. It is known that rodents do 20-hour fasting every day, which causes ketogenesis. The health benefits of intermittent fasting are not related to weight loss only. There is significant change in metabolism with free radical production. All the body organs during intermittent fasting respond so that better homeostasis is achieved. Periods of fasting cause ketogenesis. There is decreased insulin, decreased mammalian target of rapamycin (mTOR) and decreased protein synthesis. Along with, there is increased autophagy, mitochondrial stress resistance, and increased DNA repair. So, the cells become more competent to handle metabolic oxidative and ischemic stress. These changes cause long-term adaptations like increased insulin sensitivity, reduced inflammation, blood pressure, and abdominal fat.

Intermittent fasting can be done by any of the three regimens—daily fasting for 16 hours and food for 8 hours, alternate day fasting, or fasting for two days in a week. Intermittent fasting has health benefits in diabetes, cardiac diseases, obesity, cancer, and some neurological diseases. With the large amount of data, which is available, medical students should be taught intermittent fasting patterns and physicians should include these in their prescriptions. There are wide range health benefits of intermittent fasting since there is significant metabolic adaptation. There is depletion of liver glycogen and greater damage of free fatty acids in the fat tissues. Hence, intermittent fasting and caloric restriction improve stress resistance, lipid and glucose metabolism, autophagy, mitochondrial biogenesis, and consequently improved cell survival. This has significant generalized health benefits.

"Start the practice of self-control with penance, begin with fasting."
—**Bhagwan Mahavira**

COMMENT

Intermittent fasting (IF) has been propagated in India since ancient times. Our forefathers wrote in our scriptures that the last meal of the day should be before sunset and first meal after sunrise. Now, we have scientific evidence to support this claim. This article reviews all evidence in favor of intermittent fasting and chronicles, its effect on health and disease. The advantage of IF hinges on the concept of "Metabolic Switch". It means switching from glucose as an energy source to ketone bodies. Let us understand this in more detail.

Glucose and fatty acids are the main sources of energy in our body. After meals, glucose is used for energy, and fat is stored in adipose tissue as triglycerides (TGs). During periods of fasting, TGs are broken down to fatty acids and glycerol. The fatty acids travel to liver where they are converted to ketone bodies, which provide alternative source of energy during fasting. Ketone levels are low in blood after meals; they start rising within 8–12 hours of fasting. This is the metabolic switch from glucose to ketone bodies during periods of intermittent fasting.

In addition to providing fuel during fasting, ketone bodies act as potent signaling molecules with major effects on cell and organ functions. Ketone bodies regulate the expression and activity of many proteins and molecules that have beneficial effects on health and aging. These benefits include improvements in glucose regulation, blood pressure, and heart rate; the efficacy of endurance training and abdominal fat loss.

Intermittent fasting can be done in 3 ways (each of them have been shown to have similar benefits) (**Table 1**):

1. Daily time-restricted feeding (eating window of 8–10 hours, fasting for 14–16 hours)
2. Alternate day fasting (restricting calories to 500–700 kcal/day on fasting days)
3. 5:2 fasting (fasting 2 days every week)

This metabolic switch, when happens repeatedly (as in the case of IF daily, alternate day or twice a week), the individual body responds by favoring maintenance and repair systems, enhancing stress resistance, recycling damaged molecules, and promoting cell survival (**Flowchart 1**). All these changes lead to improvements in health and disease resistance.

The beneficial effects of IF have documented in human studies for the following conditions:

- Obesity and diabetes mellitus
- *Cardiovascular disease*: Improves blood pressure, resting heart rate, insulin sensitivity, high-density lipoprotein (HDL) and low-density lipoprotein (LDL) and TG levels.
- *Cancer*: Clinical trials of intermittent fasting in patients with cancer have been completed or are in progress. There is published data on patients with glioblastoma suggesting that intermittent fasting can suppress tumor growth.
- Asthma and arthritis
- Neurodegenerative disorders
- Surgical tissue injury

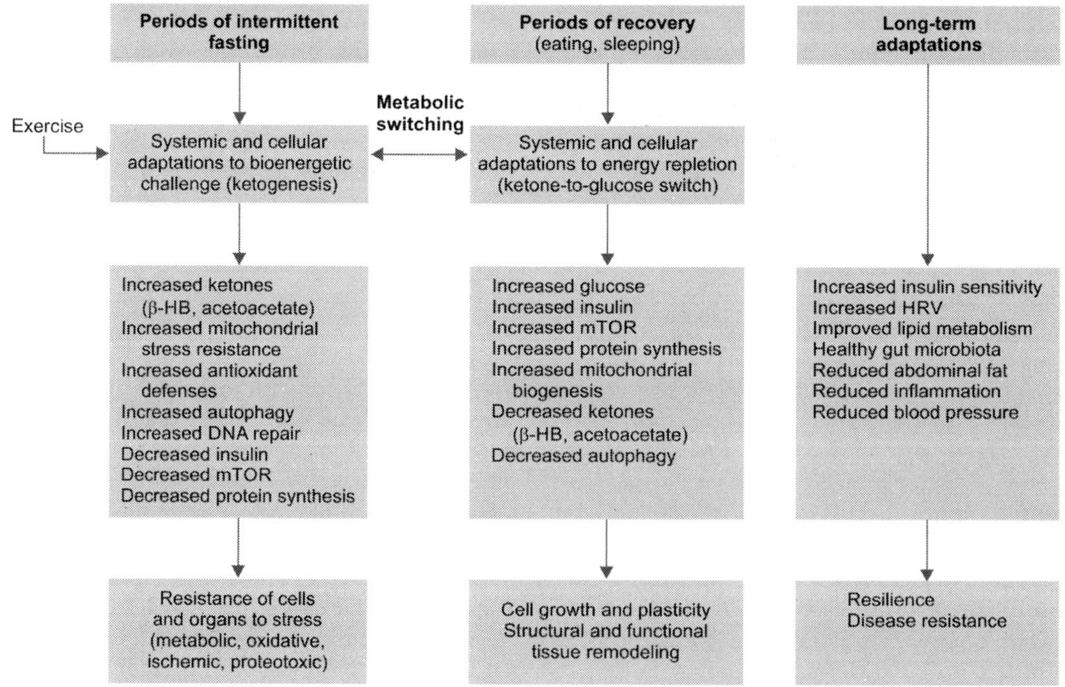

(MTOR: mammalian target of rapamycin)

FLOWCHART 1: Cellular and molecular mechanisms causing health improvement with intermittent metabolic switching.

TABLE 1: Methods to build-up intermittent fasting (IF) regimens.

Sample prescriptions			
Month	**Time-restricted feeding**	**5:2 intermittent fasting**	
Month 1	10-h feeding period 5 days/week	1,000 calories 1 day/week	Food log
Month 2	8-h feeding period 5 days/week	1,000 calories 2 days/week	Body weight
Month 3	6-h feeding period 5 days/week	750 calories 2 days/week	Glucose
Month 4 (goal)	6-h feeding period 7 days/week	500 calories 2 days/week	Ketones

Key Messages

- *Intermittent fasting (if done regularly) leads to multiple health benefits, improves various diseases, and may lead to longevity.*
- *Three regimens of intermittent fasting as described above are helpful in ameliorating many disease conditions.*

ARTICLE 10A

Drug-induced acute-on-chronic liver failure in Asian patients

Devarbhavi H, Choudhury AK, Sharma MK, Maiwall R, Mahtab MA, Rahman S, et al. Drug-induced acute-on-chronic liver failure in Asian Patients.
Am J Gastroenterol. 2019;114:929-37.

Abstract*

Objectives: Acute insults from viruses, infections, or alcohol are causes of decompensation resulting in the acute-on-chronic liver failure (ACLF). There is scarcity of information related to the drugs as triggers of ACLF. This study aimed at analyzing data related to drugs causing ACLF and evaluating clinical features, laboratory characteristics, outcome, as well as predictors of mortality among patients having drug-induced ACLF.

Methods: In the study, identification of drugs was done as precipitants of ACLF in prospective cohort of patients having ACLF from the Asian Pacific Association of Study of Liver (APASL) ACLF Research Consortium (AARC) database. Drugs were taken into consideration as precipitants following exclusion of known causes along with a temporal association between exposure and decompensation. The outcome of the study was death from decompensation.

Results: Among total 3,132 patients with ACLF, drugs were found to be the cause in 10.5% patients (n = 329, group A; mean age: 47 years; 65% men) and other non-drug causes in 89.5% patients [n = 2,803, (group B)]. The most common insults were complementary and alternative medications (in 71.7% patients) and combination antituberculosis therapy drugs in 27.3% patients. The common causes of underlying liver diseases included alcoholic liver disease in 28.6% patients, cryptogenic liver disease in 25.5%, and nonalcoholic steatohepatitis (NASH) in 16.7% patients. All the patients having drug-induced ACLF had jaundice (100%); ascites were present in 88% and encephalopathy in 46.5% patients. Drug-induced ACLF patients had high Model for End-stage Liver Disease (MELD) (30.2) and Child–Turcotte–Pugh score (12.1). As compared to the nondrug-induced ACLF, drug-induced ACLF had significantly higher overall 90-day mortality (46.5% vs. 38.8%; p = 0.007). The Cox regression model showed that arterial lactate (p < 0.001) and total bilirubin (p = 0.008) were the predictors of mortality.

Discussion: In Asia-Pacific countries, important identifiable causes of ACLF are drugs, mainly from complementary and alternative medications, followed by the anti tuberculosis drugs. In the case of drug-induced ACLF, bilirubin, encephalopathy, lactate, international normalized ratio (INR), and blood urea are predictors of mortality. *Redrafted abstract

ARTICLE 10B

Flare of autoimmune hepatitis causing acute-on-chronic liver failure: diagnosis and response to corticosteroid therapy

Anand L, Choudhury A, Bihari C, Sharma BC, Kumar M, Maiwall R, et al. Flare of autoimmune hepatitis causing acute-on-chronic liver failure: diagnosis and response to corticosteroid therapy.
Hepatology. 2019;70:587-96.

Abstract

Autoimmune hepatitis (AIH) is considered less common in the Asia-Pacific region. Due to this, AIH flare as a cause of acute-on-chronic liver failure (ACLF) is often overlooked and treatment delayed. We aimed at the defining clinical and histopathological spectrum and role of steroid therapy in AIH-ACLF. Patients with AIH-ACLF prospectively recruited and followed between 2012 and 2017 and were analyzed from the Asian-Pacific association for the Study of the Liver ACLF Research Consortium (AARC) database. Diagnosis of AIH was confirmed using International Autoimmune Hepatitis Group score or simplified AIH score with histopathological evidence. Of 2,825 ACLF patients, 82 (2.9%) fulfilled criteria of AIH (age 42.1 ± 18.1 years, 70% female). At baseline, mean bilirubin was 18.6 ± 8.2 mg/dL, Child–Turcotte–Pugh score was 11.7 ± 1.4, and Model for End-stage Liver Disease (MELD) score was 27.6 ± 6.5. Mean immunoglobulin G was 21.61 ± 7.32 g/dL, and this was elevated ≥1.1 times in 97% of cases; 49% were seronegative. Liver histology was available in 90%, with median histological activity index of 10 (interquartile range: 7–12); 90% with moderate-to-severe interface activity; 56% showing significant parenchymal necrosis (bridging and confluent necrosis); and cirrhosis in 42%. Twenty-eight (34%) patients received steroid therapy and showed shorter intensive care unit (ICU) stay (median 1.5 vs. 4 days; p < 0.001) and improved 90-day survival (75% vs. 48.1%; p = 0.02) with comparable incidence of sepsis (p = 0.32) compared to those who did not. Patients of advanced age, more severe liver disease (MELD >27; 83.3% sensitivity, 78.9% specificity, area under the receiver operating characteristic curve 0.86), presence of hepatic encephalopathy, and fibrosis grade ≥F3 had an unfavorable response to corticosteroid therapy.

Conclusion: AIH presenting as ACLF is not uncommon in Asian patients; a low threshold for liver biopsy is needed to confirm the diagnosis as nearly half the patients are seronegative; early stratification to steroid therapy or liver transplantation (MELD >27, hepatic encephalopathy in ≥F3) would reduce ICU stay and improve outcomes.

"Diagnose acute insult in ACLF—a stitch in time saves nine."

COMMENT

Acute-on-chronic liver failure (ACLF) has recently been recognized as a separate entity with a high short-term mortality. It is defined as an acute decompensation of a stable cirrhotic (previously known or unknown) with bilirubin >5 mg/dL and INR >1.5 with development of ascites and/or encephalopathy within 28 days of illness (APASL criteria). The prognosis of ACLF is poor and depends partially in the etiology of acute insult. Those insults with a possible treatment option may fair better than others, e.g., hepatitis B virus (HBV) reactivation causing acute insult may fair better than unknown cause [nucleoside analogues (NAs) can be used to treat HBV]. These two papers from India describe the outcomes of ACLF in two different groups of patients, both are important as identifying the cause of acute injury may change the line of treatment.

Drug-induced liver injury (DILI) is a common but less recognized cause of ACLF. In India, antitubercular therapy (ATT) is often responsible for DILI causing acute insult in a pre-existing cirrhotic. The authors utilized the APASL–AARC database to identify 3,132 patients with ACLF. Drugs were the cause of acute insult in 329 (10.5%) of all patients, 89.5% were due to nondrug causes. In those with drug-related ACLF, complementary and alternative medicines (CAM) (71.7%) were responsible for more cases compared to ATT (27.3%) (CAM and ATT constituting 90% of all cases with DILI). The mortality in drug-related ACLF was significantly higher than others (46.5% vs. 38.8%). However, there was no difference in severity or mortality when CAMs were compared with ATT.

This study highlights the fact that CAMs are a very important cause of liver injury (more than ATT). The prognosis is poor when drugs cause ACLF compared to nondrug causes. More efforts should go toward prevention of this injury, as no specific treatment is available.

The second article on ACLF discusses autoimmune hepatitis (AIH), a cause which is difficult to diagnose but very important as specific treatment is available (read steroids). The serum markers are often fallacious and liver biopsy (transjugular) is often required to make a diagnosis. This cohort again is derived from APASL-AARC database, diagnosis was made by International Autoimmune Hepatitis Group score or simplified AIH score with histopathological evidence (90% of patients underwent liver biopsies). Out of 2,825 ACLF patients, 82 were identified to have AIH-related ACLF. Of these 82 patients, 28 (34%) received steroid therapy. Those who received steroids had a shorter intensive care unit (ICU) and hospital stay and improved survival (75% vs. 48%). The authors also identified poor predictors of response to steroids [Model for End-stage Liver Disease (MELD) >27, advanced age, and presence of encephalopathy].

This article highlights that AIH as a cause of ACLF should be actively looked for, as it is potentially treatable with steroids. Patients with MELD >27 and advanced hepatic encephalopathy (HE) respond poorly to steroids and hence should be referred for early liver transplant.

Key Messages

- *Complementary and alternate medicines are an important cause of DILI in cirrhotics (closely followed by ATT).*
- *The prognosis of ACLF due to drug-induced injury is poorer compared to nondrug causes. No specific treatment is available except drug discontinuation.*
- *Suspected AIH-induced ACLF should be identified with a liver biopsy (transjugular). Use of steroids in AIH ACLF can lead to improvement in a substantial proportion of patients without needing liver transplant.*

Living donor liver transplantation for acute liver failure: donor safety and recipient outcome

Pamecha V, Vagadiya A, Sinha PK, Sandhyav R, Parthasarathy K, Sasturkar S, et al. Living donor liver transplantation for acute liver failure: donor safety and recipient outcome.
Liver Transpl. 2019;25:1408-21.

Abstract

In countries where deceased organ donation is sparse, emergency living donor liver transplantation (LDLT) is the only lifesaving option in select patients with acute liver failure (ALF). The aim of the current study is living liver donor safety and recipient outcomes following LDLT for ALF. A total of 410 patients underwent LDLT between March, 2011 and February, 2018, out of which 61 (14.9%) were for ALF. All satisfied the King's College criteria (KCC). Median admission to transplant time was 48 hours (range: 24–80.5 hours), and median living donor evaluation time was 18 hours (14–20 hours). Median Model for End-stage Liver Disease score was 37 (32–40) with more than two-thirds having grade 3 or 4 encephalopathy and 70% being on mechanical ventilation. The most common etiology was viral (37%). Median jaundice-to-encephalopathy time was 15 (9–29) days. Preoperative culture was positive in 47.5%. There was no difference in the complication rate among emergency and elective living liver donors (13.1% vs. 21.2%; p = 0.19). There was no donor mortality. For patients who met the KCC but did not undergo LT, survival was 22.8% (29/127). The 5-year post-LT actuarial survival was 65.57% with a median follow-up of 35 months. On multivariate analysis, postoperative worsening of cerebral edema [CE; hazard ratio (HR) 2.53; 95% confidence interval (CI) 1.01–6.31], systemic inflammatory response syndrome (SIRS; HR 16.7; 95% CI 2.05–136.7), preoperative culture positivity (HR 6.54; 95% CI 2.24–19.07), and a longer anhepatic phase duration (HR 1.01; 95% CI 1.00–1.02) predicted poor outcomes. In conclusion, emergency LDLT is lifesaving in selected patients with ALF. Outcomes of emergency living liver donation were comparable to that of elective donors. Postoperative worsening of CE, preoperative SIRS, and sepsis predicted outcome after LDLT for ALF.

"LDLT for ALF—a success story with a pinch of salt."

In contrast to acute-on-chronic liver failure (ACLF), acute liver failure (ALF) is a disease where acute hepatic insult happens on a normal pre-existing liver. The degree of injury is so massive that liver failure occurs and patient lapses into encephalopathy. Half of the patients with ALF will recover spontaneously; liver becomes normal as before the onset of disease. The other half deteriorate and die unless a life-saving liver transplant is performed. This study from India discusses the outcomes of liver transplant in this sick group of patients. It also presents the safety data of the donors who donated a part of their liver for these patients.

Over a period of 7 years at this single center in Delhi, 410 patients underwent Liver Transplant, 61 of these were for ALF. All patients who underwent

LT fulfilled Kings College Criteria (KCC). The Model for End-stage Liver Disease (MELD) score in these patients was 37. Most common cause of ALF was viral etiology, followed by antitubercular therapy (ATT) induced and indeterminate. This was a very sick group of patients [66% in grade 3–4 hepatic encephalopathy (HE), 70% on ventilator at the time of transplant]. As expected from the patient profile, complication rates were higher than for routine transplants. 21 of 61 patients died after transplant (16/21 in first 30 days after transplant). The 5-year actuarial survival was 65.6%. This is commendable considering the fact that more than 90% of these patients would have died within a few days to weeks without a transplant. More importantly, the donor safety data was excellent. There was no donor mortality, overall complication rate was 20%

(majority were grade 1–2 only). This paper tells us that living donor liver transplant is life saving even in sickest patients with ALF (those on ventilator and/or vasopressors). Despite a rapid work-up (<24 h), donor safety is not compromised, if a well-defined protocol is followed.

> ### Key Messages
>
> ⊙ *Even the sickest ALF patients are salvageable with a timely liver transplant.*
> ⊙ *Donor safety is not compromised even if the donor work-up is hurried up (as in case of ALF transplants).*

ARTICLE 12

Obeticholic acid for the treatment of non-alcoholic steatohepatitis: interim analysis from a multicentre, randomised, placebo-controlled phase 3 trial

Younossi ZM, Ratziu V, Loomba R, Rinella M, Anstee QM, Goodman Z, et al. Obeticholic acid for the treatment of non-alcoholic steatohepatitis: interim analysis from a multicentre, randomised, placebo-controlled phase 3 trial. *Lancet. 2019;394:2184-96.*

Abstract

Background: Nonalcoholic steatohepatitis (NASH) is a common type of chronic liver disease that can lead to cirrhosis. Obeticholic acid, a Farnesoid X receptor agonist, has been shown to improve the histological features of NASH. Here, we report results from a planned interim analysis of an ongoing, phase 3 study of obeticholic acid for NASH.

Methods: In this multicenter, randomized, double-blind, placebo-controlled study, adult patients with definite NASH, non alcoholic fatty liver disease (NAFLD) activity score of at least 4, and fibrosis stages F2-F3, or F1 with at least one accompanying comorbidity were randomly assigned using an interactive web response system in a 1:1:1 ratio to receive oral placebo, obeticholic acid 10 mg, or obeticholic acid 25 mg daily. Patients were excluded, if cirrhosis, other chronic liver disease, elevated alcohol consumption, or confounding conditions were present. The primary endpoints for the month-18 interim analysis were fibrosis improvement (≥1 stage) with no worsening of NASH, or NASH resolution with no worsening of fibrosis, with the study considered successful, if either primary endpoint was met. Primary analyses were done by intention to treat, in patients with fibrosis stage F2-F3 who received at least one dose of treatment and reached, or would have reached, the month 18 visit by the prespecified interim analysis cutoff date. The study also evaluated other histological and biochemical markers of NASH and fibrosis, and safety. This study is ongoing, and registered with ClinicalTrials.gov, NCT02548351, and EudraCT, 20150-025601-6.

Findings: Between December 9, 2015 and October 26, 2018, 1,968 patients with stage F1-F3 fibrosis were enrolled and received at least one dose of study treatment; 931 patients with stage F2-F3 fibrosis were included in the primary analysis (311 in the placebo group, 312 in the obeticholic acid 10 mg group, and 308 in the obeticholic acid 25 mg group). The fibrosis improvement endpoint was achieved by 37 (12%) patients in the placebo group, 55 (18%) in the obeticholic acid 10 mg group (p = 0.045), and 71 (23%) in the obeticholic acid 25 mg group (p = 0.0002). The NASH resolution endpoint was not met [25 (8%) patients in the placebo group, 35 (11%) in the obeticholic acid 10 mg group (p = 0.18), and 36 (12%) in the obeticholic acid 25 mg group (p = 0.13)]. In the safety population (1,968 patients with fibrosis stages F1-F3), the most common adverse event was pruritus [123 (19%) in the placebo group, 183 (28%) in the obeticholic acid 10 mg group, and 336 (51%) in the obeticholic acid 25 mg group]; incidence was generally mild to moderate in severity. The overall safety profile was similar to that in previous studies, and incidence of serious adverse events was similar across treatment groups [75 (11%) patients in the placebo group, 72 (11%) in the obeticholic acid 10 mg group, and 93 (14%) in the obeticholic acid 25 mg group].

Interpretation: Obeticholic acid 25 mg significantly improved fibrosis and key components of NASH disease activity among patients with NASH. The results from this planned interim analysis show clinically significant histological improvement that is reasonably likely to predict clinical benefit. This study is ongoing to assess clinical outcomes.

"A ray of hope for NASH patients with fibrosis."

COMMENT

Nonalcoholic steatohepatitis (NASH) is the second most common cause of liver disease in India (after alcoholic liver disease). Till date, only vitamin E, pioglitazone, and very recently Saroglitazar have been approved for its treatment. Interestingly, none of these three medicines have shown improvement in fibrosis in nonalcoholic fatty liver disease (NAFLD) patients. Obeticholic acid (OCA) is a new generation (precision) medicine that targets the basic pathophysiology of NAFLD. It is an agonist of Farnesoid X receptor (FXR) (nuclear receptor expressed in hepatocytes and enterocytes). FXR agonism leads to alteration in bile pool and reduces bile acid levels in the hepatocyte. This action has been proposed to decrease fat in liver and mitigate the liver injury due to NAFLD. This study published in Lancet is an interim analysis of an ongoing phase 3 trial of OCA in NASH. The trial aims to recruit 2,400 patients in total with a long-term follow-up of at least 5 years. This is an interim report of around 900 patients followed up for 18 months (liver biopsy at baseline and 18 months). Only those patients with biopsy-proven fibrosis (F2/F3 and F1 with comorbidities) were included, cirrhotics were excluded. It compares the improvement in clinical scores and histology in three groups (placebo vs. 10 mg OCA vs. 25 mg OCA). Alanine aminotransferase (ALT) levels normalized in patients on OCA compared to placebo. The fibrosis improvement was significantly higher in the 25 mg OCA arm compared to placebo (23% vs. 12%). The 10-mg OCA arm showed numerically more improvement (18% vs. 12%), but did not reach predefined significance. The side effects were seen in more than half patients in OCA arm; pruritus was most common (although mild to moderate in intensity). Although low-density lipoprotein (LDL) levels increased in a significant number of patients in the OCA arm, but were easily controlled with statin therapy. There was a higher proportion of patients in OCA arm developing gallstone-related complications (explained by alterations in bile acid pool).

In summary, OCA is an important drug that has shown any fibrosis improvement in NASH patients (**Fig. 1**). As the side effects were significant, more long-term safety data is required before this drug can be routinely recommended for use in NASH patients.

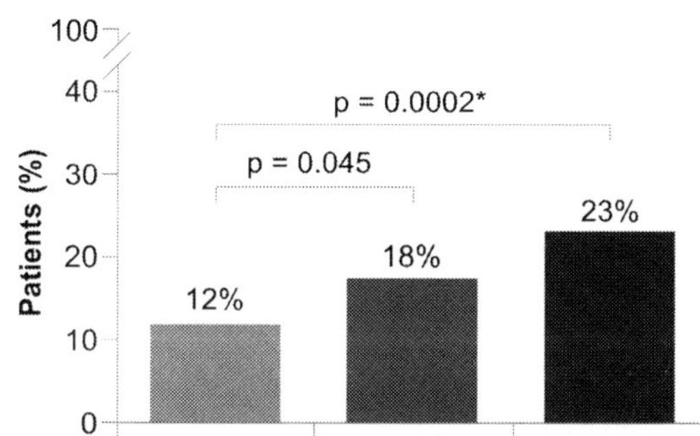

FIG. 1: Proportion of patients showing improvement in fibrosis with no worsening of nonalcoholic steatohepatitis (NASH).

Key Messages

- ⊙ *Obeticholic acid 25 mg is the first drug to show fibrosis improvement in NASH patients.*
- ⊙ *The safety profile of the drug is under question, more data is needed on safety before it can be formally approved for use in NASH patients.*

ARTICLE 13

Endoscopic or surgical myotomy in patients with idiopathic achalasia

Werner YB, Hakanson B, Martinek J, Repici A, von Rahden BHA, Bredenoord AJ, et al. Endoscopic or surgical myotomy in patients with idiopathic achalasia.
N Engl J Med. 2019;381:2219-29.

Abstract

Background: Pneumatic dilation and laparoscopic Heller's myotomy (LHM) are established treatments for idiopathic achalasia. Peroral endoscopic myotomy (POEM) is a less invasive therapy with promising early study results.

Methods: In a multicenter, randomized trial, we compared POEM with LHM plus Dor's fundoplication in patients with symptomatic achalasia. The primary endpoint was clinical success, defined as an Eckardt symptom score of 3 or less (range: 0–12, with higher scores indicating more severe symptoms of achalasia) without the use of additional treatments, at the 2-year follow-up; a noninferiority margin of −12.5 percentage points was used in the primary analysis. Secondary endpoints included adverse events, esophageal function, gastrointestinal quality of life index score (range: 0–144, with higher scores indicating better function), and gastroesophageal reflux.

Results: A total of 221 patients were randomly assigned to undergo either POEM (112 patients) or LHM plus Dor's fundoplication (109 patients). Clinical success at the 2-year follow-up was observed in 83.0% of patients in the POEM group and 81.7% of patients in the LHM group [difference: 1.4 percentage points; 95% confidence interval (CI) −8.7 to 11.4; p = 0.007 for noninferiority]. Serious adverse events occurred in 2.7% of patients in the POEM group and 7.3% of patients in the LHM group. Improvement in esophageal function from baseline to 24 months, as assessed by measurement of the integrated relaxation pressure of the lower esophageal sphincter, did not differ significantly between the treatment groups (difference: −0.75 mm Hg; 95% CI −2.26 to 0.76), nor did improvement in the score on the gastrointestinal quality of life index (difference: 0.14 points; 95% CI −4.01 to 4.28). At 3 months, 57% of patients in the POEM group and 20% of patients in the LHM group had reflux esophagitis, as assessed by endoscopy; at 24 months, the corresponding percentages were 44% and 29%.

Conclusion: In this randomized trial, POEM was noninferior to LHM plus Dor's fundoplication in controlling symptoms of achalasia at 2 years. Gastroesophageal reflux was more common among patients who underwent POEM than among those who underwent LHM. (Funded by the European Clinical Research Infrastructure Network and others; ClinicalTrials.gov number, NCT01601678.)

"Endoscopic myotomy: Need to be combined with anti-reflux measures."

COMMENT

Achalasia cardia is an esophageal motor disorder with defective relaxation of lower esophageal sphincter and disturbed esophageal peristalsis. Currently available treatments are endoscopic pneumatic dilatation, peroral endoscopic myotomy (POEM), and laparoscopic Heller's myotomy (LHM). In this multicenter, randomized noninferiority trial, POEM was compared against LHM with Dor's fundoplication. Among 221 total patients, 109 were assigned to LHM plus Dor's fundoplication and 112 to POEM. The clinical success at 2 years of follow-up was 83.0% (in POEM) and 81.7% (LHM + Dor). Serious adverse events occurred in 2.7% and 7.3% in POEM and LHM, respectively. There was no difference in improvement in esophageal function and gastrointestinal quality of life. Endoscopically defined reflux esophagitis in POEM or LHM was 57% and 20% at 3 months, and 44% and 29% at 24 months, respectively.

The POEM is noninferior to LHM plus Dor's fundoplication in symptom control. However, reflux esophagitis was more common in POEM. The likely reason being that endoscopic antireflux procedures were not combined with POEM; whereas, LHM is always done in combination with fundoplication. Though common, reflux associated with POEM is easily treated with proton pump inhibitors.

Key Message

⊙ *Symptom relief of achalasia is similar with peroral endoscopic myotomy (POEM) and laparoscopic Heller's myotomy (LHM) plus Dor's fundoplication. Although, reflux esophagitis is higher after POEM, it can be treated easily with proton pump inhibitors or prevented by endoscopic antireflux procedures.*

ARTICLE 14

Role of faecal microbiota transplantation for maintenance of remission in patients with ulcerative colitis: a pilot study

Sood A, Mahajan R, Singh A, Midha V, Mehta V, Narang V, et al. Role of faecal microbiota transplantation for maintenance of remission in patients with ulcerative colitis: a pilot study.
J Crohns Colitis. 2019;13:1311-7.

Abstract*

Objectives: This study aimed at assessing the role of fecal microbiota transplantation (FMT) in maintaining remission in the ulcerative colitis (UC).

Methods: This was a pilot study that included patients having UC in clinical remission attained following multisession FMT; patients were randomized to either maintenance FMT or placebo colonoscopic infusion every 8 weeks, for 48 weeks. In all the patients, the standard-of-care (SOC) therapy was continued. The primary endpoint of the study was maintaining steroid-free clinical remission (Mayo score ≤2, all subscores ≤1) at week 48th. The secondary endpoints included achievement of endoscopic remission (endoscopic Mayo score 0) and histological remission (Nancy grade 0 and 1) at week 48th.

Results: Among total 61 patients, randomization of 31 patients was done to receive FMT and 30 patients received placebo. The primary outcome was achieved in 87.1% (27 out of 31) patients who received FMT as compared to 66.7% (20 out of 30) patients who received placebo (p = 0.111). Significantly higher number of patients with FMT achieved secondary endpoints of endoscopic remission [FMT: 18/31 (58.1%) vs. placebo: 8/30 (26.7%); p = 0.026] and histological remission [FMT: 14/31 (45.2%) vs. placebo: 5/30 (16.7%); p = 0. 033]. Three patients on FMT (9.7%) and 8 patients who received placebo (26.7%) relapsed. Presence of no serious adverse events required discontinuation among patients on FMT. Colectomy was needed in one patient who relapsed on placebo.

Conclusion: Maintenance FMT among patients in clinical remission may aid in sustaining clinical, endoscopic, and histological remission in patients having UC. *Redrafted abstract

"Microbiome manipulation therapies: Valiant attempts, still more required."

COMMENT

Fecal microbiota transplantation (FMT) is effective and safe for maintenance of remission in patients with ulcerative colitis.

Ulcerative colitis (UC) is a chronic progressive inflammatory disease with relapsing, remitting course that requires long-term maintenance on drugs such as 5-ASA, azathioprine, or biologicals. Despite these maintenance therapies, 25–40% patients relapse annually. Anti-tumour necrosis factors (TNFs) and newer biologicals, though increasingly used for maintaining disease remission, are very expensive and have potentially serious adverse effects. Fecal microbiota transplantation (FMT) has been shown to be effective for induction of remission in patients with active UC. Sood et al. reported the results of first randomized controlled trial of FMT as maintenance therapy in patients with UC. Patients who achieved clinical remission (defined as Mayo score ≤2, with each subscore ≤1) with FMT and on stable medication regimens (5-ASA and azathioprine for 6 months) were included in the study. Around 61 patients were randomized in 1:1 ratio to receive either FMT (n = 31) or placebo (n = 30) through ileocolonoscopy every 8 weeks for next 48 weeks (at week 0, 8, 16, 24, 32, 40, and 48) along with ongoing medications. Around 100 g fecal sample diluted with 200 mL normal saline was used in the FMT group; whereas, normal saline with added food color was used as placebo. At week 48, the primary outcome (steroid free clinical remission) was achieved in 87.1% patients in FMT group versus 66.7% patients in placebo group (p = 0.111). Significantly higher proportion of patients with FMT attained secondary endpoints of endoscopic remission (58.1% vs. 26.7%; p = 0.026) and histological remission (45.2% vs. placebo: 5/30 16.7%; p = 0. 033) compared to placebo without any major adverse effects.

The study did not report the changes in microbial pattern in these patients, which contributes to its major limitation. Although the study was not powered adequately to detect efficacy of FMT, but it was a pilot study with well-designed placebo group as a comparator and it demonstrated a significant improvement in endoscopic and histological remission with lower frequency of relapse over 48 weeks of follow-up. Larger multicenter study with longer follow-up and data on serial changes in microbial pattern are needed to establish FMT as a therapeutic option for maintenance of remission in patients with UC.

Key Messages

- Multisession FMT at 8-week interval is an effective and safe maintenance therapy in patients with UC.
- Maintenance FMT resulted in increased clinical, endoscopic, and histological remission rate with lower frequency of relapse compared to placebo.

ARTICLE 15

Indian consensus on gastroesophageal reflux disease in adults: a position statement of the Indian society of gastroenterology

Bhatia SJ, Makharia GK, Abraham P, Bhat N, Kumar A, Reddy DN, et al. Indian consensus on gastroesophageal reflux disease in adults: a position statement of the Indian Society of Gastroenterology.
Indian J Gastroenterol. 2019;38:411-40.

Abstract

The Indian Society of Gastroenterology developed this evidence-based practice guideline for management of gastroesophageal reflux disease (GERD) in adults. A modified Delphi process was used to develop this consensus containing 58 statements, which were generated by electronic voting iteration as well as face-to-face meeting and review of the supporting literature primarily from India. These statements include 10 on epidemiology, 8 on clinical presentation, 10 on investigations, 23 on treatment (including medical, endoscopic, and surgical modalities), and 7 on complications of GERD. When the proportion of those who voted either to accept completely or with minor reservation was 80% or higher, the statement was regarded as accepted. The prevalence of GERD in India ranges from 7.6 to 30%, being <10% in most population studies, and higher in cohort studies. The dietary factors associated with GERD include use of spices and nonvegetarian food. *Helicobacter pylori* is thought to have a negative relation with GERD; *H. pylori* negative patients have higher grade of symptoms of GERD and esophagitis. Less than 10% of GERD patients in India have erosive esophagitis. In patients with occasional or mild symptoms, antacids and histamine H2 receptor blockers (H2RAs) may be used, and proton pump inhibitors (PPIs) should be used in patients with frequent or severe symptoms. Prokinetics have limited proven role in management of GERD.

"Made in India: Guidance statement for us based on our data."

COMMENT

There is a need for first ever consensus for treatment for gastroesophageal reflux disease (GERD) in India where prevalence ranging from 7.6 to 30%. This consensus by Indian Society of Gastroenterology (ISG) addresses the epidemiological, clinical, diagnostic, and treatment options of GERD relevant to Indian population supported by data primarily from India and also highlights the paucity of high-quality evidence to guide recommendations. In areas where there is limited data to support the evidence, the recommendations were given by experts in the clinical practice by using modified Delphi process.

This guideline emphasizes an algorithmic approach for management of patients with GERD, which can be easily followed by Physicians and Gastroenterologists in India. It is also recommended for symptom-based diagnosis of GERD rather than invasive testing and empiric treatment with proton pump inhibitor (PPI)/ H2RA. This consensus addresses the issues of management of GERD such as indications of therapeutic endoscopy and role of surgical therapy in refractory GERD based on recent evidence. Regarding surgery for GERD, guidelines recommend it is an effective alternative for long-term medical therapy and should be offered to appropriately selected patients, which was proved by a recent study. This guideline addresses the unsolved question of adverse events of proton pump inhibitor (PPI), which can be now safely used in patients supported by recent evidence and also emphasizes that unnecessary PPI should be avoided. Finally, it highlighted the need for further large studies in areas of GERD where evidence is limited and need for exclusive studies in Indian population (**Box 1**).

Box 1: Summary of the Indian consensus statement on GERD.

- GERD is common in India, in both urban and rural populations
- Obesity is a risk factor for GERD
- There is inverse association between the prevalence of *Helicobacter pylori* infection and GERD
- Eosinophilic esophagitis should be looked for in patients with refractory GERD
- GERD should be considered in patients with difficult-to-treat nonseasonal asthma and chronic cough
- Patients with GERD and those with long-standing symptoms should undergo upper gastrointestinal endoscopy at least once in their lifetime
- A standard dose PPI for 4 weeks should be the first line of therapy
- In the presence of esophageal strictures, long-term daily PPI maintenance therapy should be given
- In patients with nocturnal reflux symptoms, optimizing PPI therapy or adding an H2RA at night should be considered
- All the available PPIs in equipotent doses have similar efficacy for symptom control
- Injudicious use of long-term PPIs should be avoided

(GERD: gastroesophageal reflux disease; PPI: proton pump inhibitor)

Key Messages

⊙ *GERD should be considered in patients with difficult-to-treat nonseasonal asthma and chronic cough.*

⊙ *All the available PPIs in equipotent doses have similar efficacy for symptom control.*

ARTICLE 16

Crohn's disease exclusion diet plus partial enteral nutrition induces sustained remission in a randomized controlled trial

Levine A, Wine E, Assa A, Boneh RS, Shaoul R, Kori M, et al. Crohn's disease exclusion diet plus partial enteral nutrition induces sustained remission in a randomized controlled trial.
Gastroenterology. 2019;157:440-50.e8.

Abstract

Background and aims: Exclusive enteral nutrition (EEN) is recommended for children with mild-to-moderate Crohn's disease (CD), but implementation is challenging. We compared EEN with the CD exclusion diet (CDED), a whole-food diet coupled with partial enteral nutrition (PEN), designed to reduce exposure to dietary components that have adverse effects on the microbiome and intestinal barrier.

Methods: We performed a 12-week prospective trial of children with mild-to-moderate CD. The children were randomly assigned to a group that received CDED plus 50% of calories from formula (Modulen, Nestlé) for 6 weeks (stage 1) followed by CDED with 25% PEN from weeks 7–12 (stage 2) (n = 40, group 1) or a group that received EEN for 6 weeks followed by a free diet with 25% PEN from weeks 7–12 (n = 38, group 2). Patients were evaluated at baseline and weeks 3, 6, and 12 and laboratory tests were performed; 16S ribosomal RNA gene (V4V5) sequencing was performed on stool samples. The primary endpoint was dietary tolerance. Secondary endpoints were intention to treat (ITT) remission at week 6 (pediatric CD activity index score below 10) and corticosteroid-free ITT sustained remission at week 12.

Results: Four patients withdrew from the study because of intolerance by 48 hours, 74 patients (mean age 14.2 ± 2.7 years) were included for remission analysis. The combination of CDED and PEN was tolerated in 39 children (97.5%), whereas EEN was tolerated by 28 children (73.6%) [p = 0.002; odds ratio for tolerance of CDED and PEN: 13.92; 95% confidence interval (CI) 1.68–115.14]. At week 6, 30 (75%) of 40 children given CDED plus PEN were in corticosteroid-free remission versus 20 (59%) of 34 children given EEN (p = 0.38). At week 12, 28 (75.6%) of 37 children given CDED plus PEN were in corticosteroid-free remission compared with 14 (45.1%) of 31 children given EEN and then PEN (p = 0.01; odds ratio for remission in children given CDED and PEN: 3.77; CI 1.34–10.59). In children given CDED plus PEN, corticosteroid-free remission was associated with sustained reductions in inflammation (based on serum level of C-reactive protein and fecal level of calprotectin) and fecal Proteobacteria.

Conclusion: CDED plus PEN was better tolerated than EEN in children with mild-to-moderate CD. Both diets were effective in inducing remission by week 6. The combination CDED plus PEN-induced sustained remission in a significantly higher proportion of patients than EEN, and produced changes in the fecal microbiome associated with remission. These data support use of CDED plus PEN to induce remission in children with CD. Clinicaltrials.gov no: NCT01728870.

"You will be what you eat: No longer folklore but a scientific truth."

COMMENT

Crohn's disease exclusion diet plus partial enteral nutrition induces sustained remission in a randomized controlled trial.

Inflammatory bowel disease (IBD) is a chronic relapsing–remitting immune disorder of unknown etiology that afflicts millions of individuals around the world with debilitating symptoms. Among the various environmental factors, diet seems to play an important role in the pathogenesis of IBD. Epidemiologic studies have suggested that a diet high in fruits and vegetables and low in animal fats and sugar may decrease the risk for IBD. Exclusive enteral nutrition (EEN) has been shown to be effective than steroids in inducing remission in children, but EEN therapy limited by unpalatability and high cost. Hence, elimination diets with the exclusion of dietary components hypothesized to affect the microbiome or intestinal permeability have been developed. The Crohn's disease exclusion diet (CDED) is an exclusion diet supplemented with partial enteral nutrition (PEN) developed in Israel and has been suggested to be beneficial in children and adults with IBD. Levine et al. reported the results of a randomized, controlled trial of 78 pediatric patients with mild-to-moderate Crohn's disease comparing CDED with exclusive EEN. The intervention consisted of an initial 6-week period with CDED and 50% PEN, followed by another 6-week period with CDED and 25% PEN. The control group received exclusive EEN in the first 6 weeks followed by 25% PEN and free diet in the second 6-week period. Although both interventions were deemed to be efficacious, the CDED-PEN intervention was better tolerated than EEN, and CDED-PEN was associated with higher rates of remission at week 12. A decrease in serum C-reactive protein and fecal calprotectin was paralleled by an improvement of the fecal microbial profile in the patients that responded to both therapies, notably with a decrease of Proteobacteria. Moreover, a decrease in intestinal permeability was observed in the patients who received the CDED diet.

The major limitation of this clinical trial is lack of endoscopic evaluation for response. Furthermore, this study is only powered to assess the tolerance of two different diets and not their relative efficacy. Although higher rates of remission were seen at week 12, the calprotectin levels remained elevated in many patients. Indeed, whether the PEN is required for the CDED to be effective is unknown.

In conclusion, CDED appears to be as effective as EEN and more tolerable. Further, adequately conducted clinical research is required to explore the role of diet in treatment of IBD as monotherapy or in combination. Based on results of this study, in select patients, such as those with a short segment of inflammatory, nonpenetrating, nonstricturing Crohn's disease and mild-to-moderate symptoms, a trial of dietary therapy alone with a diet such as CDED could be attempted for a short period of time, with close follow-up, and with agreement with the patient that failure to fully respond is an indication to escalate therapy. This will be especially interesting in developing nations where increasing IBD incidence and prevalence will result in the absolute need for less costly but efficient therapeutic alternatives to biologicals.

Key Messages

- *Crohn's disease exclusion diet (CDED) plus partial enteral nutrition (PEN) is as effective and better tolerated than exclusive enteral nutrition (EEN).*
- *Reintroduction of normal diet after remission resulted in rebound inflammation and decreased remission.*
- *Exclusion of compounds in regular diet is required for persistence of change in microbiome.*

ARTICLE 17

Safety of proton pump inhibitors based on a large, multi-year, randomized trial of patients receiving rivaroxaban or aspirin

Moayyedi P, Eikelboom JW, Bosch J, Connolly SJ, Dyal L, Shestakovska O, et al. Safety of proton pump inhibitors based on a large, multi-year, randomized trial of patients receiving rivaroxaban or aspirin. *Gastroenterology. 2019;157:682-91.e2.*

Abstract

Background and aims: Proton pump inhibitors (PPIs) are effective at treating acid-related disorders. These drugs are well tolerated in the short term, but long-term treatment was associated with adverse events in observational studies. We aimed to confirm these findings in an adequately powered randomized trial.

Methods: We performed a 3 × 2 partial factorial double-blind trial of 17,598 participants with stable cardiovascular disease and peripheral artery disease randomly assigned to groups given pantoprazole (40 mg daily, n = 8,791) or placebo (n = 8,807). Participants were also randomly assigned to groups that received rivaroxaban (2.5 mg twice daily) with aspirin (100 mg once daily), rivaroxaban (5 mg twice daily), or aspirin (100 mg) alone. We collected data on development of pneumonia, *Clostridium difficile* infection, other enteric infections, fractures, gastric atrophy, chronic kidney disease, diabetes, chronic obstructive lung disease, dementia, cardiovascular disease, cancer, hospitalizations, and all-cause mortality every 6 months. Patients were followed up for a median of 3.01 years, with 53,152 patient-years of follow-up.

Results: There was no statistically significant difference between the pantoprazole and placebo groups in safety events except for enteric infections (1.4% vs. 1.0% in the placebo group; odds ratio: 1.33; 95% confidence interval: 1.01–1.75). For all other safety outcomes, proportions were similar between groups except for *C. difficile* infection, which was approximately twice as common in the pantoprazole versus the placebo group, although there were only 13 events, so this difference was not statistically significant.

Conclusion: In a large placebo-controlled randomized trial, we found that pantoprazole is not associated with any adverse event when used for 3 years, with the possible exception of an increased risk of enteric infections. ClinicalTrials.gov Number: NCT01776424.

"Innocent unless proven guilty: Long-term proton pump inhibitor use is safe except for increased enteric infections."

COMMENT

Proton pump inhibitors (PPIs) are among the most commonly prescribed drugs globally. Long-term use of PPIs has raised serious issues of drug-related adverse events and this has been based mostly on retrospective data subject to many confounding biases. Hence, the story continues to unfold.

This trial was a 3 × 2 partial factorial, multicenter, double-blind, randomized placebo-controlled trial evaluating patients with stable atherosclerotic vascular disease. Participants included were those with stable coronary or peripheral arterial disease and 65 years or older and younger atherosclerotic participants with arterial disease in at least two cardiovascular beds and/or had two additional risk factors for the disease. These were randomized to rivaroxaban 2.5 mg twice daily with aspirin 100 mg once daily, rivaroxaban 5 mg twice daily alone, or aspirin 100 mg once daily alone. Patients in each group were again randomized to receive pantoprazole 40 mg once daily or placebo. Those with continued need for PPI or H2 receptor antagonist were excluded from the PPI trial. The safety outcomes in relation to PPI use was the secondary objective of the pantoprazole trial arm. A total of 17,598 participants were randomized to pantoprazole or placebo and the median follow-up was 3 years. The study found no significant difference between the two groups in the cardiovascular outcomes, hospitalization rates, all-cause mortality, cancer incidence, fracture, gastric atrophy, and new onset chronic diseases such as diabetes mellitus, chronic kidney disease, dementia, or chronic obstructive airway disease. Among the infections, enteric infections were more common in pantoprazole group (OR 1.33; 95% CI 1.01–1.75) and no significant difference in pneumonia noted between the two groups.

This is the largest placebo controlled multi-ethnic randomized controlled trial (RCT) with relatively long-term follow-up and established the safety of PPI except for the increased risk of enteric infections, even for which the number needed to harm was very high (n = 301). Although the study was not powered to detect all the evaluated safety outcomes, there were no strong trends for these outcomes and thus additional sample size is unlikely to detect any associations. The study was conducted among the stable atherosclerotic patients and the results cannot be generalized to specific patient populations such as hospitalized patients, malnourished patients, or patients with advanced renal or cardiac failure or cirrhosis or immunosuppression. Gastric atrophy was underestimated in the study due to requirement of biopsy for diagnosis. Few potential adverse events such as micronutrient deficiencies were not measured and small changes in some endpoints such as dementia might have been missed. The long-term safety of PPIs beyond 3 years cannot be established especially for some adverse events such as dementia or malignancies, which may require longer latency periods. To sum up, the study provided the high-quality evidence that there is no increased risk for several of the previously perceived adverse effects of PPIs usage, reported predominantly from observational studies (**Table 1**).

TABLE 1: New evidence from COMPASS trial data that adds to the Expert Review and Best Practice Advice from the American Gastroenterological Association on The Risks of Long-term Use of Proton Pump Inhibitors, 2017.

Potential adverse effect with PPI (as per the Expert Review of American Gastroenterological Association, 2017)	COMPASS trial data (3 years median follow-up)
Kidney disease	No association
Dementia	No association
Bone fracture	No association
Myocardial infarction	No association
Small intestinal bacterial overgrowth	Not evaluated
Spontaneous bacterial peritonitis	Not evaluated
Clostridium difficile infection	Increased risk for enteric infections other than *Clostridium difficile* (only trend noted for *C. difficile* infection)
Pneumonia	No association
Micronutrient deficiencies	Not evaluated
Gastrointestinal malignancies	No association

Key Message

⊙ *Proton pump inhibitors can be safely used for a few years without any increased risk of adverse events including dementia, fractures, cardiovascular events, pneumonia, or death except for the increased risk of enteric infections.*

ARTICLE 18

Randomized trial of medical versus surgical treatment for refractory heartburn

Spechler SJ, Hunter JG, Jones KM, Lee R, Smith BR, Mashimo H, et al. Randomized trial of medical versus surgical treatment for refractory heartburn.
N Engl J Med. 2019;381:1513-23.

Abstract*

Background: One of the frequently encountered clinical problems is heartburn that remains in spite of proton-pump inhibitor (PPI) treatment; there are multiple potential causes of heartburn. The efficacy of treatments for PPI-refractory heartburn is still not proven; treatment focuses to control gastroesophageal reflux with either reflux-decreasing medication (such as baclofen) or antireflux surgery or on dampening visceral hypersensitivity with neuromodulators (such as desipramine).

Methods: The study included patients referred to veterans affairs (VA) gastroenterology clinics; among these, the patients with PPI-refractory heartburn were given 20 mg of omeprazole twice daily for 2 weeks, and the patients having persistent heartburn underwent esophageal biopsy, esophageal manometry, endoscopy, and multichannel intraluminal impedance-pH monitoring. If reflux-related heartburn was present in the patients, they were randomly assigned to receive either active medical treatment (omeprazole plus baclofen, with desipramine added on the basis of symptoms), surgical treatment (i.e., laparoscopic Nissen fundoplication), or control medical treatment (omeprazole with placebo). The primary outcome considered in the study was treatment success, which was defined as a reduction of ≥50% in the gastroesophageal reflux disease (GERD)-health related quality of life score (range 0–50; higher scores suggesting worse symptoms) at 1 year.

Results: Total 366 patients were included; mean age was 48.5 years; out of these, 280 were men). After pre-randomization procedures, 288 patients were excluded: during the 2-week omeprazole trial, 42 patients had relief of heartburn; trial procedures were not completed in 70 patients; 54 patients were excluded due to other reasons, 23 patients had non-GERD esophageal disorders; and functional heartburn was present in 99 patients (not because of GERD or other motility, histopathologic, or structural abnormality). Randomization was done in remaining 78 patients. The incidence of treatment success with surgery (67%, 18/27 patients) was found to be significantly superior as compared to active medical treatment (28%, 7/25 patients; p = 0.007) or control medical treatment (12%, 3/26 patients; p < 0.001). Between the active medical group and the control medical group, the difference in the incidence of treatment success was 16 percentage points (95% confidence interval −5 to 38; p = 0.17).

Conclusion: In the patients who were referred to VA gastroenterology clinics for PPI-refractory heartburn, on systematic workup, truly PPI-refractory and reflux-related heartburn were revealed in a minority of patients. In that highly selected subgroup, surgery was found to be superior as compared to medical treatment. (Funded by the Department of Veterans Affairs Cooperative Studies Program; ClinicalTrials.gov number, NCT01265550.) *Redrafted abstract

"Everything that glitters is not gold: All heartburn is not GERD."

COMMENT

Gastroesophageal reflux disease (GERD) is a very common yet a complex medical disorder with multifactorial etiology. Although acid suppression helps, about 40% are refractory in which the treatment options are limited. In a randomized, controlled trial, Spelcher et al. compared treatment success with the various therapies for refractory heartburn. These included laparoscopic

Nissen fundoplication; proton-pump inhibitor (PPI) (omeprazole) with baclofen, desipramine, or both (active medical); or omeprazole with placebo (control medical). The study population comprised patients from veterans affairs (VA) gastroenterology clinics. All had persistent refractory heartburn after a 2-week trial of omeprazole 20 mg twice daily and showed abnormal acid exposure, a positive symptom association probability (SAP), or both on ambulatory pH/impedance testing while on omeprazole. Among 366 enrolled, about 40–50% in each group had esophageal hypersensitivity alone and many others were excluded, resulting in 78 undergoing randomization. At 1 year, the primary symptom endpoint (>50% improvement in GERD-related quality of life) was met in a significantly higher percentage of surgery patients (67%) compared with the active medical group (28%) or the control medical group (12%).

This study has important implications for clinical practice. Most importantly, it showed that a majority of patient who presented with refractory heartburn were negative for the diagnosis of GERD on the basis of gold standard test of ambulatory pH testing. Hence, that is the foremost take-home point, that 50% of patients with refractory heartburn may not have GERD and need to be managed as esophageal hypersensitivity disorder rather than with acid suppressive therapies. In patients who had refractory heartburn due to GERD, surgery led to significantly higher resolution of symptoms (**Table 1**).

TABLE 1: Table showing response to Nissen fundoplication is much better than with medical therapy.

Intervention	Response n (%)	p value
Group A Surgery: Nissen fundoplication (n = 27)	18 (67%)	<0.001 (vs. Group B) 0.007 (vs. Group C)
Group B PPI + baclofen and/or desipramine (n = 25)	7 (28%)	0.17 (vs. Group C)
Group C PPI + placebo (n = 26)	3 (12%)	

(PPI: proton-pump inhibitor)

Key Messages

- *In patients with refractory heartburn, 24-hour pH metry should be done to ascertain, if the symptom is part of esophageal hypersensitivity disorder or it is part of GERD.*
- *In patients with refractory heartburn due to GERD, results with Nissen fundoplication are superior to medical therapy.*
- *Hence, understanding the pathophysiology operating in a particular patient may help in directed therapy.*

ARTICLE 19

Vedolizumab versus adalimumab for moderate-to-severe ulcerative colitis

Sands BE, Peyrin-Biroulet L, Loftus EV Jr, Danese S, Colombel JF, Törüner M, et al. Vedolizumab versus adalimumab for moderate-to-severe ulcerative colitis.
N Engl J Med. 2019;381:1215-26.

Abstract*

Background: In the patients with ulcerative colitis, biologic therapies are commonly used. There is a scarcity of head-to-head trials of such therapies in patients who have inflammatory bowel disease.

Methods: This was a phase 3b, double-blind, double-dummy, randomized trial, which was conducted at 245 centers in 34 countries. Vedolizumab was compared with adalimumab among adult patients having moderately-to-severely active ulcerative colitis for determining, if vedolizumab was superior. In up to 25% of the patients, prior exposure to a tumor necrosis factor inhibitor except adalimumab was permitted. Randomization of the patients was done to receive either infusions of 300 mg of vedolizumab on day 1 and at weeks 2, 6, 14, 22, 30, 38, and 46 (along with injections of placebo) or subcutaneous injections of 40 mg of adalimumab, with a total dose of 160 mg at week 1, 80 mg at week 2, and 40 mg every 2 weeks subsequently up to week 50 (along with infusions of placebo). In either group, dose escalation was not allowed. The primary outcome in the study was clinical remission at week 52 [which was defined as a total score of 2 or less on the Mayo scale (range 0–12; higher scores suggesting more severe disease) and no subscore >1 (range 0–3) on any of the four components of Mayo scale]. For controling type I error, analysis of efficacy outcomes was done with a hierarchical testing procedure; the variables were in the following order: Clinical remission; endoscopic improvement (which was subscore of 0 to 1 on the Mayo endoscopic component); and corticosteroid-free remission at week 52.

Results: Among 769 patients, 383 were randomized to receive at least one dose of vedolizumab and 386 patients received minimum one dose of adalimumab.

At week 52, clinical remission was present in higher proportion in vedolizumab group patients as compared to that of the adalimumab group [31.3% vs. 22.5%; difference: 8.8 percentage points; 95% confidence interval (CI) 2.5–15.0; p = 0.006]; endoscopic improvement was also present in significanlty more vedolizumab group patients (39.7% vs. 27.7%; difference: 11.9 percentage points; 95% CI 5.3–18.5; p < 0.001). Corticosteroid-free clinical remission was present in 12.6% and 21.8% of the patients in the vedolizumab group and adalimumab group, respectively (difference, −9.3 percentage points; 95% CI −18.9 to 0.4). With vedolizumab, exposure-adjusted incidence rates of infection was 23.4 events per 100 patient-years, and with adalimumab was 34.6 events per 100 patient-years. The corresponding rates for serious infection were found to be 1.6 and 2.2 events per 100 patient-years for vedolizumab and adalimumab, respectively.

Conclusion: In patients having moderately to severely active ulcerative colitis, vedolizumab was found to be superior than adalimumab in terms of achievement of clinical remission as well as endoscopic improvement; however, corticosteroid-free clinical remission was comparable (Funded by Takeda; VARSITY ClinicalTrials. gov number, NCT02497469; EudraCT number, 2015-000939-33.) *Redrafted abstract

"Vedolizumab versus adalimumab in ulcerative colitis: Head to head VARSITY trial."

COMMENT

Biologicals have become the choice of therapy in steroid-resistant ulcerative colitis. The most common biological used in this setting has been anti-tumour necrosis factor (TNF) monoclonal antibodies: Infliximab or adalimumab. Vedolizumab is a biological with a different mechanism of action. It is a lymphocyte trafficking inhibitor. It blocks the receptors on lymphocytes so that they cannot pass through the endothelium and reach the site of inflammation, which is the intestinal lamina propria. This study compared the efficacy of TNF inhibitor with gut homing lymphocyte trafficking inhibitor.

It is a randomized, double-blind double dummy active controlled trial comparing two biologic therapies vedolizumab and adalimumab in patients with ulcerative colitis. It aimed to fill a crucial knowledge gap: The comparative efficacy of treatments in ulcerative colitis. **Table 1** shows the results for outcomes of clinical remission and endoscopic improvement. In moderate-to-severe ulcerative colitis patients, vedolizumab was superior to adalimumab with respect to achievement of clinical remission and endoscopic improvement, but not corticosteroid-free clinical remission. Corticosteroid-free clinical remission occurred in 12.6% of the patients in the vedolizumab group and in 21.8% in the adalimumab group (difference, 95% CI −18.9 to 0.4).

In respect to its clinical implications, no dose intensification was permitted. However, in real-world data show that dosages are increased more often within the first year in patients who receive adalimumab (in 55–65% of patients) than in patients who receive vedolizumab (in 21%); thus, the dose of adalimumab might have been too low.

The rates of corticosteroid-free remission did not correlate with those of clinical remission among patients who received vedolizumab, in contrast to the strong correlation of these outcomes in GEMINI.

- Therefore, the superiority should be interpreted with caution, particularly in the context of high rates of continued use of corticosteroids in this trial.

TABLE 1: Results for outcomes of clinical remission and endoscopic improvement.

Total patients (769)	Clinical remission (week 52)	Endoscopic improvement
Vedolizumab (383 patients)	31.3%	39.7%
Adalimumab (386 patients)	22.5%	27.7%
95% confidence interval (CI)	2.5 to 15.0; p = 0.006	5.3 to 18.5; p < 0.001

Key Message

⊛ *In a comparison of two biologicals, patients of ulcerative colitis responded better to vedolizumab than adalimumab on clinical and endoscopic assessment.*

Section Editor: R Rajasekar

Associate Editors: Packiamary Jerome, M Ananthi

ARTICLE 1

Mortality associated with acute respiratory infections among children at home

Caballero MT, Bianchi AM, Nuño A, Ferretti AJP, Polack LM, Remondino I, et al. Mortality associated with acute respiratory infections among children at home.
J Infect Dis. 2019;219:358-64.

Abstract

Background: Numerous deaths in children aged <5 years in the developing world occur at home. Acute respiratory infections (ARIs) are thought to play an important role in these deaths. Risk factors and pathogens linked to fatal episodes remain unclear.

Methods: A case–control study among low-income children aged <5 years was performed in Buenos Aires, Argentina to define risk factors and viral pathogens among those who died of ARI at home.

Results: A total of 278 families of children aged <5 years (of whom 104 died and 174 were healthy controls) participated in the study. A total of 87.5% of ARI-associated deaths occurred among infants aged <12 months. The estimated mortality rate due to ARI among infants was 5.02 deaths/1,000 live births. Dying at home from ARI was associated with living in a crowded home [odds ratio (OR) 3.73; 95% confidence interval (CI) 1.41–9.88], having an adolescent mother (OR 4.89; 95% CI 1.37–17.38), lacking running water in the home (OR 4.39; 95% CI 1.11–17.38), incomplete vaccinations for age (OR 3.39; 95% CI 1.20–9.62), admission to a neonatal intensive care unit (OR 7.17; 95% CI 2.21–23.27), and no emergency department visit during the ARI episode (OR 72.32; 95% CI 4.82–1085.6). The at-home death rate due to respiratory syncytial virus (RSV) infection among infants was 0.26 deaths/100 live births and that due to influenza was 0.07 deaths/1,000 live births.

Conclusions: Social vulnerabilities underlie at-home mortality due to ARI. Mortality rates due to RSV and influenza virus infection are high among infants at home and are similar to those reported for hospitalized children.

"Acute respiratory infection and at home mortality."

COMMENT

The infant mortality is high in the developing countries and most of the deaths occur at home. Acute respiratory infections (ARIs) are the most common cause of infant deaths. The etiological agent is not the only cause for the demise of the child. Environmental, constitutional, and other social factors also play a critical role.

This study aims to define the risk factors and viral pathogens among those who died of ARI at home.

■ AT-HOME MORTALITY RATE (FIG. 1)

- *Infants*: 5.0 deaths/1,000 live births
- *<5 years*: 1.13 deaths/1,000 children

■ FACTORS ASSOCIATED WITH INCREASED MORTALITY

Home Environment

The families of cases dying of ARI were living in mud houses/precarious tins, crowded areas with lack of running water.

Maternal Factors

Maternal age <18 years, incomplete primary education, lack of prenatal healthcare, and lack of immunization were high in cases and controls, but these are not statistically significant.

Biological Risk Factors

The study revealed no difference in gestational age at birth, prematurity, sex, birth weight, or with mothers having asthma. Previous neonatal intensive care unit (NICU) admission has an independent role of mortality. In infants, breastfeeding was found to be a factor protective against at-home mortality.

Healthcare use during Fatal ARI

The child who has not visited a healthcare provider during the last episode of illness has a higher mortality. The study also reveals that factors beyond medical care also influence the outcome of the illness. The perception of disease severity was similar in both the groups. Lack of healthcare use during the fatal case of ARI was strongly associated with a poor outcome.

■ RESPIRATORY PATHOGENS AND ARI

Human rhinoviruses were detected throughout the year in nasopharyngeal swabs, with no statistic difference between both groups. Respiratory syncytial virus (RSV) was detected in 11 cases. The other viruses documented are H1N1 (influenza A), parainfluenza type 3. The at-home mortality associated with RSV was estimated at 0.26 deaths/1,000 live births and due to influenza A, it was 0.07 deaths/1,000 live births.

■ LIMITATIONS

The study is analyzed by verbal autopsies; it has its own inherent weakness. Nasopharyngeal swabs cannot access distal airways.

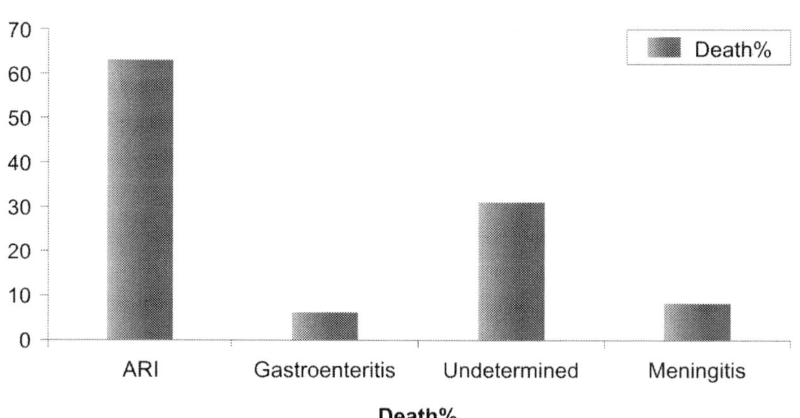

(ARI: acute respiratory infection)

FIG. 1: Causes of at-home mortality.

Key Messages

- ⊙ *Respiratory syncytial virus is the most common cause of at-home mortality associated with ARI.*
- ⊙ *Social vulnerabilities underlie at home mortality.*

ARTICLE 2

Comparison of whole-genome sequences of *Legionella pneumophila* in tap water and in clinical strains, Flint, Michigan, USA, 2016

Garner E, Brown CL, Schwake DO, Rhoads WJ, Arango-Argoty G, Zhang L, et al. Comparison of Whole-Genome Sequences of Legionella pneumophila in Tap Water and in Clinical Strains, Flint, Michigan, USA, 2016. *Emerg Infect Dis. 2019;25:2013-20.*

Abstract*

Two Legionnaires' disease outbreaks occurred in Genesee County, Michigan, during the water crisis in Flint, Michigan, USA (2014–2015). In this study, whole-genome sequences of 10 clinical isolates of *Legionella pneumophila* (which were submitted to one of the laboratories in Genesee County during the second outbreak) were compared with 103 water isolates collected in the following year. In this study, genetically diverse range of strains of *L. pneumophila* across clinical as well as water isolates were documented. Isolates that belong to 1 clade (three water isolates from a Flint hospital, three clinical isolates, one water isolate from a Flint residence, and the reference Paris strain) showed high degree of similarity (i.e., 2–1,062 single-nucleotide polymorphisms), all *L. pneumophila* sequence type 1, serogroup 1. In Flint hospital water samples, serogroup 6 isolates that belong to sequence type 2,518 were extensive but had no similarity to available clinical isolates. The *L. pneumophila* strains present in Flint tap water following the outbreaks were diverse and alike to some of the disease-causing strains. *Redrafted abstract

"Whole genome sequences of Legionella pneumophila."

COMMENT

Legionnaire's disease is a severe form of pneumonia caused by inhalation of virulent species of aerosolized Legionella bacteria. There were two outbreaks documented in Flint between June, 2014 and October, 2015. These outbreaks occur because of the change of water system from Flint River without any corrosion control measures. This leads to elevated lead in tap water, which leads to disruption in water quality and the growth of *L. pneumophila*.

This study aims to use next-generation DNA sequencing to compare *L. pneumophila* from Flint tap water and with tap water isolates from outside of Flint. WGS (whole-genome sequencing) was also used to compare isolates in terms of sequence type, average nucleotide identity, and single nucleotide polymorphisms. The study identified *L. pneumophila* isolates belonging to serogroup 1 via detection of *wzm* gene in WGS. The unknown serogroups were determined using fluorescein isothiocyanate conjugated antibodies.

The 16S ribosomal RNA genes mined from WGS indicate that all isolates except 8 were *L. pneumophila*. Serogrouping done identified all isolates belong to serogroup 1 and 6. Serogroup 1 was designated as ST2513 and serogroup 6 was designated as ST2518. Most hospital isolates belonged to ST2518 and residential tap water belonged to ST192.

Isolates were classified into distinct clades according to SNP. ST1 clade was verified by 2-1062 SNP. Clinical isolate 3 shared the highest degree of similarity with Flint tap water isolates. The SNPs were confirmed by phylogenetic analysis and average nucleotide identity comparison.

Few clinical sputum isolates were collected from the outbreaks, limiting the ability to track the source of infection. The wider collection of clinical and environmental isolates is not possible in this study due to limited availability of water isolates. The single strain of *Legionella* can colonize buildings and persists for many years. High degree of similarity was identified in ST1 isolates of water and clinical isolates. The presence of multiple clades of pneumophila suggests that no single strain is responsible for the outbreak.

The ST1 levels are conserved at the nucleotide level, thus causing difficulty in linking clinical and environmental sources. *L. pneumophila* has a high growth rate in hot conditions, but in this study, it is also evidenced in cold water systems. The final message is that multiple strains were associated with multiple sources of exposure.

Key Message

⊙ *Whole-genome sequencing-based characterization found a high degree of similarity and also identified variety of strains of L. pneumophila.*

ARTICLE 3

Dolutegravir-based or low-dose efavirenz-based regimen for the treatment of HIV-1

Kouanfack C, Mpoudi-Etame M, Bassega PO, Eymard-Duvernay S, Leroy S, Boyer S, et al. Dolutegravir-based or low-dose efavirenz-based regimen for the treatment of HIV-1.
N Engl J Med. 2019;381:816-26.

Abstract*

Background: Until June, 2018, the World Health Organization's preferred first-line treatment for human immunodeficiency virus type 1 (HIV-1) infection was an efavirenz-based regimen (in addition to a 600-mg dose of efavirenz, called as EFV600). In resource-limited settings, due to concerns related to the side effects, dolutegravir-based and low-dose efavirenz-based combinations are considered to be the first-line treatments for HIV-1.

Methods: This was an open-label, multicenter, randomized, phase-3 noninferiority trial conducted in Cameroon. Study population included adults who have HIV-1 infection and not received antiretroviral therapy and with an HIV-1 RNA level (viral load) of minimum 1,000 copies/mL; patients were randomized to receive either dolutegravir or the reference treatment of low-dose efavirenz (a 400-mg dose, called as EFV400), in combination with lamivudine and tenofovir. The primary endpoint considered in the study was the number of participants with a viral load of <50 copies/mL at week 48, based on the snapshot algorithm of Food and Drug Administration. Calculation of the difference between treatment groups was done; noninferiority was evaluated with a margin of 10 percentage points.

Results: Total 613 participants were included, who received minimum one dose of the assigned regimen. At week 48, a viral load of <50 copies/mL was present in 74.5% (231/310) participants in the dolutegravir group and in 69.0% (209/303) participants in the EFV400 group, with a difference of 5.5 percentage points [95% confidence interval (CI) −1.6 to 12.7; p < 0.001 for noninferiority]. In the participants who had a baseline viral load of minimum 100,000 copies/mL, a viral load of <50 copies/mL was observed in 66.2% (137/207) participants in the dolutegravir group and in 61.5% (123/200) participants in the EFV400 group, with a difference of 4.7 percentage points (95% CI −4.6 to 14.0). Virologic failure (i.e., viral load of >1,000 copies/mL) was present in three participants in the dolutegravir group (with none of the patients acquiring drug-resistance mutations) and in 16 patients in the EFV400 group. There was significantly more weight gain in the dolutegravir group as compared to the EFV400 group (median weight gain 5.0 kg vs. 3.0 kg, incidence of obesity 12.3% vs. 5.4%).

Conclusions: It can be concluded that in adults infected with HIV-1 in Cameroon, a dolutegravir-based regimen was found to be noninferior as compared to an EFV400-based reference regimen in terms of viral suppression at week 48. In participants with a viral load of minimum 100,000 copies/mL on the initiation of antiretroviral therapy, viral suppression was present in less number of participants than expected. (Funded by UNITAID and the French National Agency for AIDS Research; NAMSAL ANRS 12313 ClinicalTrials.gov number, NCT02777229.) *Redrafted abstract

"Dolutegravir versus low-dose efavirenz in HIV."

COMMENT

Efavirenz (600 mg) is the most preferred treatment for human immunodeficiency virus (HIV) along with the standard regimen till 2018. In view of the side effect profile and resistance pattern, dolutegravir, and low-dose efavirenz-based combinations have been considered the first-line treatment.

This study compares the efficacy and side effects of dolutegravir and low-dose efavirenz-based regimen in the treatment of HIV-1. The primary endpoint in this study is the decrease in viral load <50 copies/mL at 48 weeks of treatment.

DRUG PROFILE

Dolutegravir is an integrase inhibitor with a favorable profile for viral suppression. It has a high genetic barrier to resistance, low cost, and easily available in fixed dose combinations.

Efavirenz is a non-nucleoside reverse transcriptase inhibitor. It has a low genetic barrier to resistance, which leads to increased drug resistance mutations and increased mortality.

VIRAL LOAD (FIG. 1)

In this study, the viral load of <50 copies/mL was observed in 74.5% in dolutegravir group and 69.0% in the efavirenz group, thus meeting the criteria of noninferiority. The percentage differs among those with a baseline viral load of at least 100,000 copies/mL. It is around 61.5% in EF400 group and 66.2% among dolutegravir group, thus showing noninferiority. In patients with viral threshold of <200 copies/mL, 89.0% of dolutegravir group and 83.5% of EF400 group showed viral suppression. Virological failure (viral load of >1000 copies/mL)

was observed in 3 participants in dolutegravir group and 16 participants in EF400 group.

DRUG RESISTANCE

The prevalence of drug resistance mutations was well balanced between the two groups. The important factor associated with drug resistance was a baseline viral load of at least 100,000 copies/ mL. High level of integrase polymorphism was observed that leads to decreased efficacy of integrase inhibitor.

Thirteen patients died in the study group and >98% related to HIV-related illness.

Twenty-five patients became pregnant during the course of treatment. All the children were born alive and without any congenital abnormalities.

High glucose, weight gain, and insomnia are common in dolutegravir group. High cholesterol is seen in both groups.

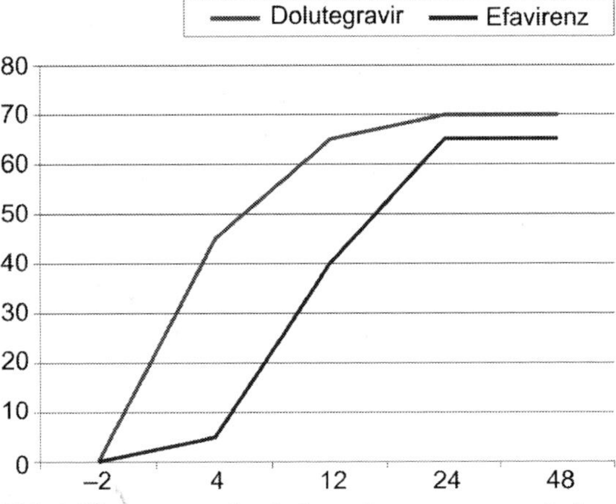

FIG. 1: Viral suppression in intention to treat population.

Key Messages

- *Dolutegravir was noninferior to efavirenz in the treatment of HIV. There is a low risk of acquiring drug-resistant mutations in dolutegravir.*
- *High baseline viral load is associated with impaired viral suppression.*
- *Early diagnosis and treatment are essential.*

ARTICLE 4

Persistence of immunity when using different human papillomavirus vaccination schedules and booster-dose effects 5 years after primary vaccination

Lazcano-Ponce E, Torres-Ibarra L, Cruz-Valdez A, Salmerón J, Barrientos-Gutiérrez T, Prado-Galbarro J, et al. Persistence of immunity when using different human papillomavirus vaccination schedules and booster-dose effects 5 years after primary vaccination.
J Infect Dis. 2019;219:41-9.

Abstract*

Background: Data related to the duration of immunity caused by different vaccination schedules of human papillomavirus (HPV) as well as the immunogenicity of a booster dose of both bivalent HPV vaccine (bHPV) and quadrivalent HPV vaccine (qHPV) is scarce.

Methods: This study included follow-up of a nonrandomized clinical trial for assessing the 5-year antibody persistence of the bHPV among girls (9–10 years of age) and women (18–24 years of age). The study compared noninferiority of the two-dose with three-dose schedule in girls at months 54 (in 639 patients) and 64 (in 990 patients). In girls who were vaccinated with a two-dose schedule of bHPV/qHPV, a booster dose of either vaccine was given at month 61. Virus-like particle-based enzyme-linked immunosorbent assay was used for measuring immunogenicity. Estimation of geometric mean titers (GMTs) for HPV16/18 was done following stratification by age group as well as vaccination schedule.

Results: At months 54 and 64, as compared to three-dose schedule, the two-dose schedule was noninferior. Up to 64 months, GMTs persisted above natural infection levels in all of the age groups. After the booster, there was an exponential increase in the anti-HPV16/18 GMTs in the same pattern, irrespective of the type of vaccine administered. With the booster dose, no safety concerns were noted.

Conclusion: Among girls, two-dose schedule is highly immunogenic, which indicates a high immune memory. Therefore, a booster dose seems to be unprofitable, given the low global coverage of immunization.

Clinical trials registration: NCT01717118. *Redrafted abstract

"Long-lasting humoral immunity and HPV vaccination."

COMMENT

Human papillomavirus (HPV) causes HPV infection, cervical precancer, and invasive cancer. Because of the high immunogenicity of HPV vaccines, the disease spectrum is reduced. WHO recommended two-dose regimen for girls between 9 and 14 years.

This study was done to analyze the duration of immunity produced by HPV vaccine and the immunogenicity of a booster dose of both bivalent (bHPV) and quadrivalent (qHPV) vaccine. They created three vaccination schedules. Doses of bHPV at months 0 and 6, two doses of bHPV and a booster dose of bHPV at month 61, and two doses of bHPV and a booster dose of qHPV at month 61. HPV16 and HPV18 antibodies were assessed using enzyme-linked immunosorbent assay (ELISA).

A high rate of seropositivity was observed for both HPV vaccine types. The result analysis demonstrates that the immune response of the two-dose schedule was noninferior to that of the three-dose schedule. There is an exponential increase in the geometric mean titers, regardless of the vaccine type (**Fig. 1**). No serious adverse effects reported except for pain in the injection site. Though there are no detectable antibodies, protective effect of HPV vaccine is maintained for 10–12 years.

This study proves that two-dose vaccination schedule is safe and produces a dramatic immune response. The antibody levels for both the vaccines remained stable for >5 years. The antibody levels of two-dose schedule remain much higher than that of a natural infection with good stability lasting for up to 64 months.

This is the first study to determine the immunogenic status and safety of both vaccine booster administered 5 years after the first dose. The booster has an exponential increase when compared to the titers after second dose of HPV. The antibody response produced by bHPV is higher than qHPV over a 5-year follow-up. The two-dose response has numerous advantages including low cost, flexibility in dosage interval, and increase coverage. This regimen has been adopted in 65% of the national immunization programs. The long-term persistence of immunity provides the data that there is a strong stimulation of memory B cells, which are responsible for the long-lasting humoral immunity.

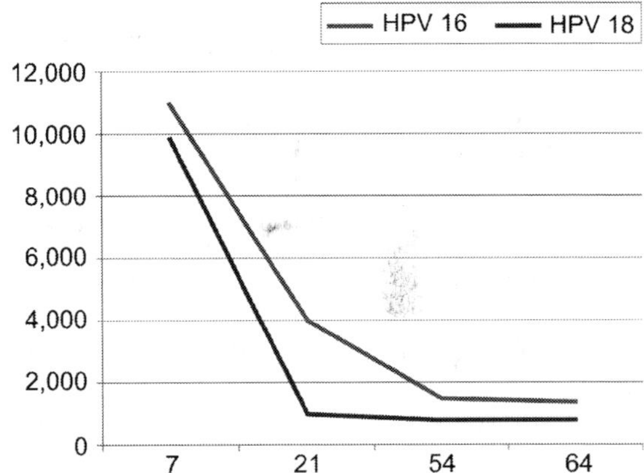

FIG. 1: Geometric mean titers of human papillomavirus (HPV)-16 and HPV-18 at different weeks.

Key Messages

⊙ *Two-dose regimen is noninferior to three-dose regimen of HPV vaccine.*

⊙ *There is no need of a booster dose, as the antibody level after the second dose itself lasts for longtime.*

ARTICLE 5

Augmented Zika and dengue neutralizing antibodies are associated with Guillain–Barré syndrome

Lynch RM, Mantis G, Encinales L, Pacheco N, Like G, Porras A, et al. Augmented Zika and dengue neutralizing antibodies are associated with Guillain–Barré syndrome.
J Infect Dis. 2019;219:26-30.

Abstract*

The role of neutralizing antibodies in Guillain–Barré syndrome (GBS) caused by Zika virus (ZIKV) is still not studied. This was a case–control study in which sera from the 2016 Zika epidemic in Colombia was used for determining the activity of neutralizing antibody against ZIKV as well as dengue virus serotype 2 (DENV2). In this study, enhanced neutralizing antibody titers were noted against DENV2 in ZIKV-infected individuals as compared to the uninfected controls and higher titers to both ZIKV and DENV2 in ZIKV-infected patients diagnosed with GBS in comparison to non-GBS ZIKV-infected controls. The findings indicated that high neutralizing antibody titers to DENV and to ZIKV were found to be associated with GBS during ZIKV infection.
*Redrafted abstract

“Guillain–Barré syndrome and Zika virus.”

COMMENT

Zika virus (ZIKV) belongs to a group of Flavivirus. The vector for this disease is *Aedes aegypti* mosquito. The most dreaded manifestation is microcephaly in babies born to infected mothers and Guillain–Barré syndrome (GBS) in adults.

Guillain–Barré syndrome is disorder of the peripheral nervous system with rapid onset of motor and sensory symptoms. The exact etiology of GBS is unknown. But, it can be triggered by viral/bacterial infection or by vaccination. The most common pathogen commonly encountered is *Campylobacter jejuni*. The antibody produced against the infection cross-reacts with the ganglioside surface of peripheral nerves. This study is used to investigate the role of Zika antibodies with GBS.

The common manifestations of ZIKV include arthralgias, fever, and myalgia. The median time to onset of neurological symptoms was 10 days from the onset of ZIKV symptoms. The neurological manifestations are lower extremity weakness, inability to walk, and paresthesias. Nearly 50% had breathing difficulty with 38% requiring intubation for respiratory failure. The mainstay of treatment was plasmapheresis and immunoglobulins. None of the patients received steroids.

In this study, neutralizing antibodies were compared between Zika-related GBS (ZGBS) and controls. The mean reciprocal titers against ZIKV were highly elevated in ZGBS cases. There was a significant elevated titers of dengue virus serotype 2 (DENV2) also. The high levels of antibody titers can represent an indirect effect that results from high viral load.

The high values of DENV2 antibodies in ZIKV-infected patients explain that DENV B cells are activated after ZIKV infection. This is an anamnestic response characterized by dengue response first, followed by de novo ZIKV response. The development of GBS happens in two ways. One is by the cross-reactivity of virus-specific antibodies (ZIKV/DENV) with nerve cells by molecular mimicry. The other possibility is by the indirect effects such as high-viral loads or high-immune activation secondary to association between neutralizing antibodies.

Key Message

⊙ *High levels of neutralizing antibody titers to DENV and ZIKV are associated with GBS during ZIKV infection.*

ARTICLE 6

Inhaled liposomal ciprofloxacin in patients with non-cystic fibrosis bronchiectasis and chronic lung infection with *Pseudomonas aeruginosa* (ORBIT-3 and ORBIT-4): two phase 3, randomised controlled trials

Hawarth CS, Bolton D, Chalmers JD, Davis AM, Froehlich J, Honda I, et al. Inhaled liposomal ciprofloxacin in patients with non-cystic fibrosis bronchiectasis and chronic lung infection with Pseudomonas aeruginosa (ORBIT-3 and ORBIT-4): two phase 3, randomised controlled trials.
Lancet Respir Med. 2019;7:213-26.

Abstract

Background: In patients with noncystic fibrosis bronchiectasis, lung infection with *Pseudomonas aeruginosa* is associated with frequent pulmonary exacerbations and admission to hospital for treatment, reduced quality of life, and increased mortality. Although inhaled antibiotics are conditionally recommended for long-term management of noncystic fibrosis bronchiectasis with frequent exacerbations, there is no approved therapy. We investigated the safety and efficacy of inhaled liposomal ciprofloxacin (ARD-3150) in two phase-3 trials.

Methods: ORBIT-3 and ORBIT-4 were international, randomized, double-blind, placebo-controlled, phase-3 trials run concurrently in similar geographical regions. Eligible patients had noncystic fibrosis bronchiectasis, had at least two pulmonary exacerbations treated with antibiotics in the previous 12 months, and had a history of chronic *P. aeruginosa* lung infection. Patients were randomly assigned (2:1) to receive either ARD-3150 or placebo. ARD-3150 (3 mL liposome encapsulated ciprofloxacin 135 mg and 3 mL free ciprofloxacin 54 mg) or 6 mL placebo (3 mL dilute empty liposomes mixed with 3 mL of saline) was self-administered once daily for six 56-day treatment cycles, for 48 weeks. The primary endpoint was time to first pulmonary exacerbation from the date of randomization to week 48. We did primary and secondary efficacy, safety, and microbiology analyses on the full analysis population, which comprised all randomized patients who received at least one dose of study drug. ORBIT-3 and ORBIT-4 are registered with ClinicalTrials.gov, numbers NCT01515007 and NCT02104245, respectively.

Findings: Between March 31, 2014 and August 19, 2015, we screened 514 patients in ORBIT-3 and 533 patients in ORBIT-4. The full analysis populations consisted of 278 patients in ORBIT-3 (183 patients received at least one dose of ARD-3150 and 95 received placebo) and 304 patients in ORBIT-4 (206 patients received at least one dose of ARD-3150 and 98 received placebo). In ORBIT-4, the median time to first pulmonary exacerbation was 230 days in the ARD-3150 group compared with 158 days in the placebo group, a statistically significant difference of 72 days [hazard ratio (HR) 0.72 (95% confidence interval (CI) 0.53–0.97), p = 0.032]. In ORBIT-3, the median time to first pulmonary exacerbation was 214 days in the ARD-3150 group and 136 days in the placebo group, a nonstatistically significant difference of 78 days [HR 0.99 (95% CI 0.71–1.38), p = 0.97]. In a pooled analysis of data from both ORBIT-3 and ORBIT-4, the median time to first pulmonary exacerbation was 222 days in the ARD-3150 group and 157 days in the placebo group, a nonstatistically significant difference of 65 days [0.82 (0.65–1.02), p = 0.074]. The numbers of adverse events and serious adverse events were similar in both groups in ORBIT-3 and ORBIT-4.

Interpretation: In patients with noncystic fibrosis bronchiectasis and chronic *P. aeruginosa* lung infection requiring antibiotic therapy in the preceding year, ARD-3150 led to a significantly longer median time to first pulmonary exacerbation compared with placebo in ORBIT-4, but not in ORBIT-3 or the pooled analysis. Inconsistency between the trials suggests further research is needed into the heterogeneity of noncystic fibrosis bronchiectasis and optimal outcome measures for inhaled antibiotics.

Funding: Aradigm Corporation.

"Bronchiectasis and pulmonary Pseudomonas aeruginosa—RCT."

COMMENT

Noncystic fibrotic bronchiectasis and pneumonia due to *Pseudomonas aeruginosa* are chronic lung infections causing frequent exacerbations, persistent cough, hospital admissions, and decreased quality of life.

Two phase-3 randomized controlled trials (RCTs) were done—ORBIT-3 and ORBIT-4 in two geographic locations with similar baseline patient population. Patients >18 years of age with noncystic fibrosis bronchiectasis confirmed by CT chest with forced expiratory volume in 1 second (FEV1) >25%, and who had at least two pulmonary exacerbations in the preceding 12 months and sputum culture showing pseudomonas aeruginosa included in the study. Patients require antibiotic treatment for lung infection within 28 days of the study. Chronic obstructive pulmonary diseases (COPDs) associated with smoking, allergic bronchitis, tuberculosis (TB), etc., are excluded from the study.

Randomization was done by computer-generated random sequence as 2:1 to receive either ARD-3150. Inhalational ciprofloxacin 6 mL self-administrable nebulizer or 6 mL saline placebo was recommended. The trial was carried out for six cycles of 56-day trial, which comprised of 28 days of nebulization trial and followed by treatment-free 28 days and the outcome was monitored.

The endpoints of the study are acute pulmonary exacerbations with increased sputum, cough, breathlessness, wheezing, or FEV1 decreases of 10% from the baseline spirometry values or radiological evidence of new pulmonary changes.

All the data obtained were analyzed by Kaplan–Meier analyses and calculations were done with SAS version 9.4 or later.

■ RESULTS

Both groups, ORBIT-3 and ORBIT-4, have similar patient compliance of >90% and higher treatment completion rate. Demographic data were also similar in both groups.

However, the latency to first pulmonary exacerbation and frequency of pulmonary exacerbations are favorable with ARD-3150 compared to placebo in ORBIT-4 (**Table 1**). Yet, this difference is absent in ORBIT-3 trial. ARD-8250 also has reduced sputum consistency in *Pseudomonas aeruginosa*.

TABLE 1: Time in days to first pulmonary exacerbation.

Study	ARD-3150	Placebo
ORBIT-3	214	136
ORBIT-4	230	158
Pooled analysis	222	157

Key Messages

⊙ *Liposomal ciprofloxacin—ARD-3150 decreases pulmonary exacerbation intensity and frequency in noncystic fibrosis bronchiectasis and pulmonary Pseudomonas aeruginosa, and improves lung functions and quality of life of these patients.*

⊙ *Inhalational ciprofloxacin avoids quinolones toxicity that can be seen in oral and intravenous administration.*

ARTICLE 7

Lassa virus circulating in Liberia: a retrospective genomic characterization

Wiley MR, Fakoli L, Letizia AG, Welch SR, Ladner JT, Prieto K, et al. Lassa virus circulating in Liberia: a retrospective genomic characterisation.
Lancet Infect Dis. 2019;19:1371-8.

Abstract

Background: An alarming rise in reported Lassa fever cases continues in West Africa. Liberia has the largest reported per capita incidence of Lassa fever cases in the region, but genomic information on the circulating strains is scarce. The aim of this study was to substantially increase the available pool of data to help foster the generation of targeted diagnostics and therapeutics.

Methods: Clinical serum samples collected from 17 positive Lassa fever cases originating from Liberia (16 cases) and Guinea (one case) within the past decade were processed at the Liberian Institute for Biomedical Research using a targeted-enrichment sequencing approach, producing 17 near-complete genomes. An additional 17 Lassa virus sequences (two from Guinea, seven from Liberia, four from Nigeria, and four from Sierra Leone) were generated from viral stocks at the US Centers for Disease Control and Prevention (Atlanta, GA) from samples originating from the Mano River Union (Guinea, Liberia, and Sierra Leone) region and Nigeria. Sequences were compared with existing Lassa virus genomes and published Lassa virus assays.

Findings: The 23 new Liberian Lassa virus genomes grouped within two clades (IV-A and IV-B) and were genetically divergent from those circulating elsewhere in West Africa. A time-calibrated phylogeographic analysis incorporating the new genomes suggests Liberia was the entry point of Lassa virus into the Mano River Union region and estimates the introduction to have occurred between 300 and 350 years ago. A high level of diversity exists between the Liberian Lassa virus genomes. Nucleotide percent difference between Liberian Lassa virus genomes ranged up to 27% in the L segment and 18% in the S segment. The commonly used Lassa Josiah-MGB assay was up to 25% divergent across the target sites when aligned to the Liberian Lassa virus genomes.

Interpretation: The large amount of novel genomic diversity of Lassa virus observed in the Liberian cases emphasizes the need to match deployed diagnostic capabilities with locally circulating strains and underscores the importance of evaluating cross-lineage protection in the development of vaccines and therapeutics.

Funding: Defense Biological Product Assurance Office of the US Department of Defense and the Armed Forces Health Surveillance Branch and its Global Emerging Infections Surveillance and Response Section.

"Genomic diversity of Lassa virus in Liberia."

COMMENT

Lassa fever is caused by Lassa virus, belonging to the family of Arenaviridae. It is endemic in West Africa and caused 300,000 infections annually with 5,000 deaths. As 80% of the cases have mild symptoms without diagnosis, the accurate number of cases is lacking. It may lead to serious hemorrhagic disease. The estimated case fatality rate for all infections is 1%. There is a lack of surveillance as well as diagnostic measures to assess the overall burden of Lassa fever.

In order to overcome this, immunoassays have been developed. Immunoassays are not as sensitive as polymerase chain reaction (PCR), and severe infections can have false-negative results due to the suppression of immunoglobulin (Ig) M and IgG responses. Molecular diagnostic tests are highly sensitive, but false-negative results are common due to high genetic diversity. In order to study the genetic diversity, they generated large (L) and small (S) level coding sequence alignments covering at least 80% of the protein coding portions of either L or S genome segment.

Seventeen samples from positive patients and 17 samples from viral stocks have been evaluated. On assessment, they found that nucleotide diversity ranged up to 27% in the L segment and 18% in the S segment. Segment level phylogenetics indicated that all Liberian genomes belong to lineage IV, with one exception 807978-P28 (appears to be a reassortant, with S segment from clade IV and L segment does not fall into IV or V). They were further classified into two major clades: IV-A and IV-B.

The time of most recent common ancestors (tMRCA) for the large clade in lineage IV and lineage V were in line with estimates 150 years ago. Liberia was the most likely location for the MRCA lineages IV and V, and it is the most likely entry point for Lassa virus into the other areas. Although L and S segment lineages were consistent, they differed substantially in their tMRCA estimates. The above findings suggest that the genetic diversity of Lassa virus is undersampled.

■ REVERSE TRANSCRIPTASE PCR ASSAYS

- Lassa Josiah MGB assay—detects lineage IV and targets glycoprotein precursor gene on the S genome segment.
- LAV assay (Nikisins)—Pan Lassa assay, targets RNA dependent, RNA polymerase.

Among the L segment assays, Nikisins assay is the best and among S segment assays, Bowen and Coulibaly B assays are best.

Further sampling is needed to capture all the genetic diversity of Lassa virus. It is ideal to switch to multiple Pan enzyme-linked immunosorbent assay (ELISA) assays to eliminate false-negative results.

Key Message

⊙ *More rapid tests and multiple pan ELISA assays are to be done to identify the genetic diversity of Lassa virus.*

ARTICLE 8

Imaging spectrum of H1N1 influenza from a tertiary liver hospital in India: first ever experience

Laroia ST, Gupta E, Kumar S, Kumar G, Sarin SK. Imaging spectrum of H1N1 influenza from a tertiary liver hospital in India: first ever experience.
J Assoc Physicians India. 2019;67:37-41.

Abstract

Aim: To review the imaging spectrum, clinical profile, and disease outcome of patients with H1N1 influenza at a tertiary liver hospital.

Settings and design: A retrospective analysis of imaging findings of 21 patients with H1N1 flu, admitted to our hospital from September, 2014 to March, 2015, was done.

Materials and methods: All patients with H1N1 virus infection were included. Mode of hospital admission, concomitant liver disease, clinical findings, liver function tests, and viral markers for hepatitis B and C infections were studied. Chest imaging findings on chest X-ray (CXR) or high-resolution CT (HRCT) were analyzed. Correlation with chronic lung disease (CLD), clinical course, mortality, and morbidity was reviewed.

Statistical analysis used: Analysis was performed with SPSS version. Mean ± standard deviation (SD), number and percentage, chi-square or Fisher exact test, t-test, and odds ratio were calculated as appropriate.

Results: The mean age was 43.52 ± 14.2 years (18 males and 3 females). Positive CXR and HRCT findings were found in 14/21 (66.7%) and 19/21 (90.5%), respectively. Most common abnormalities observed were bilateral consolidation and ground–glass opacities (9/21, 42.9% each). Mid-zone distribution was seen in 15/21 (71.4%). Underlying CLD was seen in 14/21 (66.7%) with positive findings in 11/14 (78.6%) on CXR and 13/14 (92.9%) on HRCT. Presence of pleural effusion (PE) (57.1%) and lymphadenopathy (50%) were statistically significant ($p < 0.05$). Median length of hospital stay was longer: 12 days [interquartile range (IQR) 1–30] with significant mortality rate in this group.

Conclusion: Imaging profile of patients with H1N1 influenza revealed that patients with underlying CLD were more likely to have imaging findings, pleural effusion, and lymphadenopathy, and receive intensive care and longer hospital stay with increased risk for mortality.

"H1N1 imaging and chronic liver disease."

COMMENT

The H1N1 strain of influenza A was first identified in Mexico. World Health Organization (WHO) declared it as a pandemic in 2009. After that, the disease has spread all over the world. The disease has a resurgence on and off since 2014. The causes for this surge are the temperature, host immunity, vaccination status, and the antigenic drift of the virus.

This study was conducted to review the imaging spectrum, clinical profile, and disease outcome of H1N1 patients with chronic liver disease.

In this study, more number of male (92.9%) patients were found to be H1N1 positive, with a mean age of 43.52. H1N1 patients with chronic liver disease (CLD) were older than the patients without CLD. Majority of intensive care unit (ICU) admissions with H1N1 positivity were associated with underlying CLD.

Chest X-ray was positive in 66% of the study population, of which 78% had underlying CLD.

High-resolution CT was positive in 82% of the study population, of which majority had underlying CLD. Bilateral lung consolidation was more common in CLD group, followed by ground glass opacities. This study has a peculiar involvement of mid zone in the CLD group, when compared to others, which showed upper and lower zone preponderance. The presence of pleural effusion and mediastinal lymphadenopathy was statistically significant in the CLD group.

In this study, symptomatic, reverse transcriptase polymerase chain reaction (RT-PCR)-proven H1N1 patients without any imaging findings constitute around 36% in the CLD group and 57% in the non-CLD group. Progressive disease in radiographs is high in CLD patients. This emphasizes that lung changes are more common in the CLD group (**Fig. 1**).

Complications of H1N1 such as pneumothorax, bronchiectasis, and lung cavitation are reported in some studies. The small study population is one limitation.

The average stay in the hospital was prolonged in the CLD group when compared to non-CLD group. The overall mortality is around 43%, and all patients had underlying CLD.

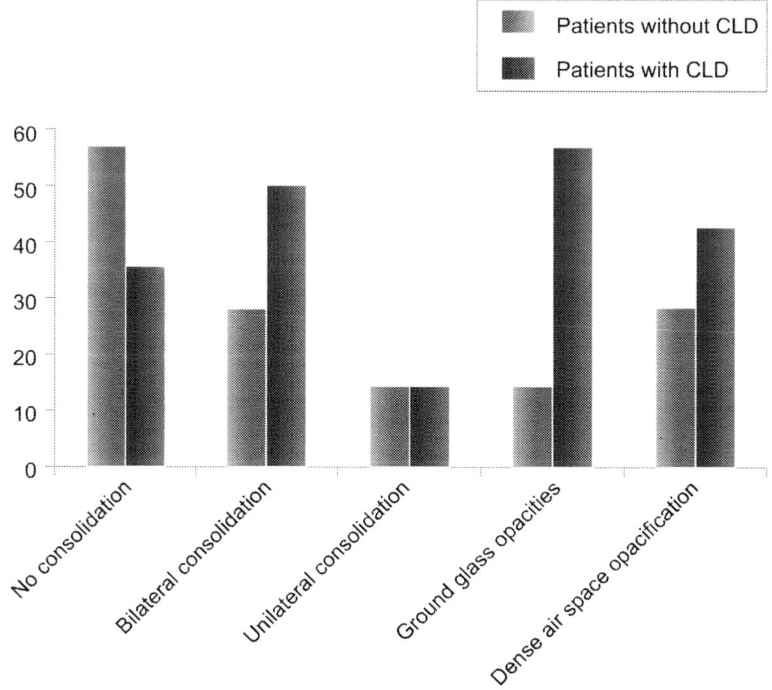

FIG. 1: Imaging pattern of H1N1 patients with chronic liver disease (CLD).

Key Messages

- *Chronic liver disease patients are more likely to have a prolonged illness with high mortality when infected with H1N1, despite intensive management in the ICU.*
- *Chronic liver disease patients have a varied presentation in imaging when infected by H1N1.*

ARTICLE 9

Etiology of classic fever of unknown origin (FUO) among immunocompetent Indian adults

Rupali P, Garg D, Viggweswarupu S, Sudarsanam TD, Jeyaseelan V, Abraham OC. Etiology of classic fever of unknown origin (FUO) among immunocompetent Indian adults.
J Assoc Physicians India. 2019;67:21-6.

Abstract

Background: Fever of unknown origin (FUO) has been a vexing problem for physicians for decades. The advent of imaging, functional scans, guided procedures, and advanced molecular techniques has made many of the hitherto undiagnosed diseases easily diagnosable. FUO epidemiology can be geographically unique varying from country to region. Studies done in India are scarce, with variable definitions.

Methods: This prospective observational cohort study recruited 300 consecutive patients presenting with classic FUO as defined by Durack and Street. Potential diagnostic clues (PDCs) were identified and workup proceeded toward establishing a confirmatory diagnosis.

Results: Among the 300 classic FUO in our series, infections, neoplasms, and noninfectious inflammatory diseases (NIIDs) contributed to 48%, 21.6%, and 20.6% of the cases. Tuberculosis and melioidosis were the most important infections. Hematological malignancies like non-Hodgkin's lymphoma, Hodgkin's lymphoma, and Leukemia contributed to 78% of neoplasms causing FUO; whereas, solid organ malignancies contributed to 18% of the cases. Among the NIIDs, systemic lupus erythematosus, granulomatous diseases, and vasculitis contributed to 26%, 18%, and 14.5%, respectively. Diagnostic tests of utility included image-guided biopsies (100%), CT scan of abdomen and/or thorax (92.4%), and lymph node biopsies at 72%. Mortality was 5%. A boot strapping analysis was done on PDCs contributing to each specific diagnostic category and algorithms were developed.

Conclusion: This is the largest series of FUO from South India. Systematic sequence of investigations without start of empirical therapy led to a diagnosis in 99.4%, which is the highest in described literature.

"Classic fever of unknown origin—etiology."

COMMENT

Fever of unknown origin (FUO) is a nightmare for physicians. The causes of FUO are diverse. Unless a deep understanding of the etiology is not possible, it is difficult to arrive at a diagnosis.

■ DEFINITION

- Petersdorf and Beeson (1961):
  - Fever >38.3°C on several occasions
  - Duration >3 weeks
  - Uncertain diagnosis after 1 week of inpatient investigations
- Durack and Street:
  - Fever >38.3°C on several occasions
  - Duration >3 weeks
  - Not able to arrive at a diagnosis after three outpatient (OP) visits or 3 days as an inpatient

■ TYPES OF FUO

- Classic FUO
- Neutropenic FUO
- Nosocomial FUO
- HIV associated FUO

■ CLINICAL FEATURES

The mean duration of fever in this study is 148 days (21–1,460). More than 65% are males. The common symptoms are anorexia, weight loss, cough, dyspnea, and musculoskeletal pain. The clinical signs include pallor, hepatosplenomegaly, lymphadenopathy, focal deficits, etc.

■ ETIOLOGY (FIG. 1)

- *Infections*: The infections are the most common cause of FUO. Nearly 48% is contributed by infections. In this study, tuberculosis (TB) accounts for 61% of FUO. Pulmonary TB (14%), extrapulmonary TB (33%), disseminated TB (45%), and occult TB contribute to 8%. Lymph node involvement is around 70% in extrapulmonary TB. Melioidosis is the second most common fever in this study accounting for around 10% and common among diabetes. The other infective causes of FUO are endocarditis, visceral abscess, enteric, brucellosis, leishmaniasis, etc.

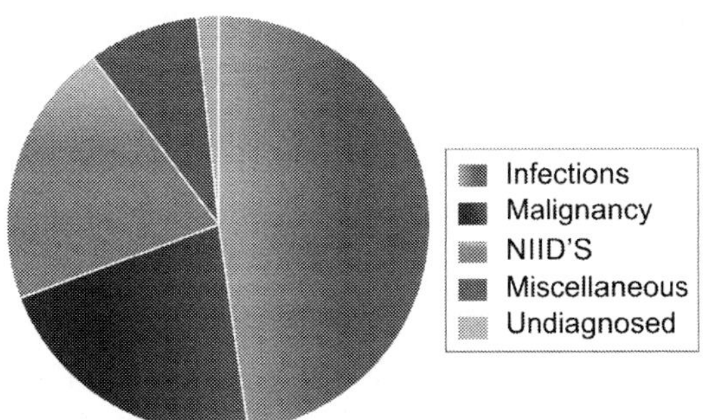

(NIID: noninfectious inflammatory disease)

FIG. 1: Etiology of fever of unknown origin (FUO).

- *Neoplasms*: Malignancy contributes to 21.6% of causes of FUO in this study. This is the second most common cause of FUO in adults >50 years. Hematological malignancies account for 78% and solid organ malignancies around 18%. Non-Hodgkin's and Hodgkin's lymphoma are the major components.
- *Noninfectious inflammatory diseases (NIIDs)*: This spectrum of disease accounts for 20.6% of the etiology of FUO. This is the second most common cause of FUO in people <50 years [systemic lupus erythematosus (26%), granulomatous diseases (18%), and vasculitis around 14.5%].
- *Miscellaneous*: 8.6%
- *Undiagnosed*: 1.6%

■ INVESTIGATION

- Erythrocyte sedimentation rate (ESR) and C-reactive protein (CRP) will be elevated. The elevation of alkaline phosphatase (ALP) occurs in 56.5% of the study population.
- Invasive procedures with tissue biopsies yield a 100% results. Image-guided biopsies are the mainstay of diagnosis. In this study, lymph node biopsy helps in arriving at a prompt diagnosis in around 63% of the people.
- CT revealed the diagnosis in 72.4%, ultrasonography (USG) and positron emission tomography (PET) contribute around 67%. Only 3% of the study population is diagnosed by only clinical diagnosis.

Key Messages

- ⊙ *Infections are the most common cause of FUO and aggressive diagnostic approach can avoid empiric therapy as much as possible.*
- ⊙ *Invasive tests yield a 100% diagnostic accuracy.*

ARTICLE 10

Association between plasma antibody responses and risk for *Cryptococcus*-associated immune reconstitution inflammatory syndrome

Yoon HA, Nakouzi A, Chang CC, Kuniholm MH, Carreño LJ, Wang T, et al. Association between plasma antibody responses and risk for *Cryptococcus*-associated immune reconstitution inflammatory syndrome.
J Infect Dis. 2019;219:420-8.

Abstract*

Background: In individuals infected with human immunodeficiency virus (HIV) and cryptococcal meningitis (CM), initiation of antiretroviral therapy (ART) puts them at risk for C-IRIS, i.e., *Cryptococcus*-associated immune reconstitution inflammatory syndrome. The association between antibody immunity and C-IRIS risk has still not been studied.

Methods: In this study, we compared plasma levels of immunoglobulin, *Cryptococcus neoformans* glucuronoxylomannan (GXM) capsule-specific and laminarin (Lam)-binding immunoglobulin (Ig)M and IgG, and percentages of peripheral blood total and memory B cells between total 27 patients infected with HIV and CM who developed C-IRIS and 63 who did not developed C-IRIS. The associations of these parameters were assessed with risk of C-IRIS.

Results: Before initiation of ART, as compared to those who did not developed C-IRIS, plasma IgM, Lam-binding IgM (Lam-IgM), Lam-IgG, and GXM-IgM levels were significantly lower among patients who developed C-IRIS. On multivariate analysis, it was observed that there was significant inverse associations between C-IRIS and IgM (p = 0.0003); Lam-IgM (p = 0.0005); Lam-IgG (p = 0.002); and GXM-IgM (p = 0.002) independent of age, sex, HIV viral load, CD4+ T-cell count, and cerebrospinal fluid fungal burden. No associations were noted between C-IRIS and total or memory B cells.

Discussion: Antibody profiles consisting of plasma IgM, Lam-IgM, Lam-IgG, and/or GXM-IgM may play a role in furthering our knowledge of C-IRIS pathogenesis; it also has potential as biomarkers of C-IRIS risk.
*Redrafted abstract

"Plasma antibody response and risk for Cryptococcus-associated immune reconstitution syndrome."

COMMENT

Cryptococcal meningitis is one of the most severe opportunistic infection in human immunodeficiency virus (HIV) patients causing 18,100 deaths in 2014. During antifungal treatment, individuals with cryptococcal meningitis have a high risk for *Cryptococcus*-associated immune reconstitution syndrome (C-IRIS) due to the immune response of the host.

■ RISK FACTORS FOR C-IRIS

- Persistent *Cryptococcus* in cerebrospinal fluid (CSF).
- Poor CD4 recovery after antiretroviral therapy (ART).
- Increased interleukin (IL)-5, IL-7 levels in plasma.
- Paucity of cerebrospinal fluid (CSF) inflammation prior to ART initiation.

Glucuronoxylomannan (GXM) is present in the capsule of *Cryptococcus*. In HIV-infected individuals and in those who developed cryptococcosis, the levels of GXM binding immunoglobulin (Ig)M were low. GXM–IgG was higher in patients with risk for cryptococcal meningitis with HIV infection.

The levels of plasma immunoglobulin, IgM, laminarin IgM and lam IgG, GXM IgM, GXM IgG, pustulan IgM and pustulan IgG along with peripheral blood B-cell subtypes are assessed in this study to find out the relationship between C-IRIS and antibody immunity. HIV patients with first episode of cryptococcal meningitis are included in the study. They received induction therapy with amphotericin B mg/kg for 14 days followed by consolidation therapy with fluconazole 400 mg for 8–12 weeks. ART was initiated on day 8 of antifungal therapy. Around 27 out of 90 patients developed C-IRIS.

The parameters were measured at baseline, week 4, and week 12. Plasma immunoglobulins were measured by Luminex, antibodies to GXM, lam and pustulan measured by enzyme-linked immunosorbent assay (ELISA), and peripheral B cells were determined by flow cytometry. The patients who developed C-IRIS had lower levels of antibodies like IgM, lam IgM/IgG, GXM IgM, and pustulan IgM/IgG. The higher levels of these antibodies at baseline were associated with a low risk of C-IRIS. There was no difference in the number of B cells between both groups.

The natural antibody response mediates host benefit against *Cryptococcus neoformans* by enhancing phagocytosis and dampening of inflammation. Reduced levels of natural antibody that reacts with β-glucans can deserve further consideration as a potential biomarker for risk of C-IRIS at ART initiation. Lam antibodies were associated with a better prognosis in patients with candidiasis. *Cryptococcus neoformans* β-glucosylceramide-binding antibodies from patients with cryptococcosis inhibited *C. neoformans*. The higher level of antibodies contributes to lower fungal burdens in C-IRIS groups. Higher levels of GXM–IgG were associated with an active cryptococcosis in HIV patients.

Key Messages

- ⊙ *The antibodies may in the future be used as a biomarker for C-IRIS in patients on antifungal therapy.*
- ⊙ *C-IRIS has a lethal effect on the life of the patients. So, early prediction of C-IRSIS would improve the care and management of CM patients.*

ARTICLE 11

Once-daily plazomicin for complicated urinary tract infections

Wagenlehner FME, Cloutier DJ, Komirenko AS, Cebrik DS, Krause KM, Keepers TR, et al. Once-Daily Plazomicin for Complicated Urinary Tract Infections.
N Engl J Med. 2019;380:729-40.

Abstract*

Background: In gram-negative uropathogens, increasing multidrug resistance requires novel treatments for serious infections. One of the aminoglycosides is plazomicin, which has bactericidal activity against multidrug-resistant (consisting of carbapenem-resistant) enterobacteriaceae.

Methods: Total 609 patients who had complicated urinary tract infections (UTIs), as well as acute pyelonephritis, were randomly assigned in a 1:1 ratio to receive either intravenous (IV) plazomicin (15 mg/kg of body weight once daily) or meropenem (1 g every 8 hours), along with optional oral step-down therapy following at least 4 days of IV therapy, for a duration of 7–10 days of therapy. The study's primary objective was to demonstrate the noninferiority of plazomicin to meropenem in the complicated UTIs treatment, as well as acute pyelonephritis, with a noninferiority margin of 15 percentage points. The primary endpoints considered in the study were composite cure (i.e., clinical cure as well as microbiologic eradication) at day 5 and at the test-of-cure visit (15–19 days following initiation of therapy) in the microbiologic modified intention-to-treat population.

Results: Plazomicin was found to be noninferior to meropenem in terms of the primary efficacy endpoints. At day 5, composite cure was noted in 168 of 191 patients (88.0%) in the plazomicin group and in 180 of 197 patients (91.4%) in the meropenem group [difference −3.4 percentage points; 95% confidence interval (CI) −10.0 to 3.1]. At the test-of-cure visit, composite cure was noted in 156 of 191 patients (81.7%) and 138 of 197 patients (70.1%), respectively (difference 11.6 percentage points; 95% CI 2.7–20.3). At the test-of-cure visit, it was observed that significantly more patients in the plazomicin group as compared to meropenem group had microbiologic eradication, as well as eradication of enterobacteriaceae non-susceptible to aminoglycosides (78.8% vs. 68.6%) and enterobacteriaceae producing extended-spectrum β-lactamases (82.4% vs. 75.0%). At late follow-up (24–32 days following initiation of therapy), less number of patients in the plazomicin group compared to the meropenem group had clinical relapse (1.6% vs. 7.1%) or microbiologic recurrence (3.7% vs. 8.1%). Increases in level of serum creatinine ≥0.5 mg/dL (≥40 μmol/L) above baseline were present in 7.0% and 4.0% of patients in the plazomicin group and meropenem group, respectively.

Conclusion: In the treatment of complicated UTIs as well as acute pyelonephritis that is caused by enterobacteriaceae, including multidrug-resistant strains, once-daily plazomicin was found to be noninferior to meropenem. (Funded by Achaogen and the Biomedical Advanced Research and Development Authority; EPIC ClinicalTrials.gov number, NCT02486627.) *Redrafted abstract

"Role of plazomicin in complicated urinary tract infections."

COMMENT

Complicated urinary tract infections are UTIs in patients with underlying anatomical abnormalities or with risk factors such as indwelling urinary catheters. The most common pathogen responsible for complicated UTI is enterobacteriaceae. The emergence of multidrug resistance within this family is the main concern present days. They receive inappropriate antibiotics, with a longer hospital stay at high cost. Delay in treatment may lead to septic shock and death.

The treatment group of drugs includes ciprofloxacin and cephalosporins. Due to the emergence of resistance, carbapenems gained importance, as resistance has been documented in that group also. Need of a new class of drug is essential. Aminoglycosides play a major role in this scenario. Plazomicin is an aminoglycoside, which has the activity of maintaining its function by resisting all the mechanism that can lead to resistance to enterobacteriaceae. It is technically prepared in such a way that it evades modification by aminoglycoside-modifying enzymes.

In this study, patients with complicated UTI were randomly assigned to two groups. One group received plazomicin 15 mg/kg body weight once daily and the other group meropenem 1 g every 8 hours intravenously with the option for oral step-down dose after a minimum of 4 days, for a total of 7–10 days. Levofloxacin was the oral agent used. Creatinine clearance was serially monitored.

The mean duration of intravenous (IV) therapy was 5.5 days in both groups. *Escherichia coli* was the most common pathogen identified, followed by *Klebsiella*. Nearly 28% had extended spectrum β-lactamase type, 30% had multidrug-resistant pathogens and 26% were not susceptible to other aminoglycosides.

The composite cure was established in 88% in plazomicin and 91% in meropenem group at day 5. The cure rate at the test of cure visit was observed in 81.7% in plazomicin group and 70.1% in meropenem group. The addition of oral therapy did not offer any benefit. The microbiological eradication was same in both groups at day 5, but it is increased in plazomicin group at the end of IV therapy. Clinical relapse occurred in 1.6% and 7.1% and microbiological recurrence occurred in 3.7% and 8.1% respectively in plazomicin and meropenem group (**Fig. 1**).

The decline in renal function was seen in 3.6% in plazomicin and 1.3% in meropenem group. No deaths were documented during the trial period. All the above findings prove that plazomicin was noninferior to meropenem in the treatment of complicated UTI.

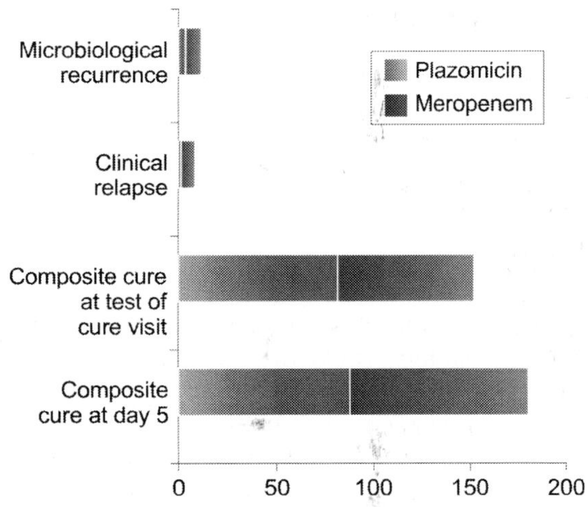

FIG. 1: Primary and additional efficacy endpoints.

Key Messages

- *Plazomicin can be used as a once daily regimen for complicated UTI.*
- *Renal function should be monitored at regular intervals.*

ARTICLE 12

Evaluation of the relationship between IL-12, IL-13 and TNF-α gene polymorphisms with the susceptibility to brucellosis: a case control study

kazemi S, Vaisi-Raygani A, Keramat F, Saidijam M, Soltanian AR, Alahgholi-Hajibehzad M, et al. Evaluation of the relationship between IL-12, IL-13 and TNF-α gene polymorphisms with the susceptibility to brucellosis: a case control study.
BMC Infect Dis. 2019;19:1036.

Abstract

Background: The cytokine gene polymorphism is important for the genetic susceptibility of infectious diseases. The aim of the present study was to investigate the relationship between tumor necrosis factor (TNF)-α, interleukin (IL)-12, and IL-13 gene polymorphisms and predisposition to brucellosis.

Methods: In this study, 107 patients with brucellosis and 107 healthy individuals were evaluated. The single-nucleotide polymorphisms (SNPs) of TNF-α (−238 G/A) and IL-12 (+1,188 A/C) were done by amplification refractory mutation system-polymerase chain reaction (ARMS-PCR), and IL-13 genotyping at positions −1,512 (A/C) and −1,112 (C/T) was analyzed by restriction fragment length polymorphism-polymerase chain reaction (RFLP-PCR) methods. IL-12, IL-13, and TNF-α serum levels were measured by a sandwich enzyme-linked immunosorbent assay (ELISA).

Results: IL-13 (−1,512 A/C) was associated with brucellosis risk in dominant model [OR (95% CI) = 2.17 (1.02–4.62)], p-value = 0.041. However, there was no difference in allele and genotype frequencies of TNF-α (−238 G/A), IL-12 (+1,188 A/C) and IL-13 [−1,512 (A/C) and −1,112 (C/T)] between patients and controls. Serum levels of IL-12 and TNF-α were significantly more frequent in the patients than in the control groups.

Conclusion: The IL-13 gene polymorphism can be used as a biomarker for detecting susceptibility to *Brucella* disease.

"Gene polymorphisms of interleukins and brucellosis."

COMMENT

Brucellosis is caused by *Brucella species*, a gram-negative, nonspore-forming, nonmotile, intracellular bacterium. The use of unpasteurized dairy products and inhalation of contaminated aerosols are the common modes of transmission. It causes diseases in both humans and animals. Active brucellosis in humans is characterized by fever, sweating, weight loss, arthralgia, hepatosplenomegaly, and endocarditis. It causes abortion, placental retention, and infertility in animals. It is diagnosed by clinical features, positive blood culture, as well as by polymerase chain reaction (PCR).

There are multiple factors involved in the pathogenesis of infectious diseases. It includes immunity, environment, and genetics. The genetic polymorphisms of cytokines play a key role in the genetic susceptibility of infectious diseases. This study helps in finding a relationship between interleukin (IL)-12, IL-13, and tumor necrosis factor (TNF)-α gene polymorphisms and their serum concentrations and its susceptibility to brucellosis.

■ ROLE OF CYTOKINES

Cytokines set the main pathway for adaptive immunity. The increased or decreased expression of cytokines plays a major role in the pathogenicity.

TH1 cells are essential for disease prevention and TH2 cells are responsible for disease progression. When the infection sets in, phagocytes are activated with release of proinflammatory cytokines. IL-12 stimulates TH1 cells, activates macrophages, and promotes intracellular killing of bacteria. IL-13 downregulates TH1 cells, promoting infection. Genomic deoxyribonucleic acid (DNA) was extracted, processed, and genotyping done. Serum levels are analyzed by enzyme-linked immunosorbent assay (ELISA).

Interleukin-13 was associated with brucellosis risk in dominant model. Alleles and genotypic frequencies of IL-12, IL-13, and TNF α were not statistically significant. The serum levels of IL-12 and TNF-α show a statistically significant correlation between cases and controls. This study also highlights that there is no significant associations between serum levels of interleukins and gene polymorphisms (**Table 1**).

In other studies, TNF-α, GG genotype was a protective factor and GA genotype were a risk factor against developing brucellosis.

In this study, patients had elevated serum levels of IL-12 and TNF-α compared to controls. Also, there is no documented evidence of association of IL-13 polymorphisms and infectious diseases except for brucellosis. The study with higher population is needed for better accuracy in the future.

TABLE 1: Serum levels of interleukins with brucellosis patients and controls.

Interleukin (pg/mL)	Patients	Controls	p value
TNF	15.20	1.34	<0.001
IL-12	4.39	2.68	<0.001
IL-13	4.23	2.30	<0.308

(IL: interleukin; TNF: tumor necrosis factor)

Key Message

◉ *Interleukin-13 gene polymorphism can be used as a biomarker for detecting susceptibility to Brucella disease.*

ARTICLE 13

Low serum estradiol levels are related to *Mycobacterium avium* complex lung disease: a cross-sectional study

Uwamino Y, Nishimura T, Sato Y, Tamizu E, Asakura T, Uno S, et al. Low serum estradiol levels are related to *Mycobacterium avium* complex lung disease: a cross-sectional study.
BMC Infect Dis. 2019;19:1055.

Abstract

Background: The risk factors for *Mycobacterium avium* complex lung disease (MAC-LD) are not well known. We hypothesized that low serum estradiol (E2) levels are related to MAC-LD, as most patients with MAC-LD are postmenopausal women.

Methods: This cross-sectional study compared patients with MAC-LD and healthy controls. Study subjects were postmenopausal women aged 65 years or younger. Serum testosterone, dehydroepiandrosterone sulfate (DHEA-S), and E2 levels were measured and categorized as high or low based on median levels. We performed multivariate analysis, receiver operating characteristic (ROC) curve analysis, and age- and body mass index (BMI)-matched subgroup analysis to evaluate the association between low serum E2 levels and MAC-LD. Additionally, using blood samples obtained for other clinical studies, the levels of sex steroid hormones were compared between age- and BMI-matched MAC-LD and bronchiectasis female patients without nontuberculosis mycobacterial infections (non-NTM BE).

Results: Forty-two patients with MAC-LD and 91 healthy controls were included. The median E2 (2.20 pg/mL vs. 15.0 pg/mL, p < 0.001), testosterone (0.230 ng/L vs. 0.250 ng/L, p = 0.005), and DHEA-S (82.5 µg/dL vs. 114.0 µg/dL, p < 0.001) levels were lower in the MAC-LD group than in the control group. Multivariate analysis revealed that low serum E2 [adjusted odds ratio (OR) 34.62; 95% confidence interval (CI) 6.02–199.14) was independently related to MAC-LD, whereas, low DHEA-S and testosterone were not. ROC analysis illustrated a strong relationship between low serum E2 levels and MAC-LD (area under the curve 0.947; 95% CI 0.899–0.995). Even the age- and BMI-matched subgroup analysis of 17 MAC-LD patients and 17 healthy controls showed lower serum E2 in MAC-LD patients than in healthy controls. Additionally, serum E2 levels of 20 MAC-LD patients were lower than plasma E2 levels of 11 matched non-NTM BE patients (1.79 pg/mL vs. 11.0 pg/mL, p < 0.001).

Conclusion: Low serum E2 levels were strongly related to MAC-LD in postmenopausal women.

"Serum estradiol and Mycobacterium avium complex lung disease."

COMMENT

Mycobacterium avium complex lung disease (MAC-LD) is the most common pulmonary nontuberculous mycobacterial (NTM) infection in US and Japan. MAC-LD is a chronic, refractory, and respiratory infection with unclear pathogenesis and unclear risk factors. This study is done to determine the role of serum estradiol levels in the causation of MAC-LD, as most of the patients with this disease are postmenopausal women. Glycopeptidolipid (GPL) is a specific antigen that is present in the cell wall of MAC. The presence of anti-GPL antibodies against the lipid antigen glycopeptidolipid is specific for MAC infection. These antibodies are more common in middle-aged and elderly women. This finding is a factor for the hypothesis of this study implicating that decrease in sex hormone levels might represent a risk factor for MAC infection.

■ SERUM ESTRADIOL AND MAC

Long-term estradiol administration

↓

↑ Interleukin-1 beta secretion

↓

Release of nitric oxide synthase

↓

Enhance the killing of intracellular mycobacteria by macrophages

The above mechanism indicates that estradiol plays a protective role in MAC infection indicating that low levels of estradiol is an independent risk factor for MAC infection. The number of years after menopause strongly correlated with age.

They also compared the serum sex steroid hormone levels of MAC-LD patients with plasma sex steroid hormone levels of bronchiectasis patients without NTM infections in order to prove that sex steroid hormone levels were specifically associated with MAC-LD (**Table 1**).

Serum E2, testosterone, and DHEA-S levels were significantly lower in the MAC-LD group than in the control group. According to logistic regression analysis, low serum E2 levels were independently related to MAC-LD. There is a great difficulty in diagnosing MAC-LD without microbiology and imaging. The results of this study indicate that low E2 levels may be used as a predictor for MAC infection.

This study has some limitations. The circadian rhythm variation may affect the levels of hormones especially testosterone. Further studies with a large population are needed to assess whether low serum E2 is associated with other chronic lung infection. It is still unclear whether the decline in E2 levels precedes MAC-LD or MAC-LD reduces the concentration of E2 level.

TABLE 1: Serum levels of sex hormones.

Serum levels	MAC-LD	Control
Serum E2	2.20 pg/mL	15.0 pg/mL
Testosterone	0.23 ng/L	0.25 ng/L
DHEA-S	82.5 µg/dL	114.0 µg/dL

(E2: estradiol; MAC-LD: *Mycobacterium avium* complex lung disease; DHEA-S: dehydroepiandrosterone sulfate)

Key Message

⊙ *Low serum E2 levels were independently related to MAC-LD in middle-aged and presenile postmenopausal women.*

ARTICLE 14

Outcomes of bedaquiline treatment in patients with multidrug-resistant tuberculosis

Mbuagbaw L, Guglielmetti L, Hewison C, Bakare N, Bastard M, Caumes E, et al. Outcomes of bedaquiline treatment in patients with multidrug-resistant tuberculosis.
Emerg Infect Dis. 2019;25:936-43.

Abstract*

World Health Organization recommends bedaquiline for the multidrug-resistant (MDR) and extensively drug-resistant (XDR) tuberculosis (TB) treatment. Data from five cohorts of patients (who were treated with bedaquiline in Armenia, France, Georgia, and South Africa and in a multicountry study) was pooled in this study. The rate of culture conversion to negative at 6 months (by the end of 6 months of treatment) was 78% [95% confidence interval (CI) 73.5% to 81.9%], and the treatment success rate was 65.8% (95% CI 59.9% to 71.3%). The death rate was 11.7% (95% CI 7.0% to 19.1%). In 91.1% (95% CI 82.2% to 95.8%) of the patients, >1 adverse events were present, and serious adverse event was noted in 11.2% (95% CI 5.0% to 23.2%) patients. Lung cavitations were found to be consistently associated with unfavorable outcomes. In MDR and XDR-TB treatment regimens, use of bedaquiline seems to be effective as well as safe in different settings; however, the certainty of evidence was found to be very low. *Redrafted abstract

"Role of bedaquiline in MDR TB."

COMMENT

Tuberculosis accounts for 10 million new cases worldwide. Out of that, 558,000 were multidrug-resistant (MDR) tuberculosis (TB). MDR-TB caused 230,000 deaths worldwide.

- *MDR TB*: It refers to resistance to rifampicin and isoniazid, with or without resistance to other first-line drugs.
- *Extensively drug-resistant TB (XDR-TB)*: It refers to MDR-TB with additional resistance to any fluoroquinolones and to any of the three second-line injectables.

The treatment of MDR and XDR-TB is complex with multiple drugs, costly with long duration of treatment and its adverse effects. Bedaquiline was recommended by WHO in the treatment of MDR-TB in 2018, including children >6 years of age. Bedaquiline belongs to the group of diarylquinoline class used to treat MDR-TB.

This study shows an overall culture conversion rate of 78.0% with bedaquiline along with standard regimen for a period of 6 months. The cure rate was 60.1%, treatment success 65.8%, death rate 11.7%, treatment failure 5.1%, and lost to follow-up 14.8% (**Fig. 1**). The culture conversion rate was less in patients with more severe resistance profile,

FIG. 1: Death rate before and after bedaquiline.

with lung cavitations and in those with human immunodeficiency virus (HIV) infection.

Around 11% experienced serious adverse events. The data in this study indicates absence of bedaquiline effect on QT prolongation and highlights the low rates of cardiotoxicity. There was no correlation between QT prolongation and extended bedaquiline use. The lower death rate supports the use of bedaquiline in MDR-TB.

The routine use of bedaquiline for >6 months in MDR-TB is not advisable by WHO. It can be used beyond 24 weeks, if the regimen is unlikely to cure the disease or with a high risk of drug resistance. The absence of certain statistic variables and absence of comparative data with non-bedaquiline patients limit the inferences. The findings are taken from a generalized population, which is a big strength to this study.

Key Messages

⊙ *Bedaquiline is safe and effective for MDR-TB along with standard regimen.*

⊙ *Poor outcomes in patients with severe drug resistance and with lung cavitations.*

ARTICLE 15

A randomized, controlled trial of Ebola virus disease therapeutics

Mulangu S, Dodd LE, Davey RT Jr, Mbaya OT, Proschan M, Mukadi D, et al. A randomized, controlled trial of Ebola virus disease therapeutics.
N Engl J Med. 2019;381:2293-303.

Abstract*

Background: Presently, many experimental therapeutics for Ebola virus disease (EVD) are developed; however, there is a need for assessment of safety and efficacy of the most promising therapies in a randomized controlled trial.

Methods: In the study, a trial was conducted in the Democratic Republic of Congo (where an outbreak began in August, 2018) including four investigational therapies for EVD. Study population included patients (of any age) with positive result for Ebola virus ribonucleic acid (RNA) on reverse transcriptase polymerase chain reaction (RT-PCR) assay. Standard care was provided to all patients, who were randomly assigned in a 1:1:1:1 ratio to either intravenous administration of the triple monoclonal antibody ZMapp (i.e., control group), or the antiviral agent remdesivir (which is the single monoclonal antibody MAb114), or the triple monoclonal antibody REGN-EB3. In a later version of the protocol, addition of the REGN-EB3 group was done; therefore, data of such patients were compared with ZMapp group patients who were enrolled at or after the time the additon of REGN-EB3 group was done (i.e., ZMapp subgroup). The primary endpoint considered in the study was death at 28 days.

Results: From November 20th, 2018 to August 9th, 2019, total 681 patients were enrolled; at this time, it was ribonucleic acid (RNA) by the data and safety monitoring board that patients should be assigned only to the MAb114 and REGN-EB3 groups for remaining duration of trial. This recommendation was based on the findings of an interim analysis, which demonstrated superiority of these groups to ZMapp and remdesivir in terms of mortality. At 28 days, 35.1% (61/174) patients died in the MAb114 group, in comparison to 49.7% (84/169) in the ZMapp group (p = 0.007), and 33.5% (52/155) patients in the REGN-EB3 group died, in comparison to 51.3% (79/154) in the ZMapp subgroup (p = 0.002). Improved survival was associated with a shorter duration of symptoms before admission and reduced baseline values not only for viral load, but also for serum creatinine and aminotransferase levels. The four serious adverse events found in patients were considered to be potentially associated with the trial drugs.

Conclusion: MAb114 and REGN-EB3 were found to be superior to ZMapp in decreasing mortality from EVD. During disease outbreaks, scientifically and ethically sound clinical research can be carried out, which can help in informing about the outbreak response. (Funded by the National Institute of Allergy and Infectious Diseases and others; PALM ClinicalTrials.gov number, NCT03719586.) *Redrafted abstract

"Ebola virus disease therapeutics."

COMMENT

Ebola virus outbreak is more common in Democratic Region of Congo. In order to prevent further outbreaks, they conducted the following trial of four investigational therapies—its safety and efficacy.

The persons with positive reverse transcriptase polymerase chain reaction (RT-PCR) within 3 days before screening were included in the study. The primary endpoint of this study was death at 28 days.

■ TRIAL AGENTS AND THEIR DOSAGE

- ZMapp—50 mg/kg body weight every third beginning on day 1 (total 3 doses).
- Remdesivir—200 mg for adults, loading dose on day 1, followed by maintenance dose 100 mg starting on day 2, and continuing for 9–13 days.
- MAb114—50 mg/kg, administered as a single infusion on day 1.
- REGN–EB3—150 mg/kg, as a single infusion on day 1.

The common symptoms encountered in this group were diarrhea, fever, abdominal pain, headache, and vomiting. Around 25% of the patients had received ZEBOV-GP vaccine.

The mean baseline creatinine and aspartate aminotransferase values were higher in the ZMapp and remdesivir group. The overall mortality was around 43%. The patients with high viral load have a high mortality. The percentage of patients died in the MAb114 and REGN-EB3 was lower when compared to other groups. The time to the first negative result was shorter in the MAb114 and REGN-EB3 group than in the ZMapp group. In the remdesivir group, the estimated mortality exceeded 50%. Patients who received vaccination have a lower mortality.

■ PROGNOSTIC INDICATORS OF DEATH

- Higher viral loads
- Higher values of creatinine.
- Increased aspartate aminotransferase (AST)/ alanine aminotransferase (ALT).
- Long duration of symptoms at enrollment.
- Baseline nucleoprotein cycle threshold (Ct) value.

Four adverse events have been documented leading to death—two in the ZMapp group and one in the remdesivir group. But, cause of death could not be readily distinguished from underlying fulminant Ebola virus disease (EVD). The delay in treatment, i.e., receiving full dose of regimen, influences the disease outcome. Early diagnosis and treatment are associated with increased survival. The baseline values of creatinine and aminotransferases were high in the ZMapp and remdesivir groups, which imply the patients in that group are already sick, which would have accounted for the difference in outcome.

Key Message

⊛ *The efficacy of these drugs, rather than safety, may provide rationale use of these drugs in the future.*

ARTICLE 16

Safety and immunogenicity of the oral, inactivated, enterotoxigenic *Escherichia coli* vaccine ETVAX in Bangladeshi children and infants: a double-blind, randomised, placebo-controlled phase 1/2 trial

Qadri F, Akhtar M, Bhuiyan TR, Chowdhury MI, Ahmed T, Rafique TA, et al. Safety and immunogenicity of the oral, inactivated, enterotoxigenic Escherichia coli vaccine ETVAX in Bangladeshi children and infants: a double-blind, randomised, placebo-controlled phase 1/2 trial.
Lancet Infect Dis. 2020;20:208-19.

Abstract

Background: Enterotoxigenic *Escherichia coli* causes diarrhea, leading to substantial mortality and morbidity in children, but no specific vaccine exists. This trial tested an oral, inactivated, enterotoxigenic *E. coli* vaccine (ETVAX), which has been previously shown to be safe and highly immunogenic in Swedish and Bangladeshi adults. We tested the safety and immunogenicity of ETVAX, consisting of four *E. coli* strains overexpressing the most prevalent colonization factors (CFA/I, CS3, CS5, and CS6) and a toxoid (LCTBA) administered with or without a double-mutant heat-labile enterotoxin (dmLT) as an adjuvant, in Bangladeshi children.

Methods: We did a randomized, double-blind, placebo-controlled, dose-escalation, age-descending, phase 1/2 trial in Dhaka, Bangladesh. Healthy children in one of three age groups (24–59 months, 12–23 months, and 6–11 months) were eligible. Children were randomly assigned with block randomization to receive either ETVAX, with or without dmLT, or placebo. ETVAX [half (5.5×10^{10} cells), quarter (2.5×10^{10} cells), or eighth (1.25×10^{10} cells) adult dose], with or without dmLT adjuvant (2.5 µg, 5.0 µg, or 10.0 µg), or placebo were administered orally in two doses 2 weeks apart. Investigators and participants were masked to treatment allocation. The primary endpoint was safety and tolerability, assessed in all children who received at least one dose of vaccine. Antibody responses to vaccine antigens, defined as at least a two-time increase in antibody levels between baseline and post-immunization, were assessed as secondary endpoints. This trial is registered with ClinicalTrials.gov, NCT02531802.

Findings: Between December 7, 2015 and January 10, 2017, we screened 1,500 children across the three age groups, of whom 430 were enrolled and randomly assigned to the different treatment groups (130 aged 24–59 months, 100 aged 12–23 months, and 200 aged 6–11 months). All participants received at least one dose of vaccine. No solicited adverse events occurred that were greater than moderate in severity, and most were mild. The most common solicited event was vomiting [10 (8%) of 130 patients aged 24–59 months, 13 (13%) of 100 aged 12–23 months, and 29 (15%) of 200 aged 6–11 months; mostly of mild severity], which appeared related to dose and age. The addition of dmLT did not modify the safety profile. Three serious adverse events occurred, but they were not considered related to the study drug. Mucosal IgA antibody responses in lymphocyte secretions were detected against all primary vaccine antigens (CFA/I, CS3, CS5, CS6, and the LCTBA toxoid) in most participants in the two older age groups; whereas, such responses to four of the five antigens were less frequent and of lower magnitude in infants aged 6–11 months than in older children. Fecal secretory IgA immune responses were recorded against all vaccine antigens in infants aged 6–11 months. Around 78 (56%) of 139 infants aged 6–11 months who were vaccinated developed mucosal responses against at least three of the vaccine antigens versus 14 (29%) of 49 of the infants given placebo. Addition of the adjuvant dmLT enhanced the magnitude, breadth, and kinetics (based on number of responders after the first dose of vaccine) of immune responses in infants.

Interpretation: The encouraging safety and immunogenicity of ETVAX and benefit of dmLT adjuvant in young children support its further assessment for protective efficacy in children in enterotoxigenic *E. coli*-endemic areas.

Funding: PATH (Bill and Melinda Gates Foundation and the UK's Department for International Development), the Swedish Research Council, and The Swedish Foundation for Strategic Research.

"Safety and immunogenicity of ETVAX in children and infants."

COMMENT

Escherichia coli is one of the most common bacteria causing diarrhea in children. The mortality and morbidity are high. Till now, no vaccine exists. This study is done to emphasize the safety, largest tolerable dose, and immunogenicity of ETVAX (enterotoxigenic *E. coli* vaccine) in children. This vaccine has already been tested in adults and found to have a good safety profile.

They divided the children into three groups (4–59 months, 1–3 months, and 6–11 months). They were randomly immunized with oral doses of ETVAX at 2 weeks interval with or without double-mutant heat-labile enterotoxin (dmLT). The primary endpoint was safety and tolerability of vaccine. The secondary endpoint was to assess the antibody responses to primary antigens (CFA/I, CS3, CS5, and CS6 LTB) before and postvaccination.

All patients received at least one dose of the vaccine. There are only three severe adverse events documented, which are not related to the trial. The most common event is vomiting, which is mild and improved without treatment within 1 day. This vomiting is inversely related to the dose and age of the child. Around 7% had mild fever, which is also transient.

The antibody responses in mucosa, feces, serum, and plasma have been estimated. The mucosal IgA response against lymphocyte secretions (ALS) is high in older children and it was detected for all the primary vaccine antigens, somewhat lower for CS6. The response decreases, as the age decreases. Fecal secretary IgA responses were significantly high in all primary antigens in infants 6–11 months. Fecal lactoferrin levels were also measured in order to rule out breast milk contamination. The addition of dmLT to the schedule has no effect on safety, but it enhanced the immune responses in infants. The ALS responses are analyzed by highly sensitive electrochemiluminescence assay (**Fig. 1**).

The IGg responses were also induced, but of lower magnitude. No difference of immunogenicity was observed between different

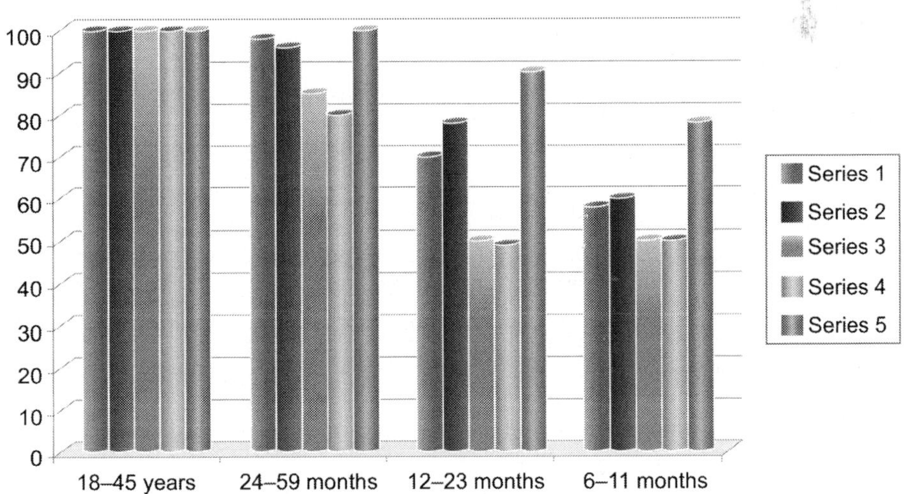

FIG. 1: Mucosal antibody responses against five primary antigens in different age groups.

doses of vaccine or with and without dmLT. The frequency of responders to different antigens was greater in ALS and fecal samples than in plasma samples. The immunological effect of reduced dosage of vaccine might be mitigated by the coadministration of dmLT. The use of electrochemiluminescence for assay is the main strength of this study.

Key Messages

- ⊙ *The largest tolerable dose of ETVAX was assessed significantly in this study for different age population.*
- ⊙ *The vaccine was safe, without any adverse effects.*

ARTICLE 17

Evaluation of GeneXpert MTB/RIF system performances in the diagnosis of extrapulmonary tuberculosis

Mechal Y, Benaissa E, Mrimar NE, Benlahlou Y, Bssaibis F, Zegmout A, et al. Evaluation of GeneXpert MTB/RIF system performances in the diagnosis of extrapulmonary tuberculosis.
BMC Infect Dis. 2019;19:1069.

Abstract

Background: Tuberculosis represents a serious public health problem and a significant diagnostic and therapeutic challenge worldwide. Molecular diagnostic techniques are crucial in the World Health Organization's new tuberculosis control strategy. This study aims to evaluate the performance of GeneXpert *Mycobacterium tuberculosis* (MTB)/rifampicin (RIF) (Cepheid Sunnyvale, CA, United States) in diagnosis of extrapulmonary tuberculosis then compare its performance in detecting RIF resistance to genotype MTBDRplus (HAIN Life Sciences, Nehren, Germany).

Methods: Samples from pulmonary and/or extrapulmonary origins were analyzed in a 21-month retrospective study. Samples were sent to the bacteriology laboratory for *Mycobacterium tuberculosis* detection using conventional bacteriological and molecular methods (GeneXpert MTB/RIF and MTBDRplus). Sensitivity and specificity were calculated for the stained smear and GeneXpert according to culture (Gold Standard) as well as for GeneXpert MTB/RIF in both negative and positive microscopy tuberculosis cases. Data's statistical analysis was performed with SPSS13.0 software.

Results: Seven hundred fourteen patients' samples were analyzed; the average age was 47.21 ± 19.98 years with a male predominance (66.4%). Out of 714 samples, 285 were from pulmonary and 429 were from extrapulmonary origins. The positivity rates for microscopy, GeneXpert MTB/RIF, and culture were 12.88, 20.59, and 15.82%, respectively. These rates were 18.9, 23.85, and 20.35% for pulmonary samples and 9.71, 18.41, and 12.82% for extrapulmonary samples, respectively. The sensitivity and specificity of GeneXpert MTB/RIF were almost the same in both pulmonary and extrapulmonary samples [(78.2 and 90.4%) and (79.3 and 90.3%)], respectively. RIF resistance rate found by GeneXpert MTB/RIF was 0.84%. Comparison of RIF resistance obtained by GeneXpert MTB/RIF and genotype MTBDRplus showed 100% agreement between the two techniques for studied samples.

Conclusion: This confirms GeneXpert MTB/RIF advantage for tuberculosis diagnosis, particularly extrapulmonary tuberculosis with negatively stained smear. The performance of GeneXpert and genotype MTBDRplus are similar in detection of RIF resistance. However, variability of detection performance according to tuberculosis endemicity deserves more attention in the choice of screening techniques of RIF resistance, hence, the interest of conducting comparative studies of detection performance under low and medium endemicity on large samples of tuberculosis populations.

"Role of GeneXpert MTB/RIF in the diagnosis of extrapulmonary tuberculosis."

COMMENT

Tuberculosis (TB) is a global problem worldwide. There are 10.4 million new cases of TB and 1.7 million deaths related to TB worldwide. Extrapulmonary TB contributes around 14%. The diagnosis of extrapulmonary TB is a really challenging task for the clinicians. The variable clinical presentation and difficult accessibility for samples with paucibacillary samples, all reduce the sensitivity of conventional diagnostic tests.

At present, TB is diagnosed by culture methods using clinical samples such as sputum, bronchial aspirations, bronchoalveolar lavage (BAL), cerebrospinal fluid (CSF), and tissue samples. It has several disadvantages such as operator dependency, need for specialized laboratories, high cost, and long duration for reporting. The use of molecular diagnostic tests can increase the diagnostic accuracy and reduce time consumption. This study helps in the evaluation of the performance of GeneXpert in the diagnosis of extrapulmonary TB and to compare with genotype MTBDRplus in detecting rifampicin (RIF) resistance.

◼ MOLECULAR TESTS

- *GeneXpert Mycobacterium tuberculosis (MTB)/ RIF*: The only molecular test approved by WHO. It can detect the presence of TB as well as the presence of mutations responsible for RIF resistance. Result can be obtained within hours.
- *Genotype MTBDRplus*: It is a multiplex deoxyribonucleic acid (DNA) amplification test. It is also used for detection of mycobacteria as well as drug resistance to RIF and isoniazid in a single test. Reports can be obtained within few hours.

The positivity rates for microscopy, GeneXpert MTB/RIF, and culture were 12.88, 0.59, and 15.82%, respectively (**Fig. 1**).

In culture-negative patients, GeneXpert identified 9.65% of TB. The lymph node samples of GeneXpert yield a high rate of positivity in culture and microscopy negative samples.

The detection of RIF resistance by GeneXpert is 0.84%, which showed a 100% agreement with MTBDRplus. GeneXpert has 20% more sensitive than microscopy for extrapulmonary samples. This makes the clinician to arrive at an early diagnosis and treatment. The reports may vary according to endemicity and the nature of the site sampled. The negative predictive value of GeneXpert MTB/RIF exceeds 99%, making it possible to exclude with assurance the diagnosis.

The performance determination of GeneXpert MTB/RIF is related to the nature of probes used for the detection of mutations. The adjustment of detection probes is essential for the reliability of GeneXpert.

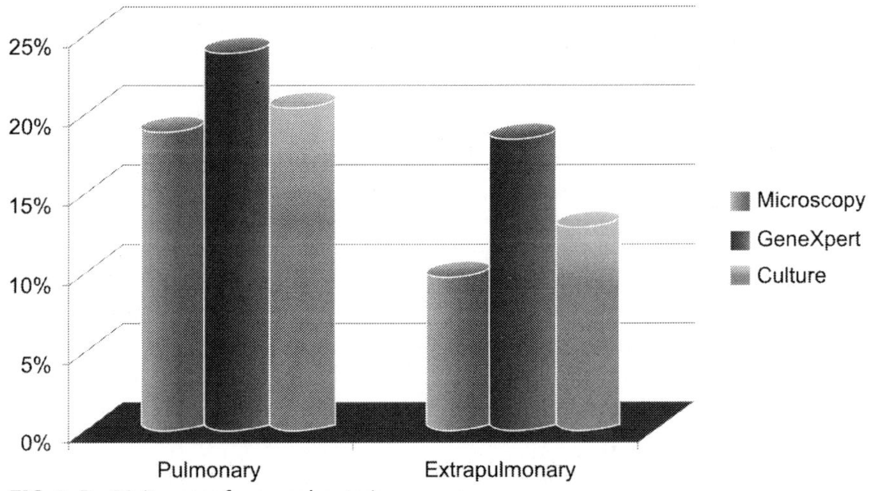

FIG. 1: Positivity rates for mycobacteria.

Key Message

- GeneXpert is a test of choice for the diagnosis of extrapulmonary TB, especially in culture- or microscopy-negative samples.

ARTICLE 18

Systemic RAGE ligands are upregulated in tuberculosis individuals with diabetes co-morbidity and modulated by antituberculosis treatment and metformin therapy

Kumar NP, Moideen K, Nancy A, Viswanathan V, Shruthi BS, Sivakumar S, et al. Systemic RAGE ligands are upregulated in tuberculosis individuals with diabetes co-morbidity and modulated by anti-tuberculosis treatment and metformin therapy. *BMC Infect Dis. 2019;19:1039.*

Abstract

Background: Ligands of the receptor for advanced glycation end products (RAGE) are key signaling molecules in the innate immune system, but their role in tuberculosis-diabetes comorbidity (TB-DM) has not been investigated.

Methods: We examined the systemic levels of soluble RAGE (sRAGE), advanced glycation end products (AGE), S100A12, and high mobility group box 1 (HMGB1) in participants with either TB-DM, TB, DM, or healthy controls (HC).

Results: Systemic levels of AGE, sRAGE, and S100A12 were significantly elevated in TB-DM and DM in comparison to TB and HC. During follow-up, AGE, sRAGE, and S100A12 remained significantly elevated in TB-DM compared to TB at 2nd month and 6th month of anti-tuberculosis treatment (ATT). RAGE ligands were increased in TB-DM individuals with bilateral and cavitary disease. sRAGE and S100A12 correlated with glycosylated hemoglobin levels. Within the TB-DM group, those with known diabetes (KDM) revealed significantly increased levels of AGE and sRAGE compared to newly diagnosed DM (NDM). KDM participants on metformin treatment exhibited significantly diminished levels of AGE and sRAGE in comparison to those on nonmetformin regimens.

Conclusion: Our data demonstrate that RAGE ligand levels reflect disease severity and extent in TB-DM, distinguish KDM from NDM and are modulated by metformin therapy.

"Systemic RAGE ligands are upregulated in TB-DM individuals and modulated by ATT and metformin therapy."

COMMENT

Ligands of RAGE (receptors of advanced glycation end products) are the key signaling molecules in innate immune system. But, their receiver operating characteristic (ROC) in tuberculosis (TB) with diabetes mellitus (DM) has not been coinvestigated so far.

Diabetes worsens both innate and adaptive immunity, which increases risk of poor TB outcome, poorer clinical presentation, and increases TB mortality.

The RAGE ligands are known to accumulate more in DM and in chronic inflammatory conditions like TB.

In our study, we segregated the subjects into four groups as TB-DM, TB alone, DM alone, and healthy controls. We evaluated the systemic levels of RAGE ligands:

- At baseline and with antituberculosis treatment (ATT).
- At 2 months after completion of intensive phase of ATT.
- At 6 months after completion of ATT.

The data collected in the study were analyzed and completed using GraphPad PRISM version.

Activated glycation end products (AGEs) are elevated in DM with or without TB and it is much more elevated in the presence of TB infection with DM. Known diabetics with high glycosylated hemoglobin (HbA1c) show elevated levels of AGE and patients who are on treatment with metformin for DM show relatively low RAGE. This elevated age is consistent in the baseline, at 2 months and even after 6 months endpoints. This shows age to relate more to DM rather than TB alone and metformin tends to modulate age.

Soluble receptor for advanced glycation end products (sRAGE) is similar to age and is elevated in TB-DM than TB alone or DM alone. It is proportional to the amount of TB infection as evident by high levels in diabetics, bilateral disease, and cavitatory TB. It is also modulated by metformin. Another ligand scoo is also upregulated in the similar way and modulated by metformin treatment in TB-DM.

Key Messages

- *Diabetic patients who acquire TB exhibit profound elevation of RAGE ligands—RAGE, AGE, sRAGE, scoo, and HMGBb1—which in turn elevates proinflammatory cytokines leading to severe form of TB infection with poor outcome.*
- *Diabetic patients with good control of glycemia with metformin show better results and lesser complicated TB owing to downregulation of RAGE ligands.*

ARTICLE 19

Efficacy and risk of harms of repeat ivermectin mass drug administrations for control of malaria (RIMDAMAL): a cluster-randomised trial

Foy BD, Alout H, Seaman JA, Rao S, Magalhaes T, Wade M, et al. Efficacy and risk of harms of repeat ivermectin mass drug administrations for control of malaria (RIMDAMAL): a cluster-randomised trial.
Lancet. 2019;393:1517-26.

Abstract

Background: Ivermectin is widely used in mass drug administrations for controlling neglected parasitic diseases, and can be lethal to malaria vectors that bite treated humans. Therefore, it could be a new tool to reduce *Plasmodium* transmission. We tested the hypothesis that frequently repeated mass administrations of ivermectin to village residents would reduce clinical malaria episodes in children and would be well tolerated with minimal harms.

Methods: We invited villages (clusters) in Burkina Faso to participate in a single-blind (outcomes assessor), parallel-assignment, two-arm, cluster-randomized trial over the 2015 rainy season. Villages were assigned (1:1) by random draw to either the intervention group or the control group. In both groups, all eligible participants who consented to the treatment and were at least 90 cm in height received single oral doses of ivermectin (150–200 µg/kg) and albendazole (400 mg), and those in the intervention group received five further doses of ivermectin alone at 3-week intervals thereafter over the 18-week treatment phase. The primary outcome was cumulative incidence of uncomplicated malaria episodes over 18 weeks (analyzed on a cluster intention-to-treat basis) in an active case detection cohort of children aged 5 years or younger living in the study villages. This trial is registered with ClinicalTrials.gov, number NCT02509481.

Findings: Eight villages agreed to participate, and four were randomly assigned to each group. Around 2,712 participants [1,333 (49%) males and 1,379 (51%) females; median age 15 years (IQR 6–34)], including 590 children aged 5 years or younger, provided consent and were enrolled between May 22 and July 20, 2015 (except for 77 participants enrolled after these dates because of unavailability before the first mass drug administration, travel into the village during the trial, or birth), with 1,447 enrolled into the intervention group and 1,265 into the control group. Around 330 (23%) participants in the intervention group and 233 (18%) in the control group met the exclusion criteria for mass drug administration. Most children in the active case detection cohort were not treated because of height restrictions. Around 14 (4%) children in the intervention group and 10 (4%) in the control group were lost to follow-up. Cumulative malaria incidence was reduced in the intervention group (648 episodes among 327 children; estimated mean 2.00 episodes per child) compared with the control group [647 episodes among 263 children; 2.49 episodes per child; risk difference −0.49 (95% CI −0.79 to −0.21), p = 0.0009, adjusted for sex and clustering]. The risk of adverse events among all participants did not differ between groups [45 events (3%) among 1,447 participants in the intervention group vs. 24 events (2%) among 1,265 in the control group; risk ratio 1.63 (1.01–2.67); risk difference 1·21 (0.04–2.38), p = 0.060], and no adverse reactions were reported.

Interpretation: Frequently repeated mass administrations of ivermectin during the malaria transmission season can reduce malaria episodes among children without significantly increasing harms in the populace.

Funding: Bill and Melinda Gates Foundation.

"Ivermectin mass drug trial for control of malaria."

COMMENT

Malaria is one of the most dreaded tropical diseases. At present, there are several control measures for malaria, which include treatment with antimalarials, vector control with insecticidal mosquito nets, and indoor spraying of insecticides. Even with effective measures, artemisinin-resistant *Plasmodium* and resistance among *Anopheles* vectors threaten the spread in endemic areas. The main target now is to prevent the residual transmission of malaria in order to eliminate malaria.

This study uses ivermectin as a repeated mass drug trial in endemic area. It targets ligand-gated chloride channels leading to disruption of neuromuscular transmission and kills the malaria vector, which fed on treated people. It also helps in inducing transmission-blocking activity against *Plasmodium* in surviving mosquitoes. They targeted children <5 years, as they are at high risk for diseases in endemic areas with impaired immunity. They received ivermectin

(150–200 g/kg) and albendazole 400 mg on day 1, followed by ivermectin alone at 3 weekly intervals for next 5 doses.

The primary outcome of the study states that there was a lower incidence of malaria episodes per child in then intervention group. The proportion of children with zero malaria episodes was more than twice in the intervention group. The median time to malaria episode was also longer (**Fig. 1**).

The entomological data such as human biting rate, weekly entomological inoculation rate, and proportion of parous mosquitoes did not differ between two groups. The patients received fewer mosquito bites during the trial period, evidenced by the lower values of serological reactivity to an *Anopheles* salivary gland. The adverse events have been documented in only 2% of the trail group. This includes vomiting, pruritus, tremors, and edema of limbs, which resolved over the course of time. The mortality was around 20 persons. But, none were related to intervention. The children who suffered multiple episodes of malaria in spite of ivermectin had multiple risk factors. The risk factors are not using mosquito nets, being outside in the evening, failure of artemisinin therapy, incomplete treatment, genetics, and resistance.

The results of the study suggests that repeated mass drug administration of ivermectin has reduced the incidence of malaria in endemic areas among the targeted population with potentially no harm related to drug.

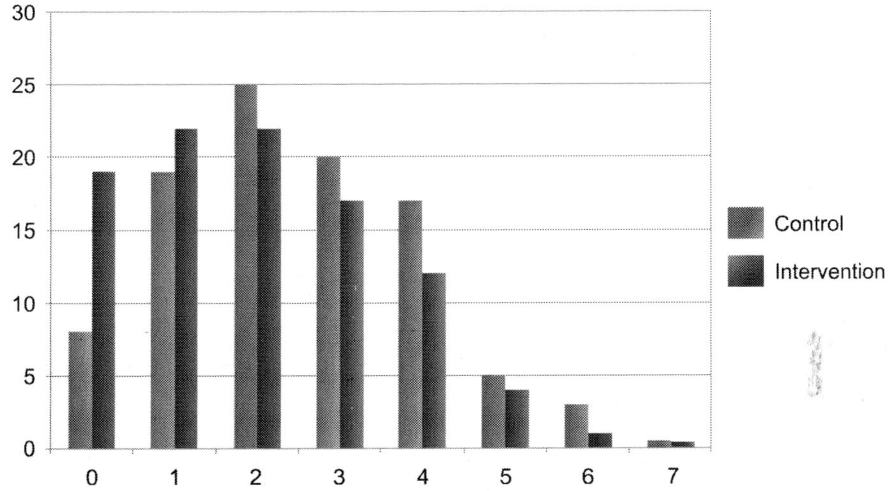

FIG. 1: Frequency distribution of malaria episodes.

Key Messages

⊙ *Ivermectin helps in the reduction of malaria incidence in endemic areas thereby making it a better chemoprophylactic drug.*

⊙ *Drug safety is better with reduced side effects and mortality.*

ARTICLE 20

Vancomycin-resistant *Staphylococcus aureus*: formidable threat or silence before the storm?

Kest H, Kaushik A. Vancomycin-resistant *Staphylococcus aureus*: formidable threat or silence before the storm? *J Infect Dis Epidemiol. 2019;5:1-9.*

Abstract

Globally, *Staphylococcus aureus* (*S. aureus*), notably methicillin-resistant *S. aureus* (MRSA), is a leading cause of morbidity and mortality. Vancomycin is considered a drug of last resort for severe MRSA and other resistant gram-positive infections. Vancomycin enjoyed a high level of success for decades following MRSA outbreaks until recent reports of increasing *S. aureus* minimum inhibitory concentrations (MICs) culminating in high-level vancomycin-resistant *S. aureus* (VRSA), first reported in 2002. Since then, there have been selected case reports of VRSA disease in the US and other countries. The resistance mechanism of VRSA is mediated by the vanA operon carried on the mobile genetic element Tn1546 acquired from vancomycin-resistant *Enterococcus* (VRE); co-infections with VRE have occurred in all cases. There has been no documented person-to-person VRSA transmission. The prolonged interval between exposure to vancomycin and VRSA development and the limited number of cases are reassuring; whether this translates to the needed extended period of clinical quiescence before a global epidemic is unknown. According to the World Health Organization (WHO), *S. aureus* pathogenicity and resistance patterns pose a significant threat to human health worldwide; MRSA, vancomycin intermediate-resistant *S. aureus* (VISA), and VRSA are currently classified as bacteria of high priority with potential to cause significantly devastating worldwide mortality in the absence of effective containment and therapeutic solutions. There are limited choices of drugs that are effective against VRSA; several promising therapeutic options are in research and development phases. VISA and VRSA have also been isolated in animal husbandry from pigs, goats, and cattle.

We review VRSA history and evolution, clinical spectrum, and management. We also speculate on future trends.

"Biography of vancomycin-resistant Staphylococcus aureus."

COMMENT

Staphylococcus aureus is a fascinating bacterium because of its unique spread, disease manifestations, and its peculiar behavior of adaptation to any antibiotic including development of resistance before or immediately following extensive use.

■ RESISTANCE CHRONOLOGY (TABLE 1)

- Penicillin resistance—by the production of penicillinase, potent plasma-encoded beta lactam ring hydrolyzer.
- Methicillin-resistant *S. aureus (MRSA)*—this strain was isolated even without prior exposure to methicillin. This initially occurred in hospitals.
  - *CA-MRSA*: Community-acquired MRSA. Better antimicrobial susceptibility
  - *HA-MRSA*: Healthcare-acquired MRSA. Multidrug resistant

TABLE 1: Timeline of *Staphylococcus aureus* resistance.

Antibiotic	Year introduced	Year resistance identified
Penicillin	1943	1940
Methicillin	1960	1962
Linezolid	2000	2001
Vancomycin	1972	2002
Ceftaroline	2010	2011

- *VISA: Vancomycin intermediate-resistant S. aureus—*
  - MRSA with increased minimum inhibitory concentration (MIC) (4–8 µg/mL) to vancomycin.
- *VRSA: Vancomycin-resistant S. aureus—* Vancomycin is the last resort treatment for MRSA. During the initial days, it was used logically because of the narrow therapeutic window. Later due to the emergence of multiple resistant pathogens with severe diseases, the use of vancomycin increased leading to mutations and the emergence of VRSA. The MIC >16 µg/mL to vancomycin was termed as VRSA.

■ MECHANISM OF RESISTANCE

It is mediated by the vanA operon carried on the mobile genetic element TN1546 acquired from vancomycin-resistant *Enterococcus faecalis*. Horizontal spread can occur through bacterial conjugation. Polymicrobial infections with VRE and MRSA in the hospitals have been an essential factor in VRSA infections. So far, 14 VRSA strains have been documented without any person-to-person transmission.

■ CLINICAL AND LABORATORY STANDARD INSTITUTE (2009)

Breakpoints of *S. aureus* and vancomycin are MIC <2 µg/mL, MIC <4–8 µg/mL and

MIC >16 µg/mL respectively for vancomycin-susceptible, intermediate, and resistant *S. aureus*.

■ MANAGEMENT

- Immunization to promote individual and herd immunity against preventable infections.
- Safe food handling and preparation.
- Handwashing
- Judicious use of antibiotics.
- Strict adherence to infection control guidelines.
- Monitoring and surveillance.

Antibiotics

Refer to **Table 2**.

TABLE 2: List of antibiotics used in vancomycin-resistant *Staphylococcus aureus* (VRSA).

1. Linezolid	2. Daptomycin
3. Tedizolid	4. Telavancin
5. Quinupristin	6. Oritavancin
7. Dalfopristin	8. Ceftaroline

■ FUTURE OF VRSA

The prolonged interval between VRSA use and the emergence of resistance is promising. It is currently classified as a bacterium of high priority with the potential to cause significant mortality.

Key Messages

- *Vancomycin-resistant Staphylococcus aureus is a global threat, currently quite. But, at any time, it may re-emerge and cause a major catastrophe.*
- *Judicious use of antibiotics is essential in reducing the resistance among pathogens.*

ARTICLE 21

Determinants of AIDS and non-AIDS related mortality among people living with HIV in Shiraz, Southern Iran: a 20-year retrospective follow-up study

Gheibi Z, Shayan Z, Joulaei H, Fararouei M, Beheshti S, Shokoohi M. Determinants of AIDS and non-AIDS related mortality among people living with HIV in Shiraz, southern Iran: a 20-year retrospective follow-up study.
BMC Infect Dis. 2019;19:1094.

Abstract

Background: Human immunodeficiency virus (HIV) infection has become a global concern. Determining the factors leading to death among HIV patients helps in controlling acquired immune deficiency syndrome (AIDS) epidemic. Up to now, little is known about mortality and its determinants among people living with HIV in the Middle East and North Africa (MENA) region, including Iran. The purpose of this study was to assess the risk factors of AIDS-related mortality (ARM) and non-AIDS-related mortality (NARM) among people with HIV in Iran.

Methods: This 20-year retrospective study was conducted on 1,160 people with HIV whose data were collected from 1997 to 2017. The association of the study outcomes (ARM and NARM) with various study variables, including demographic status at the time of diagnosis and clinical indexes during the follow-up, was examined to define the predictors of mortality among the patients. Regarding, Cox proportional hazard and competing risk models were fitted and adjusted hazard ratios (AHR), sub-distribution hazard ratio (SHR), and the 95% confidence intervals (CI) were reported.

Results: During the follow-up period, 391 individuals (33.7%) died with 86,375 person-years of follow-up. Of the total deaths, 251 (64.2%) and 140 (35.8%) were ARM and NARM, respectively. Rates of the mortality caused by AIDS and non-AIDS were 3.2 and 4.5 per 1,000 person-months, respectively. Responding to combined antiretroviral treatment (cART) 6 months after initiation, receiving pneumocystis pneumonia (PCP) prophylaxis, and higher CD4 count at diagnosis, reduced the hazard of ARM and NARM. However, older age, late HIV diagnosis, and last HIV clinical stages increased the hazard of AIDS related to mortality. Additionally, male gender, older age, incarceration history, and last HIV clinical stages increased the non-AIDS mortality.

Conclusions: Mortality caused by AIDS and non-AIDS remains high among people with HIV in Iran, particularly among males and those with late diagnosis. It seems that applying effective strategies to identify infected individuals at earlier stage of the infection, and targeting individuals with higher risk of mortality can decrease the mortality rate among HIV-infected people.

"Determinant of mortality in HIV-infected patients—a retrospective study."

COMMENT

Human immunodeficiency virus (HIV) has become a global problem and determining the causes of mortality in patients living with HIV and acquired immune deficiency syndrome (PLHA) may enhance their survival rate.

A 20-year retrospective study from 1997–2017 was conducted on 1,160 people with HIV in Shiraz Southern Iran. Patients who are pregnant and under 16 years of age are excluded from the study.

Causes of death of HIV were classified as ARM— acquired immune deficiency syndrome (AIDS)-related mortality, if occurred due to opportunistic diseases, cervical cancer, and HIV-related causes, and NARM—non-AIDS-related mortality, if it is due to CVS, liver diseases, carcinoma not related to HIV, drug abuse, and accident.

If CD4 counts were recorded 6 months prior to death, it would be classified as ARM, if <200, and NARM, if >200 cells/mm^3.

Other variables such as gender, age of HIV detection, educational and marital status, employment, mode of infection, CD4 counts, access to antiretroviral treatment (ART), pneumocystis pneumonia (PCP) prophylaxis, any other coinfections, tuberculosis (TB), stage of HIV on detection were also recorded.

All data are analyzed and compiled by Cox-model and competing risk analysis method. On analyzing the data, the cumulative incidence of ARM was more when compared to NARM. ARM shows a variable pattern depending on the ART program implemented by the government over the period of 20 years, whereas NARM remained fairly stable (**Fig. 1**).

AIDS-related mortalities were mainly contributed by male gender, late detection of HIV, old age, low CD4 count at the time of detection, associated opportunistic infections, TB, drug addiction, etc.

Non-AIDS-related mortality is mainly due to drug overdose, malignancies unrelated to HIV, accidents, smoking, hepatitis, etc.

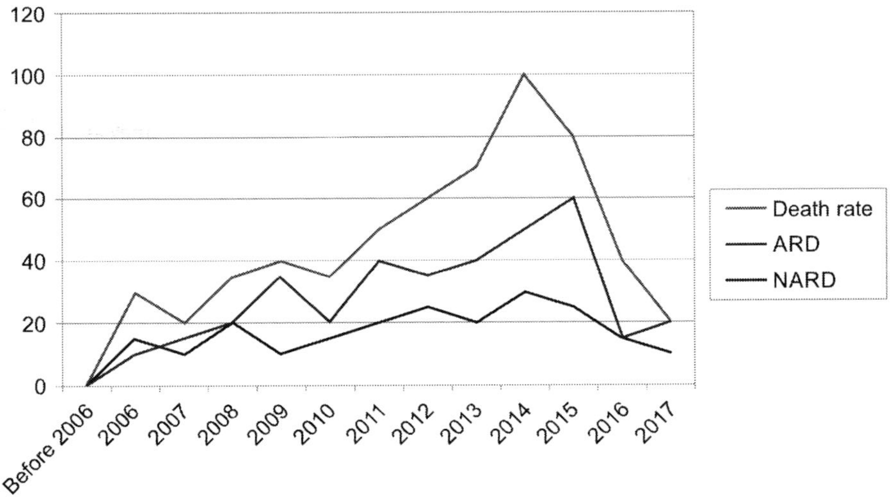

(ARD: AIDS-related death; NARD: non-AIDS-related death)

FIG. 1: Mortality percentage during study period.

Key Messages

- *Early detection of HIV, giving more attention to males who need to avoid drug abuse, and effective implementation of highly active antiretroviral therapy (HAART) may contribute to reduce ARM.*
- *Effective planning, awareness among public on HIV, access to ART, and proper follow-up contribute to reduce mortality in the long run.*

ARTICLE 1

Cabazitaxel versus abiraterone or enzalutamide in metastatic prostate cancer

de Wit R, de Bono J, Sternberg CN, Fizazi K, Tombal B, Wülfing C, et al. Cabazitaxel versus abiraterone or enzalutamide in metastatic prostate cancer.
N Engl J Med. 2019;381:2506-18.

Abstract*

Background: The treatment options for patients with metastatic castration-resistant prostate cancer showing progression within 12 months of treatment with docetaxel include cabazitaxel, a microtubule inhibitor and abiraterone or enzalutamide. The limited data comparing the safety and efficacy of two treatment regime exists.

Methods: We randomly assigned, in a 1:1 ratio, patients who had previously received docetaxel and abiraterone or enzalutamide, were given cabazitaxel (at a dose of 25 mg/m^2 body-surface area intravenously every 3 weeks, plus prednisone daily and granulocyte colony-stimulating factor) or either of the two androgen-signaling-targeted inhibitors (either 1,000 mg of abiraterone plus prednisone daily or 160 mg of enzalutamide daily). Imaging-based progression-free survival was the primary endpoint, while survival, response, and safety were the secondary endpoints.

Results: Of the total of 255 patients, imaging-based progression or death was reported in 95 of 129 patients (73.6%) in the cabazitaxel group, as compared with 101 of 126 patients (80.2%) in the group that received an androgen-signaling-targeted inhibitor [hazard ratio 0.54; 95% confidence interval (CI) 0.40–0.73; p < 0.001], after a median follow-up of 9.2 months. The median imaging-based progression-free survival and the median overall survival were 8.0 months and 13.6 months with cabazitaxel, respectively. These values for the androgen-signaling-targeted inhibitors were 3.7 months and 11.0 months, respectively. The median progression-free survival was 4.4 months with cabazitaxel and 2.7 months with an androgen-signaling-targeted inhibitor (hazard ratio for progression or death 0.52; 95% CI 0.40–0.68; p < 0.001). A prostate-specific antigen response occurred in 35.7% and 13.5% of the patients, respectively (p < 0.001), and tumor response was noted in 36.5% and 11.5% (p = 0.004). Around 56.3% of patients receiving cabazitaxel and in 52.4% of those receiving an androgen-signaling-targeted inhibitor reported adverse events of grade 3 or higher.

Conclusion: In patients with metastatic castration-resistant prostate cancer, previously treated with docetaxel and androgen-signaling-targeted inhibitor agents, cabazitaxel was associated with improved clinical outcomes, when compared with abiraterone or enzalutamide. (Funded by Sanofi; CARD ClinicalTrials. gov number, NCT02485691.) *Redrafted abstract

"Once you choose hope, anything is possible."

—**Christopher Reeve**

COMMENT

Prostate cancer is the second leading cause of cancer-related death in men in the US and has the third position in Europe. Metastatic castration-resistant prostate cancer has four lines of medical treatment, including taxanes (docetaxel and cabazitaxel), androgen-signaling-targeted inhibitors (abiraterone and enzalutamide), immunotherapy (sipuleucel-T), and a bone-targeted radiopharmaceutical agent (radium-223 dichloride) signifying that the ideology of treatment is more toward life-extending therapies during earlier stages of the disease. Docetaxel, abiraterone, enzalutamide, and apalutamide, in combination with androgen deprivation therapy, prolonged survival among patients with metastatic hormone-sensitive prostate cancer. Androgen-signaling-targeted inhibitors have also prolonged metastasis-free survival, as compared with placebo, among patients with nonmetastatic castration-resistant prostate cancer. Cabazitaxel is a next-generation taxane that has been approved for the treatment of metastatic castration-resistant prostate cancer in patients who have previously been treated with a docetaxel-containing regimen because of its retention of activity and better safety profile (lower incidence of alopecia, peripheral neuropathy, peripheral edema, and nail disorders). Studies suggest that patients may not have a response to abiraterone or enzalutamide after their disease progresses, while they are receiving an androgen-signaling-targeted inhibitor (abiraterone or enzalutamide) and also that partial cross-resistance may develop between androgen-signaling-targeted inhibitors and docetaxel. The CARD trial investigated whether cabazitaxel would be superior to an androgen-signaling-targeted inhibitor in patients who had previously been treated with docetaxel and the alternative androgen-signaling-targeted agent (abiraterone or enzalutamide).

Cabazitaxel had more than doubled the imaging-based progression-free survival in all groups regardless of timing of androgen-signaling-targeted inhibitors before or after docetaxel. All key secondary endpoints (overall survival, progression-free survival, PSA response, and tumor response) also favored cabazitaxel. The chance of developing resistance was less in taxanes owing to their different mechanism of action and cabazitaxel had more tumor penetration and hence did not lose its activity like docetaxel. The incidence of adverse events of grade 3 or higher was similar in the two treatment groups while the incidence of adverse events leading to death during the trial was twice as high with an androgen-signaling-targeted inhibitor as with cabazitaxel.

This was an open-label trial with no central review of the standard imaging, although a previous study has suggested little variance between local and central imaging review in this population. No preplanned analysis of the influence of the sequence of abiraterone–enzalutamide (or vice versa) was undertaken.

The trial results prospectively confirmed that patients with metastatic castration-resistant prostate cancer who had previously been treated with docetaxel and had disease progression within 12 months while receiving an androgen-signaling-targeted inhibitor (abiraterone or enzalutamide) had longer imaging-based progression-free survival and overall survival when treated with cabazitaxel than when treated with the other androgen-signaling-targeted inhibitor (abiraterone in patients who had previously received enzalutamide, or enzalutamide in those who had previously received abiraterone).

Key Messages

⊙ *Cabazitaxel led to longer imaging-based progression-free survival than abiraterone or enzalutamide among patients with metastatic castration-resistant prostate cancer who had previously received docetaxel and the alternative androgen-signaling-targeted inhibitor (abiraterone or enzalutamide).*

⊙ *All key secondary endpoints (overall survival, progression-free survival, PSA response, and tumor response) were also favored by cabazitaxel.*

ARTICLE 2

A cross-sectional observational study of geriatric dermatoses in a tertiary care hospital of Northern India

Agarwal R, Sharma L, Chopra A, Mitra D, Saraswat N. A cross-sectional observational study of geriatric dermatoses in a tertiary care hospital of Northern India.
Indian Dermatol Online J. 2019;10:524-9.

Abstract

Introduction: Geriatric dermatoses are one of the most common reasons for day-to-day consultation in the elderly. Over the past few years, understanding of the pathophysiology of skin changes in the geriatric age group has improved and has paved the way for better therapeutic options. There are only a few studies conducted in India about the geriatric dermatoses. This article reviews the various physiological and pathological changes of aging, dwelling on the role of intrinsic and extrinsic factors in the pathogenesis of aging skin thus better understanding of this emerging branch in dermatology leading to enhance resource management for elderly population.

Materials and methods: This is a cross-sectional observational study carried out on 500 consecutive patients aged 60 years and above in Department of Dermatology of a tertiary care hospital of Northern India after meeting the inclusion and exclusion criteria.

Results: Out of 500 patients studied with male-to-female ratio of 1.4, wrinkles followed by cherry angiomas were the most common physiological cutaneous manifestations, and infective dermatoses followed by allergic contact dermatitis were the most common pathological conditions seen. Few rare cases were also seen during the study such as cutis marmorata, delusion of parasitosis, and sweet syndrome in case of acute myeloid leukemia.

Conclusion: Geriatric dermatology is an emerging branch in dermatology, and an update on this, will go a long way to effectively manage these patients. A thorough knowledge of the epidemiology as well as gender distribution of dermatological diseases in geriatric population in the tertiary care hospital will help in assessing health status and healthcare needs related to skin for better allocation of resources, distribution of material and manpower, and help healthcare providers in better decision-making resulting in higher clientele satisfaction.

"I will remember that there is art to medicine as well as science, and that warmth, sympathy, and understanding may outweigh the surgeon's knife or the chemist's drug."

—Hippocrates

COMMENT

Aging is a natural process in which molecular changes over time lead to progressive decline in function and anatomical organization of multiple systems and organs. Similarly, physiological and structural changes in human skin lead to decline in the normal functioning; predominantly, its capacity to repair DNA changes, healing, and immune response making the elderly person susceptible to various skin disorders. With aging, flattening of dermoepidermal junction, reduction of the number of interdigitations, and melanocytes give pale appearance to the skin and hair. Also, there is a reduction in bulk of dermis and accumulation of a brown-colored pigment lipofuscin, a marker of cell damage. All these changes give rise to various dermatoses such as pruritus, eczema, xerosis, etc., and fatal-like skin malignancies which lead to significant morbidity and impairment of quality of life. The geriatric population is afflicted with a great many dermatology concerns, not only because of normal aging process but also the additional stressors acquired from the environmental causes. The long-term effect of the exterior causes such as UV radiation, chemical irritants, temperature, humidity, dryness, pathogens, and so forth are compounded for those who have had to endure longer. Geriatric dermatoses are a very challenging job for the clinician in terms of diagnosis, management, and follow-up. As the skin of the elderly population is going through a lot of changes from both an intrinsic and extrinsic point of view, it is imperative for the physician to have a better understanding of the pathophysiology of geriatric skin disorders and their specific management, which differs slightly from an adult population.

Key Messages

- *The various geriatric dermatoses are due to structural and physiological changes along with the cumulative effect of sun exposure during lifetime.*
- *The prevalence of dermatoses in elderly is increased due to presence of associated systemic diseases and drug resistance due to indiscriminate use of antibiotics.*

ARTICLE 3

Prevalence, risk factors, circumstances for falls and level of functional independence among geriatric population: a descriptive study

Pitchai P, Dedhia HP, Bhandari N, Krishnan D, D'Souza NRJ, Bellara JM. Prevalence, risk factors, circumstances for falls and level of functional independence among geriatric population: a descriptive study.
Indian J Public Health. 2019;63:21-6.

Abstract*

Introduction: In the elderly population, falls are the commonly encountered problems; in India, the research is centered predominantly on recognizing and managing risk factors. However, there is a lack of research related to circumstances of the fall and the factors associated with it. The primary objective of the present study is to evaluate the prevalence of fall, risk factors, and circumstances for falls, and level of functional independence among the elder individuals. The secondary objective is to assess the fear of fall (FOF) as well as association of demographic factors with FOF among elderly population.

Materials and methods: This cross-sectional study included 2,049 elderly individuals of ≥60 years age; sample population was recruited by one-stage cluster sampling technique within three cities of Maharashtra, i.e., Panvel, Thane, and Mumbai. A questionnaire, Barthel Index, Kuppuswamy Scale, and Fall Efficacy Scale-International were used for collecting data. SPSS software was used for obtaining responses. Descriptive statistics as well as Chi-square test were employed.

Results: The prevalence of falls was 24.98%. There was a significant association of demographic characteristics, including age group, education, marital status, and socioeconomic status, with elder individuals (p < 0.05). In morning, 44.92% of the falls happened; most of the falls, i.e., 65.43% happened indoors. Slips were reported by 56.45% fallers; sustained injuries were noted in 60.55% fallers. FOF was present in 34.70% fallers; reduction of functional activities was reported by 23.67% fallers and affection in activities of daily living was present in 18.06% fallers.

Conclusion: Findings of the present study demonstrated that fall is an important health problem and offers information about the risk factors that influence the falls in elderly population. *Redrafted abstract

"Alas, our frailty is the cause, not we! For such as we are made of, such we be."
—**William Shakespeare**

COMMENT

Falls account for significant morbidity and mortality among the elderly population. The causes of falls in the elderly are multifactorial and it includes disturbance in balance and gait, visual and motor reaction time problems, visual impairment, cardiovascular disorders, and cognitive problems. Falls may also be due to some extrinsic factors such as poor lighting, low friction floor surfaces, poorly fitted clothing, or lack of aids/equipment. Till date, research has largely focused on identification and management of risk factors, but the situation of fall and its associated factors are sparsely researched.

A cross-sectional study was carried out among 2,049 elderly population of 60 years and above from Mumbai, Panvel, and Thane cities, Maharashtra. The primary objective of the study was to find the prevalence of fall, investigate risk factors, circumstances of fall, and the level of functional independence in elderly population. The secondary objective was to find out fear of fall (FOF) and its association of demographic factors on elderly population. The prevalence of fall in this study was found to be 24.98%. Demographic factors such as age group, education, marital status, and socioeconomic status had demonstrated a significant association with older adults ($p < 0.05$); 44.92% of falls occurred in the morning, the majority of falls (65.43%) occurred indoors, 56.45% of the fallers reported to have slips and 60.55% of the fallers had sustained injuries. From the total participants, 34.70% of the fallers reported FOF, 23.67% of the fallers expressed reduced functional activities, and 18.06% of the fallers demonstrated affection in activities of daily living.

Falls are essentially preventable and hence focus should be to evaluate falls and recognize the risk factors, which are of utmost importance in falls prevention programs. Developing and providing a comprehensive care of preventive, curative, and rehabilitative services to the elderly is the need of the hour. Extensive education, communication, and awareness program regarding fall events and preventive measures need to be undertaken. Guidelines for the prevention and treatment of fallers should be developed and training of health workers, physicians, and caregivers in fall prevention programs should be undertaken.

Key Messages

⊙ *Falls in the elderly are preventable and recurrent falls in the geriatric population should be appropriately addressed as falls contribute to significant morbidity and mortality among the elderly population.*

⊙ *Proper education, widespread awareness campaign, and training healthcare providers form the key in the fall prevention programs.*

ARTICLE 4

Old subjects with sepsis in the emergency department: trend analysis of case fatality rate

Fabbri A, Marchesini G, Benazzi B, Morelli A, Montesi D, Bini C, et al. Old subjects with sepsis in the emergency department: trend analysis of case fatality rate.
BMC Geriatr. 2019 Dec 23;19:372.

Abstract

Background: The burden of sepsis represents a global healthcare problem. We aimed to assess the case fatality rate (CFR) and its predictors in subjects with sepsis admitted to a general Italian hospital from 2009 to 2016, stratified by risk score.

Methods: We performed a retrospective analysis of all sepsis-related hospitalizations after Emergency Department (ED) visit in a public Italian hospital in an 8-year period. A risk score to predict CFR was computed by logistic regression analysis of selected variables in a training set (2009–2012), and then confirmed in the whole study population. A trend analysis of CFR during the study period was performed dividing patient as high-risk (upper tertile of risk score) or low-risk.

Results: Two thousand four hundred ninety-two subjects were included. Over time, the incidental admission rate (number of sepsis-related admissions per 100 total admissions) increased from 4.1% (2009–2010) to 5.4% (2015-2016); p < 0.001, accompanied by a reduced CFR (from 38.0 to 18.4%; p < 0.001). A group of 10 variables (admission to intensive care unit, cardiovascular dysfunction, HIV infection, diabetes, age ≥80 years, respiratory diseases, number of organ dysfunction, digestive diseases, dementia and cancer) were selected by the logistic model to predict CFR with good accuracy: AUC 0.873 (0.009). Along the years, CFR decreased from 31.8% (2009-2010) to 25.0% (2015-2016); p = 0.007. The relative proportion of subjects ≥80 years (overall 52.9% of cases) and classified as high-risk did not change along the years. CFR decreased only in low-risk subjects (from 13.3 to 5.2%; p < 0.001), and particularly in those aged ≥80 (from 18.2–6.6%; p = 0.003), but not in high-risk individuals (from 69.9 to 64.2%; p = 0.713).

Conclusion: Between 2009 and 2016, the incidence of sepsis-related hospitalization increased in a general Italian hospital, with a downward trend in CFR, only limited to low-risk patients and particularly to subjects ≥80 years.

"The line between life and death is not thicker than an eyelid."

—**Eiji Yoshikawa**

COMMENT

Sepsis is a life-threatening condition caused by the body's overwhelming response to an infection leading to tissue damage, organ failure, and death. Sepsis occurs when the chemicals released by the immune system to fight an infection causes inflammation throughout the entire body, thereby leading to blood clots and leaky vessels. The decreased blood flow further damages different organs of the body by depriving them of nutrients and oxygen. Sepsis can lead to septic shock, which is a medical emergency condition. Any infection in the body can trigger sepsis and it is seen more commonly in elderly population, immunocompromised patients, and in persons with comorbidities such as kidney disease, diabetes, hypertension, and cancer. Since the immune system gets weakened with age, elderly population are more vulnerable to sepsis. Pneumonia and urinary tract infection remain the two most common causes of sepsis among the elderly population.

A study was conducted to assess the case fatality rate (CFR) and its predictors in subjects with sepsis admitted to a general Italian hospital from 2009 to 2016, stratified by risk score. A retrospective analysis of all sepsis-related hospitalizations was performed after Emergency Department (ED) visit in a public Italian hospital in an 8-year period. Two thousand four hundred ninety-two subjects were included. Over time, the incidental admission rate (number of sepsis related admissions per 100 total admissions) increased from 4.1% (2009–2010) to 5.4% (2015–2016); p < 0.001, accompanied by a reduced CFR (from 38% to 18.4%; p < 0.001). A group of 10 variables (admission to intensive care unit, cardiovascular dysfunction, HIV infection, diabetes, age ≥80 years, respiratory diseases, number of organ dysfunction, digestive diseases, dementia, and cancer) were selected by the logistic model to predict CFR with good accuracy: AUC 0.873 (0.009). Along the years, CFR decreased from 31.8% (2009–2010) to 25% (2015–2016); p = 0.007. The relative proportion of subjects ≥80 years (overall 52.9% of cases) and classified as high-risk did not change along the years. CFR decreased only in low-risk subjects (from 13.3 to 5.2%; p < 0.001) and particularly in those aged ≥80 (from 18.2 to 6.6%; p = 0.003), but not in high-risk individuals (from 69.9 to 64.2%; p = 0.713).

Sepsis causes significant morbidity and mortality and all efforts should be made to prevent sepsis. Vaccinations against pneumonia, flu, and other potential infections should be done and good hygiene should be practiced.

Key Messages

- *Sepsis should be aggressively managed, as it causes significant morbidity and mortality especially in high-risk individuals.*
- *Elderly and high-risk individuals should be educated adequately regarding symptoms and signs of sepsis and measures to prevent it.*

ARTICLE 5

A prospective study of hepatic safety of statins used in very elderly patients

Guo M, Zhao J, Zhai Y, Zang P, Lv Q, Shang D. A prospective study of hepatic safety of statins used in very elderly patients. *BMC Geriatr. 2019;19:352.*

Abstract

Background: Statins play an important role in the care of patients with cardiovascular disease and have a good safety record in clinical practice. Hepatotoxicity is a barrier that limits the ability of primary care physicians to prescribe statins for patients with elevated liver transaminase values and/or underlying liver disease. However, limited population-based data are available on the use of statin therapy and on the hepatotoxicity of statins in very elderly patients. This prospective study evaluated the liver enzyme elevation during statin therapy in very elderly patients (≥80 years old).

Methods: Patients with hypercholesterolemia (LDL-C levels ≥3.4 and <5.7 mmol/L), atherosclerosis, coronary heart disease (CHD), or a CHD-risk equivalent were enrolled and received once daily statin treatment. Multivariate logistic regression models were used to study the impact of age, gender, hepatitis B infection, fatty liver disease, biliary calculus, other chronic diseases, drug kinds, alcohol abuse, statin variety, and statin dose variables.

Results: A total of 515 consecutive patients ranging from 80 to 98 years old were included in the analysis. These patients were treated with simvastatin, fluvastatin, pravastatin, rosuvastatin, or atorvastatin. Twenty-four patients (4.7; 95% CI 2.7–6.6) showed an increase in their hepatic aminotransferase levels. No significant difference of hepatic aminotransferase elevation rates was observed in different statin treatment groups. The incidence of mild, moderate, and severe elevation of aminotransferase levels was 62.5% (15/24), 29.2% (7/24), and 8.3% (2/24), respectively. None of the patients developed hepatic failure. Nine patients with moderate or severe aminotransferase elevations discontinued therapy. The time of onset of hepatic aminotransferase elevation ranged from 2 weeks to 6 months after statin treatment. The onset of hepatic aminotransferase elevation was within 1 month for 70.8% of patients. The patients took 2 weeks to 3 months to recover their liver function after statin therapy cessation. Multivariate analysis identified chronic hepatitis B infection and alcohol consumption as independent factors associated with the hepatic response to statins—odd ratio (OR) 12.83; 95% CI (4.36–37.759) and OR 2.736; 95% CI (1.373–5.454), respectively.

Conclusion: The prevalence of elevated transaminases was higher than published data in very elderly patients. Overall, statin treatment is safe for patients ≥80 years old.

"A good physician treats the disease, the great physician treats the patient who has the disease."

—William Osler

COMMENT

Statins are β-hydroxy β-methylglutaryl-CoA (HMG-CoA) reductase inhibitors, which are used to lower low-density lipoprotein cholesterol (LDL-C) and so are commonly used for the primary prevention in persons at high risk of cardiovascular disease and secondary prevention for those who have already developed cardiovascular disease including atherosclerosis. Side effects of statins mainly include abnormal blood levels of liver enzymes and muscle pain. Different types of statins include atorvastatin, pravastatin, rosuvastatin, simvastatin, and fluvastatin.

Patients with hypercholesterolemia (LDL-C levels ≥3.4 and ≤5.7 mmol/L), atherosclerosis, coronary heart disease (CHD), or a CHD-risk equivalent were enrolled and received once daily statin treatment. Multivariate logistic regression models were used to study the impact of age, gender, hepatitis B infection, fatty liver disease, biliary calculus, other chronic diseases, drug kinds, alcohol abuse, statin variety, and statin dose variables.

A total of 515 consecutive patients ranging from 80 to 98 years old were included in the analysis. These patients were treated with simvastatin, fluvastatin, pravastatin, rosuvastatin, or atorvastatin. 24 patients [4.7; 95% confidence interval (CI) 2.7–6.6] showed an increase in their hepatic aminotransferase levels. No significant difference of hepatic aminotransferase elevation rates was observed in different statin treatment groups. The incidence of mild, moderate, and severe elevation of aminotransferase levels was 62.5% (15/24), 29.2% (7/24), and 8.3% (2/24), respectively. None of the patients developed hepatic failure. Nine patients with moderate and severe aminotransferase elevations discontinued therapy. The time of onset of hepatic aminotransferase elevation ranged from 2 weeks to 6 months after statin treatment. The onset of hepatic aminotransferase elevation was within 1 month for 70.8% of patients. The patients took 2 weeks to 3 months to recover their liver function after statin therapy cessation. Multivariate analysis identified chronic hepatitis B infection and alcohol consumption as independent factors associated with the hepatic response to statins.

Key Message

⊙ *Statins should be used with caution in patients with deranged liver function test.*

ARTICLE 6

Association between anemia and frailty in 13,175 community-dwelling adults aged 50 years and older in China

Ruan Y, Guo Y, Kowal P, Lu Y, Liu C, Sun S, et al. Association between anemia and frailty in 13,175 community-dwelling adults aged 50 years and older in China.
BMC Geriatr. 2019;19:327.

Abstract

Background: Anemia and frailty contribute to poor health outcomes in older adults; however, most current research in lower income countries has concentrated on anemia or frailty alone rather than in combination. The aim of the present study was to investigate the association between anemia and frailty in community-dwelling adults aged 50 years and older in China.

Methods: The study population was sourced from the 2007/10 SAGE China Wave 1. Anemia was defined as hemoglobin <13 g/dL for men and <12 g/dL for women. A Frailty index (FI) was compiled to assess frailty. The association between anemia and frailty was evaluated using a 2-level hierarchical logistic model.

Results: The prevalence of anemia was 31.0% (95% CI 28.4, 33.8%) and frailty 14.7% (95% CI 13.5, 16.0%). In the univariate regression model, presence of anemia was significantly associated with frailty (OR = 1.62; 95% CI 1.39, 1.90) and the effect remained consistent after adjusting for various potential confounding factors including age, gender, residence, education, household wealth, fruit and vegetable intake, tobacco use, alcohol consumption, and physical activity (adjusted OR = 1.31; 95% CI 1.09, 1.57). Each 1 g/dL increase in hemoglobin concentration was associated with 4% decrease in the odds of frailty after adjusting for several confounding variables (adjusted OR = 0.96; 95% CI 0.93, 0.99).

Conclusion: Anemia and low-hemoglobin concentrations were significantly associated with frailty. Therefore, healthcare professionals caring for older adults should increase screening, assessment of causes, and treatment of anemia as one method of avoiding, delaying, or even reversing frailty.

"Do as much as possible for the patient, and as little as possible to the patient."
—Bernard Lown

COMMENT

Anemia is defined as to be hemoglobin level <12g% in woman and <13g% in man. Frailty in adult is estimated by frailty index (FI). Frailty was defined using the deficit accumulation approach. An FI was generated as the proportion of deficits present out of 40 variables available in the SAGE database, including self-rated health, nine medically diagnosed conditions, four medical symptoms, 13 functional activities assessments, 10 activities of daily living (ADLs), body mass index [BMI, calculated as weight/height^2 (kg/m^2)], grip strength, and gait speed. Individual scores ranged from 0 (no deficits) to 1 (highest level of deficits in all variables). The FI cut-off value of 0.2 was defined as approaching a frail state.

Both anemia and frailty increase vulnerability to stressors and leads to negative outcomes such as falls, dependency, hospitalization, and death. Fried suggested a frailty phenotype identified by the presence of 3 out of 5 components, these are: Unintentional weight loss, weakness, poor endurance and energy, slowness, and low physical activity.

Anemia reduces oxygen-carrying capacity, which leads to tissue hypoxia, which causes poor outcomes and reduces submaximal and maximal aerobic capacity, failing muscle strength, and cognitive impairment. It also leads to frailty. In USA, study has shown inverse relationship between interleukin (IL)-6 and hemoglobin level in frail subjects. It suggests frail subjects having chronic inflammation has got less hemoglobin level. Some suggest age-related chronic inflammation is the explanatory reason behind the relationship of anemia and frailty. Both may show pathophysiological pathway of chronic inflammation resulting in immunosenescence-associated changes and increase oxidative stress.

Key Message

- *Frailty and anemia are significantly associated with each other, thus healthcare personnel treating adults should assess the cause and treat anemia as one of the methods for delaying and reversing frailty.*

ARTICLE 7

Cardiovascular risk factors and memory decline in middle-aged and older adults: the English Longitudinal Study of Ageing

Olaya B, Moneta MV, Bobak M, Haro JM, Demakakos P. Cardiovascular risk factors and memory decline in middle-aged and older adults: the English Longitudinal Study of Ageing.
BMC Geriatr. 2019;19:337.

Abstract

Background: We investigated the association between trajectories of verbal episodic memory and burden of cardiovascular risk factors (CVRFs) in middle-aged and older community dwellers.

Methods: We analyzed data from 4,372 participants aged 50–64 years and 3,005 persons aged 65–79 years old from the English Longitudinal Study of Ageing who were repeatedly evaluated every 2 years and had six interviews of a 10-year follow-up. We measured the following baseline risk factors: Diabetes, hypertension, smoking, physical inactivity, and obesity to derive a CVRF scores. Adjusted linear mixed effect regression models were estimated to determine the association between number of CVFRs and six repeated measurements of verbal memory scores, separately for middle-aged and older adults.

Results: Cardiovascular risk factors were not significantly associated with memory at baseline. CVFRs were significantly associated with memory decline in middle-aged (50–64 years), but not in older (65–79 years) participants. This association followed a dose-response pattern with increasing number of CVFRs being associated with greater cognitive decline. Comparisons between none versus some CVRFs yielded significant differences (p < 0.05).

Conclusion: Our findings confirm that the effect of cumulative CVRFs on subsequent cognitive deterioration is age-dependent. CVRFs are associated with cognitive decline in people aged 50–64 years, but not in those aged ≥65 years. Although modest, the memory decline associated with accumulation of CVRFs in midlife may increase the risk of late-life dementia.

> *"It is much more important to know what sort of a patient has a disease than what sort of a disease a patient has."*
>
> **—William Osler**

COMMENT

Cardiovascular risk factors (CVRFs) are highly prevalent among the geriatric population and are a leading cause of morbidity and mortality. Among them, tobacco smoking, hypertension, obesity, diabetes, chronic kidney disease, etc., are noteworthy. However, several population-based studies have also identified CVRFs as strong risk factors for cognitive decline and dementia. The cognitive decline is proposed to be driven by cardiovascular diseases (CVDs) to an extent. CVRFs might lead to inflammation and oxidative stress, cerebral small vessel diseases, cerebral hypoxia, and hypoperfusion, or neurodegeneration in the brain, which may be contributory. An age-dependent relationship is hypothesized to exist between cognitive decline and CVRF. Some studies have also demonstrated that aggregated CVRFs at midlife are associated with cognitive decline in the middle age.

The purpose of this study was to find whether this association followed a dose-response pattern by exploring the interaction between time and CVRFs. About 4,372 participants aged 50–64 and 3,005 persons aged 65–79 years old from the English Longitudinal Study of Ageing who were repeatedly evaluated every 2 years and a 10-year follow-up were evaluated. An adjusted linear mixed effect regression model was used to determine the association between number of CVFRs and six repeated measurements of verbal memory scores, separately for middle-aged and older adults. CVFRs were significantly associated with decline in memory among middle-aged (50–64 years) participants. Increasing number of CVFRs were associated with greater cognitive decline, suggesting a statistically significant dose-response relationship.

Overall, our findings suggest a greater cardiovascular risk burden on contemporaneous memory decline in midlife, but not in late-life, supporting the hypothesis that the deleterious effect of cumulative CVRFs is age-dependent. They also suggest that the effect of CVRFs follows a dose-response association with verbal episodic memory decline, which is independent of other potential confounders. It was found that greater CVRF burden was associated with faster decline in reaction time. The prospective association between cumulative CVRFs and memory in participants aged 50–64 years is dose response with the memory score getting lower for every additional CVRF. It has been suggested that CVRFs no longer act as risk factors for dementia. Overall, middle-aged participants present with better levels of health at baseline. There is also the hypothesis that the duration of the exposure to CVRFs might impact on the rate of cognitive decline.

This study supports the deleterious effect of aggregate CVRFs in midlife (50–64 years) on subsequent decline over a period of 10 years, whereas, this association was not found when CVRFs were measured in older adults (over 65 years). These differences in cognitive decline might increase with increase in age leading to greater risk for future dementia, such as AD.

Key Messages

- *The effect of cumulative CVRFs on subsequent cognitive deterioration is age-dependent.*
- *The decline in memory associated with accumulation of CVRFs in midlife may increase the risk of late-life dementia.*
- *Due to co-existence of risk factors, intervention focusing on the combined effect of multiple CVRFs is preferable.*
- *Interventions over these modifiable conditions at midlife may halt this cognitive deterioration.*

ARTICLE 8

Polypharmacy in older patients: identifying the need for support by a community pharmacist

Beuscart JB, Petit S, Gautier S, Wierre P, Balcaen T, Lefebvre JM, et al. Polypharmacy in older patients: identifying the need for support by a community pharmacist.
BMC Geriatr. 2019;19:277.

Abstract

Background: The community pharmacist is a key player in medication reviews of older outpatients. However, it is not always clear which individuals require a medication review. The objective of the present study was to identify high-priority older patients for intervention by a community pharmacist.

Methods: As part of their final-year placement in a community pharmacy, pharmacy students conducted 10 interviews each with older adults (aged 65 or over) taking at least five medications daily. The student interviewer also offered to examine the patient's home medicine cabinet. An interview guide was developed by an expert group to assess the difficulties in managing and taking medications encountered by older patients.

Results: The 141 students interviewed a total of 1,370 patients (mean age: 81.5; mean number of medications taken daily: 9.3). Of the 1,370 interviews, 743 (54.2%) were performed in the patient's home, and thus also included an examination of the home medicine cabinet. Adverse events were reported by 566 (42.0%) patients. A total of 378 patients (27.6%) reported difficulties in preparing, administering and/or swallowing medications. The inspections of medicine cabinets identified a variety of shortcomings: Poorly located cabinets (in 15.0% of inspections), medication storage problems (21.7%), expired medications (40.7%), potentially inappropriate medications (15.0%), several different generic versions of the same drug (19.9%), and redundant medications (20.4%).

Conclusion: In a community pharmacy setting, high-priority older patients for intervention by a community pharmacist can be identified by asking simple questions about difficulties in managing, administering, taking, or storing medications.

"Best clinical decisions are at the heart of appropriate care, the goal to which our system should aspire."

—Anna Reid

COMMENT

Older adults are exposed to an augmented risk of adverse drug reactions due to polypharmacy, and this has a substantial impact on mortality and the prospect of hospitalization. Quite, a lot of interventions directed at reducing this risk have been suggested, with a significant focus on detecting and easing potentially unbecoming prescriptions. These interventions require healthcare professionals to be more aware of at-risk situations and patients requiring precise assistance.

A cross-sectional study was performed in-between January 5th and June 30th, 2015, in community pharmacies in the Nord-Pas-de-Calais zone of France. One and each of the 141 sixth-year student interns was asked to engage in a dialogue 10 older patients (aged 65 and over) taking at least five medications regularly, in order to assess their home medication management. This interview could be performed at either the pharmacy or (if the patient consented) at the patient's home.

In the latter case, the interviewer had the advantage of examining the patient's home medicine cabinet and medication storage.

The 141 students interviewed an out-and-out 1,370 patients. Of the 1,370 interviews, 743 (54.2%) were executed in the patient's home, and thus also comprised of an examination of the home medicine cabinet. Adverse events were reported by 566 (42.0%) patients. A total of 378 patients (27.6%) reported hitches while preparing, administering, and/or swallowing medications. The inspections of medicine cabinets identified a variety of shortcomings such as—poorly located cabinets (in 15.0% of inspections), medication storage problems (21.7%), expired medications (40.7%), potentially inappropriate medications (15.0%), several different generic versions of the same drug (19.9%), and redundant medications (20.4%).

Key Message

- *In a community pharmacy setting, high-priority older patients for intervention by a community pharmacist can be ascertained by asking simple questions vis-à-vis difficulties in managing, administering, taking, or storing medications.*

ARTICLE 9

A randomized trial of progesterone in women with bleeding in early pregnancy

Coomarasamy A, Devall AJ, Cheed V, Harb H, Middleton LJ, Gallos ID, et al. A randomized trial of progesterone in women with bleeding in early pregnancy.
N Engl J Med. 2019;380:1815-24.

Abstract*

Background: Role of progesterone for the maintenance of pregnancy is well established. Here, we aim to evaluate its role in preventing pregnancy loss in patients with bleeding in early pregnancy and assess its effect on pregnancy outcome.

Methods: A multicenter, randomized, double-blind, placebo-controlled trial was conducted to evaluate role of progesterone in women with vaginal bleeding in early pregnancy by comparing it with placebo. Vaginal suppositories of 400 mg of progesterone or matching placebo twice daily were given randomly to the patients from the time at which they presented with bleeding through 16 weeks of gestation. The primary outcome was the birth of a live-born baby of at least 34 weeks of gestation. The primary analysis was performed on all participants for whom data on the primary outcome were available. Multiple imputations for missing data were used while performing sensitivity analysis of the primary outcome.

Results: Out of 4,153 women from 48 hospitals in the United Kingdom, 2,079 and 2,074 received progesterone and placebo, respectively. Around 97% had the available data for the primary outcome. The incidence of live births (≥34 weeks of gestation) was 75% in the progesterone group and 72% in the placebo group [relative rate 1.03; 95% confidence interval (CI) 1.00–1.07; p = 0.08]. Similar findings were observed in sensitivity analysis (relative rate 1.03; 95% CI 1.00–1.07; p = 0.08]. No statistically significant difference was noted in the incidence of adverse events between the groups.

serious complication of miscarriage surgery and occurs in up to 30% women. There is urgent need for more comprehensive evaluation of the potential role of antibiotic prophylaxis in this context.

Pelvic infection is determined by the presence of two or more of the following clinical and laboratory features:

- Purulent vaginal discharge
- Pyrexia (>38°C)
- Uterine tenderness on examination
- Total leukocyte count >12×10^9 cells/L

With no other recognized cause of infection, or only one of these four clinical features if there was a clinically identified need to administer antibiotics for the treatment of a presumed pelvic infection.

However, undue usage of prophylactic antibiotics before surgery may result in antibiotic resistance and may require unnecessary expenses, which may not be feasible in low-income countries.

Current international guidelines recommend the use of prophylactic antibiotics in abortion surgery but not in miscarriage surgery.

In low-income settings, managing miscarriage complications can involve substantial out-of-pocket expenses. Trials and studies conducted in this regard have not yielded substantial benefit for prophylactic use of antibiotics but antibiotic administration is required for prevention of postsurgery sepsis, if there is previously found source of infection and one of the clinical features of pelvis sepsis.

Key Message

⊙ *Pelvic infection is a disabling condition, especially for women of low-income group because of economic constraints. So, judicious use of antibiotics pre- and post-miscarriage surgery is required based on clinical findings in order to prevent antibiotic resistance and reduce economic burden.*

ARTICLE 11

Characteristics and obstetric outcomes in pregnant women with acute hepatitis E virus infection in tertiary care hospital of Himachal Pradesh

Kashyap R, Joshi I, Gupta D, Prashar A, Minhas S. Characteristics and obstetric outcomes in pregnant women with acute hepatitis E virus infection in tertiary care hospital of Himachal Pradesh.
J Assoc Physicians India. 2019;67:20-2.

Abstract

Background: Hepatitis E virus (HEV) infection is a major concern regarding morbidity and mortality among pregnant women especially in developing countries. The objective of this study was to determine the characteristics and obstetric outcomes in pregnant women with acute HEV infection in tertiary care hospital of Himachal Pradesh.

Methods: Prospective observational study has been done in the department of Obstetrics and Gynecology and department of Medicine and Emergency Medicine among all the pregnant women who were seropositive for hepatitis E viral marker in two consecutive years. Information regarding basic characteristics of pregnant women and obstetric outcome has been collected.

Results: Among 30 pregnant women with hepatitis E viral infection, a case fatality ratio of 8.0% for hepatitis E infection was found. About 13.3% of the pregnancies ended up as intrauterine death. Most common age group affected was below 25 years. Mode of delivery among 70% of the women was normal vaginal delivery though 30% women delivered prematurely.

Conclusion: This prospective case series of 30 pregnant women with acute hepatitis E viral infection indicates poor maternal, obstetric, and fetal outcome among pregnant women with hepatitis E viral infection.

"Neglect starts out as an infection then becomes a disease."

—Jim Rohn

COMMENT

Hepatitis E is a water-borne pathogen, which is transmitted by the fecal–oral route, mostly due to ingestion of fecally contaminated water. Hepatitis E is a single-stranded RNA virus with an incubation period ranging from 15 to 64 days. Hepatitis E infection during pregnancy, especially in the third trimester, is associated with more severe infection and may lead to fulminant hepatic failure and maternal death in up to 15–25% of cases. Though the mechanism of liver injury is not clear, it is postulated that interplay of hormonal and immunologic changes during pregnancy, along with a high-viral load of HEV, renders the women more vulnerable. During pregnancy, fetus is maintained in the maternal environment by suppression of T cell-mediated immunity, rendering pregnant woman more susceptible to viral infections such as hepatitis E virus (HEV) infection. During pregnancy, levels of estrogen, progesterone, and human chorionic gonadotropin increase as pregnancy advances. These hormones play a significant role in altering immune regulation and increasing viral replications.

A prospective observational study was done in the department of Obstetrics and Gynecology and department of Medicine and Emergency Medicine among all the pregnant women who were seropositive for hepatitis E viral marker in two consecutive years. The objective of the study was to determine the characteristics and obstetric outcomes in pregnant woman with acute HEV infection in tertiary care hospital of Himachal Pradesh. Information regarding basic characteristics of pregnant women and obstetric outcome was collected. Among 30 pregnant women with hepatitis E viral infection, a case fatality ratio of 8% for hepatitis E infection was found. About 13.3% of the pregnancies ended up as intrauterine death. Most common age group affected was below 25 years. Mode of delivery among 70% of the women was normal vaginal delivery, though 30% women delivered prematurely. This prospective case series of 30 pregnant women with acute hepatitis E viral infection indicates poor maternal, obstetric, and fetal outcome among pregnant women with hepatitis E viral infection.

There is a very high risk of vertical transmission of HEV from the mother to the fetus. HEV infection during pregnancy was associated with miscarriage, preterm delivery, stillbirth or neonatal death. Breastfeeding is considered safe in asymptomatic women infected with HEV despite the presence of anti-HEV antibodies and HEV RNA in the colostrum. To reduce the risk of contracting HEV, it is essential to maintain hygienic practices such as proper handwashing, particularly before handling food, avoiding drinking water from unknown sources, and avoiding eating unpeeled fruits and vegetables.

> ## Key Messages
>
> ◉ *Hepatitis E infection during pregnancy, especially in the third trimester, has a more fatal outcome that might lead to fulminant hepatitis, increasing maternal and fetal morbidity and mortality.*
>
> ◉ *It is safe for asymptomatic women with hepatitis E infection to breastfeed.*
>
> ◉ *Hepatitis E can be prevented by handling food appropriately, practicing good hygiene, and drinking safe water.*

ARTICLE 12

Women's psychosocial outcomes following an emergency caesarean section: a systematic literature review

Benton M, Salter A, Tape N, Wilkinson C, Turnbull D. Women's psychosocial outcomes following an emergency caesarean section: a systematic literature review.
BMC Pregnancy Childbirth. 2019;19:535.

Abstract

Background: Given the sudden and unexpected nature of an emergency cesarean section (EmCS) coupled with an increased risk of psychological distress, it is particularly important to understand the psychosocial outcomes for women. The aim of this systematic literature review was to identify, collate, and examine the evidence surrounding women's psychosocial outcomes of EmCS worldwide.

Methods: The electronic databases of EMBASE, PubMed, Scopus, and PsycINFO were searched between November, 2017 and March, 2018. To ensure articles were reflective of original and recently published research, the search criteria included peer-reviewed research articles published within the last 20 years (1998 to 2018). All study designs were included, if they incorporated an examination of women's psychosocial outcomes after EmCS. Due to inherent heterogeneity of study data, extraction and synthesis of both qualitative and quantitative data pertaining to key psychosocial outcomes were organized into coherent themes and analysis was attempted.

Results: In total 17,189 articles were identified. Of these, 208 full text articles were assessed for eligibility. One hundred forty-nine articles were further excluded, resulting in the inclusion of 66 articles in the current systematic literature review. While meta-analyses were not possible due to the nature of the heterogeneity, key psychosocial outcomes identified that were negatively impacted by EmCS included post-traumatic stress, health-related quality of life, experiences, infant-feeding, satisfaction, and self-esteem. Post-traumatic stress was one of the most commonly examined psychosocial outcomes, with a strong consensus that EmCS contributes to both symptoms and diagnosis.

Conclusion: EmCS was found to negatively impact several psychosocial outcomes for women in particular post-traumatic stress. While investment in technologies and clinical practice to minimize the number of EmCSs is crucial, further investigations are needed to develop effective strategies to prepare and support women who experience this type of birth.

"A positive attitude will always lead to positive outcomes."

—**Peter Kivista**

COMMENT

Emergency cesarean section (EmCS) is defined as an unplanned cesarean section delivery performed before or after onset of labor, which is typically urgent and is most often required due to maternal, fetal, or placental conditions (e.g., eclampsia, fetal distress, uterine rupture, placental/cord accidents, failed instrumental birth, etc.). While cesarean section has an important place in potentially saving both baby and mother from harm, it is associated with short- and long-term psychological and physical risks, which can extend many years beyond the current delivery and affect the health of the woman, her child, and future pregnancies. A series of rapid psychological adjustments may be anxiety provoking, distressing, and emotionally unsettling for women.

A systematic literature review was done, which was aimed to identify, collate, and examine the evidence surrounding women's psychosocial outcomes of emergency cesarean section worldwide. The electric databases of EMBASE, PubMed, Scopus, and PsycINFO were searched between November, 2017 and March, 2018. All study designs were included, if they incorporated an examination of women's psychosocial outcomes after emergency cesarean section. Total 17,189 articles were identified. Of these, 208 full text articles were assessed for eligibility. One hundred forty-nine articles were further excluded, resulting in the inclusion of 66 articles in the current systematic literature review. While meta-analysis was not possible due to the nature of heterogeneity, key psychosocial outcomes were identified that were negatively impacted by emergency cesarean section included post-traumatic stress, health-related quality of life, experiences, infant feeding, satisfaction, and self-esteem. Post-traumatic stress was one of the most commonly examined psychosocial outcomes, with a strong consensus that emergency cesarean section contributes to both symptoms and diagnosis.

Emergency cesarean section was found to negatively impact several psychosocial outcomes for women in particular post-traumatic stress, while investment in technologies and clinical practice to minimize the number of emergency cesarean section is crucial, further investigations are needed to develop effective strategies to prepare and support women who experience this type of birth.

The outcome of obstetric care is to ensure both mother and infant remain physically healthy, but psychosocial aspects and outcomes of maternity care and obstetrics are no less important.

Key Message

- *Psychosocial outcomes recognized and examined in the literature as potentially related to cesarean section include—mental health problems such as post-traumatic stress and anxiety; postpartum depression; the mother–infant relationship; decreased maternal satisfaction with childbirth; parent's sexual functioning and health behaviors such as infant feeding.*

ARTICLE 13

The study of Wilson disease in pregnancy management

Yu XE, Pan M, Han YZ, Yang RM, Wang J, Gao S. The study of Wilson disease in pregnancy management. *BMC Pregnancy Childbirth. 2019;19:522.*

Abstract

Introduction: Pregnancy management in women with Wilson disease (WD) remains an important clinical problem. This research was conducted to investigate how to avoid worsening of WD symptoms during pregnancy and increase pregnancy success in women with WD by identifying the best pregnancy management approaches in these patients.

Patients and methods: The clinical data of 117 pregnancies among 75 women with WD were retrospectively analyzed. Related information of the fetus was also recorded and analyzed. At the same time, regression analysis was performed for data of 22 pregnant women without WD, as normal controls.

Results: Of a total of 117 pregnancies among the 75 women with WD and 31 pregnancies among the 22 control women included in this study, there were 108 successful pregnancies and nine spontaneous abortions. Among the 108 successful pregnancies, 97 women a history of copper chelation therapy before pregnancy; all 97 women stopped anti-copper therapy during pregnancy. The nine women with spontaneous abortion had no pre-pregnancy history of copper displacement therapy. The incidence of lower limb edema was higher in the WD group than in normal controls ($p = 0.036$). Compared with the control group, there was a higher proportion in the WD group of male infants ($p = 0.022$) and lower average infant birth weight ($t = 3.514$; $p = 0.001$).

Conclusion: It is relatively safe for women with WD patients to become pregnant. The best management method for pregnancy in women with WD may be intensive pre-pregnancy copper chelation therapy and no anti-copper treatment during pregnancy.

"I believe in the sanctity of human life, from the womb to the tomb."

—Chris Smith

COMMENT

Wilson disease (WD) is an autosomal recessive genetic disorder that can be treated at present. WD is initiated by excessive deposition of ATP7B copper transporter protein, which causes a range of symptoms in different organs. Common sites of copper deposition are the liver and the brain. At present, the main treatment method involves using copper-chelating agents, such as penicillamine and trientine. Few studies have testified on pregnancy in patients with WD, and the conclusions of the prevailing research contrast considerably. A retrospective analysis was conducted in pregnant women with WD in China, focusing on how to avoid the exasperation of disease symptoms during pregnancy and increase the success rate in pregnancy of women with WD, to find the best management approach for this patient population.

The clinical data of 117 pregnancies with 75 women with WD were in retrospect analyzed. Relevant information of the fetus was also documented and analyzed. At the same time, regression analysis was implemented for data of 22 pregnant women without WD, as standard controls.

Out of 117 pregnancies among the 75 women with WD and 31 pregnancies amid the 22 control women encompassed in this study, there were 108 successful pregnancies and nine spontaneous abortions. Among the 108 fruitful pregnancies, 97 women had a history of copper chelation therapy before pregnancy; all 97 women stopped anti-copper therapy during pregnancy. The nine women with spontaneous abortion had no pre-pregnancy history of copper displacement therapy.

Key Message

⊚ *Women with WD have complicated concerns in pregnancy, and prospective studies in this patient population are quite lacking; all published reports, till date, are retrospective analyses. It is relatively quite safe for women with WD patients to become pregnant. The best management method for pregnancy in women with WD may be rigorous pre-pregnancy copper chelation therapy and no anti-copper treatment during pregnancy.*

ARTICLE 14

Prevalence and risk factors for postpartum depression among women seen at primary health care centres in Damascus

Roumieh M, Bashour H, Kharouf M, Chaikha S. Prevalence and risk factors for postpartum depression among women seen at primary health care centres in Damascus.
BMC Pregnancy Childbirth. 2019;19:519.

Abstract

Background: In Syria, there are no previous studies on postpartum depression (PPD). The aim of this study was to identify the prevalence of PPD and investigate its risk factors among Syrian women seen at the Primary Health Care Centres in Damascus.

Methods: This descriptive cross-sectional study was carried out between January and December, 2017 in Damascus, Syria. Postpartum women seen at a convenience sample of the largest and well-utilized primary healthcare centers in Damascus were invited to participate in the study. The Arabic version of the validated Edinburgh Postnatal Depression Scale questionnaire was used to measure PPD. A cut-off score of 13 was considered to indicate probable depression.

Results: Out of a total of 1,105 women participated in this study, 28.2% had a score of 13 (probable depression). The multivariate analysis showed that PPD was significantly associated with a reported health problem during last pregnancy [OR = 2.2; 95% confidence interval (CI) 1.4–3.5]; displacement (OR = 1.4; 95% CI 1.04–1.97); perceived exposure to a lot of life stressors (OR = 5.04; 95% CI 2.4–10.5); while antenatal care had a protective effect (OR = 0.52; 95% CI 0.36–0.75).

Conclusions: The prevalence of PPD among Syrian women in this study was relatively high, as compared to other Arab and non-Arab countries. Displacement due to the Syrian crisis among other factors was associated with PPD. Obstetricians and other professionals should be sensitized about the importance of screening for the problem for better management.

"Depression is living in a body that fights to survive, with a mind that tries to die."

—**Danny Baker**

COMMENT

The World Health Organization states that about 10% of pregnant women worldwide and 13% of women who have just delivered a baby experience a mental disorder, primarily depression. Common Perinatal Mental Disorders (CPMDs) are more widespread in low- and lower-middle-income countries; i.e., 15.6% of women in low- and lower-middle-income countries experienced a mental disorder during pregnancy and 19.8% experienced a mental disorder after childbirth.

Postpartum depression (PPD), a non-psychotic depressive disorder classified by the Diagnostic and Statistical Manual of Mental Disorders as an Episode of Major Depressive Disorder that begins within 4 weeks of childbirth, is a major disabling mood disorder that distresses women during childbearing years. Social factors that are associated with developing PPD include stressful life events, childcare stress, and prenatal anxiety. In addition, a history of the previous episode of PPD, marital conflict, and single parenthood are also predictive of PPD.

This cross-sectional, descriptive study was carried out in the months January and December, 2017 in Damascus, Syria. Postpartum women seen at a suitability sample of the largest and most well-utilized primary healthcare centers in Damascus were cordially invited to partake in the study. The Arabic version (as per the regional language) of the validated Edinburgh Postnatal Depression Scale questionnaire was used to measure PPD. A cut-off score of 13 was contemplated to indicate probable depression. Data from the field were checked for quality and entered using Excel. Data were then analyzed using the Statistical Package or the Social Sciences (SPSS), Version 22 (IBM, Chicago, Illinois, USA).

The multivariate analysis showed that PPD was ominously associated with a health problem during last pregnancy.

Key Message

⊙ *The predominance of postpartum depression among Syrian women in this study was reasonably high, as paralleled to other Arab and non-Arab countries. Displacement due to the Syrian crisis among other factors was coupled with postpartum depression. Obstetricians and other professionals should be made aware about the importance of screening for the problem for enhanced management.*

ARTICLE 15

Prevalence of gestational diabetes according to commonly used data sources: an observational study

Lawrence RL, Wall CR, Bloomfield FH. Prevalence of gestational diabetes according to commonly used data sources: an observational study.
BMC Pregnancy Childbirth. 2019;19:349.

Abstract

Background: It is well recognized that prevalence of gestational diabetes mellitus (GDM) varies depending on the population studied and the diagnostic criteria used. The data source used also can lead to substantial differences in the reporting of GDM prevalence but is considered less frequently. Accurate estimation of GDM prevalence is important for service planning and evaluation, policy development, and research. We aimed to determine the prevalence of GDM in a cohort of New Zealand women using a variety of data sources and to evaluate the agreement between different data sources.

Methods: A retrospective analysis of prospectively collected data from the Growing Up in New Zealand Study, consisting of a cohort of 6,822 pregnant women residing in a geographical area, is defined by three regional health boards in New Zealand. Prevalence of GDM was estimated using four commonly used data sources. Coded clinical data on diabetes status were collected from regional health boards and the Ministry of Health's National Minimum Dataset, plasma glucose results were collected from laboratories servicing the recruitment catchment area and coded according to the New Zealand Society for the Study of Diabetes diagnostic criteria, and self-reported diabetes status collected via interview administered questionnaires. Agreement between data sources was calculated using the proportion of agreement with 95% confidence intervals (CI) for both a positive and negative diagnosis of GDM.

Results: Prevalence of GDM combining data from all sources in the Growing Up in New Zealand cohort was 6.2%. Estimates varied from 3.8 to 6.9% depending on the data source. The proportion of agreement between data sources for presence of GDM was 0.70 (95% CI 0.65, 0.75). A third of women who had a diagnosis of GDM according to medical data reported having no diabetes in interview-administered questionnaires.

Conclusion: Prevalence of GDM varies considerably depending on the data source used. Health services need to be aware of this and to understand the limitations of local data sources to ensure service planning and evaluation; policy development and research are appropriate for the local prevalence. Improved communication of the diagnosis may assist women's self-management of GDM.

"Failing to listen to the woman is one of the biggest mistakes a practitioner can make."
— **Helen Varney**

COMMENT

The prevalence of gestational diabetes mellitus (GDM) does vary depending upon the population that is being studied and the very diagnostic criteria that are being used the source of data can also lead to significant differences in reporting of GDM prevalence but is considered scantily. The accurate and correct estimation of GDM prevalence is very important for planning services and evaluating and developing policies and research. Here, we aim to determine the prevalence of GDM in a group of New Zealand women using a varied data source and to evaluate agreement between different types of data sources.

Prospectively collected data retrospectively analyzed from Growing Up in New Zealand study consisted of 6,822 pregnant women in a geographical location determined by three regional health boards in New Zealand. The prevalence was estimated using four commonly used data sources. Regional Health Boards and the Ministry's Health National minimum dataset-provided coded clinical data on diabetes status and plasma glucose results were collected from laboratories servicing the recruitment catchment area and coded according to the New Zealand Study of Diabetes Diagnostic Criteria.

The prevalence of GDM combining data from all sources in New Zealand cohort was 6.2%. Moreover, one-third of women who had GDM reported to be non-diabetic in interview-administered questionnaires.

Appropriate and prompt management of GDM reduces the risk of adverse pregnancy outcomes. The finding that one-third of women with a diagnosis of GDM did not report having any form of diabetes when asked in interview-administered questionnaires raises the question as to whether these women received or adhered to treatment for GDM.

The findings in this study indicate that commonly used prevalence statistics may under-estimate the true prevalence of GDM.

Key Messages

- *A large proportion of women in New Zealand appear to be unaware of their diagnosis of GDM and thus self-report may underestimate the prevalence.*
- *Lack of awareness of the diagnosis of GDM may potentially have a negative impact on pregnancy outcomes for her and her baby.*

ARTICLE 16

Clinical utility of genetic testing in 201 preschool children with inherited eye disorders

Lenassi E, Clayton-Smith J, Douzgou S, Ramsden SC, Ingram S, Hall G, et al. Clinical utility of genetic testing in 201 preschool children with inherited eye disorders.
Genet Med. 2020;22:745-51.

Abstract*

Purpose: Genetic testing for inherited disorders has the ability to influence patient management and health outcomes. This study aims to assess the current clinical utility of genetic testing for inherited eye disorders (IEDs) in preschool children.

Methods: Data of 201 unrelated children (0–5 years old) with IEDs obtained from North West Genomic Laboratory Hub, Manchester, UK was collected over a 7-year period. The final cohort had 74 children with bilateral cataracts, eight with bilateral ectopia lentis, 28 with bilateral anterior segment dysgenesis, 32 with albinism, and 59 with inherited retinal disorders. A panel-based genetic testing was conducted for all participants.

Results: The panel-based genetic testing had a diagnostic yield of 64% (ranging from 39 to 91% depending on the condition). The management of 33% of probands (75% for ectopia lentis, 50% for cataracts, 33% for inherited retinal disorders, 7% for anterior segment dysgenesis, and 3% for albinism) was affected by this testing, as it prevented additional investigations and led to the introduction of personalized surveillance measures.

Conclusion: Early identification of IEDs in preschool children using genetic testing prevents additional investigations and helps in providing anticipatory guidance for their management. *Redrafted abstract

> *"Your genetics load the gun. Your lifestyle pulls the trigger."*
>
> **—Mehmet Oz**

COMMENT

An important cause of visual impairment in children and young adults is inherited eye disorder (IED). Prevailing subtypes include pediatric cataracts, inherited retinal disease (IRD), ocular anterior segment dysgenesis (ASD), as well as albinism. These disorders may manifest as isolated ophthalmic disorders (nonsyndromic forms) or as a part of multisystemic syndromes that incorporate extraocular features (syndromic forms). In the latter scenario, ocular signs are often one of the first exhibiting features of a syndrome (Marfan's syndrome presenting as ectopia lentis).

A major property to consider in all genetic tests is irrefutable clinical utility, the ability of the test to impact patient management and health outcomes. Here, we aim to assess the current clinical practicality of genetic testing in varied pediatric IEDs.

Subjects were retrospectively determined through the database of the North West Genomic Laboratory Hub, Manchester, UK. Children, diagnosed through the tertiary pediatric ophthalmic genetics' facility at Manchester University NHS Foundation Trust, Manchester, UK, were included. The families choosing to undergo genetic analysis were suggested pretest counseling and provided written informed consent.

Overall, 201 young children met the inclusion criteria for the study (**Fig. 1**). Median age at referral for genetic analysis was 3 years. Extraocular features were noted for genetic testing in 33/201 cases (16%), while a relevant family history was documented at the time of referral for genetic testing in 31/201 cases (15%).

The diagnostic crop of genetic testing for the cohort was 64% (ranging from 39 to 91% depending on the condition). The test result led to reformed management (including preventing additional investigations or resulting in the introduction of personalized surveillance measures) in 33% of probands (75% for ectopia lentis, 50% for cataracts, 33% for inherited retinal disorders, 7% for anterior segment dysgenesis, and 3% for albinism).

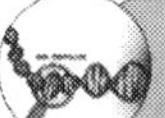
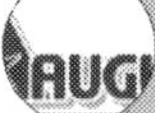
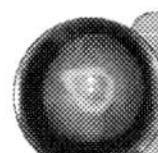

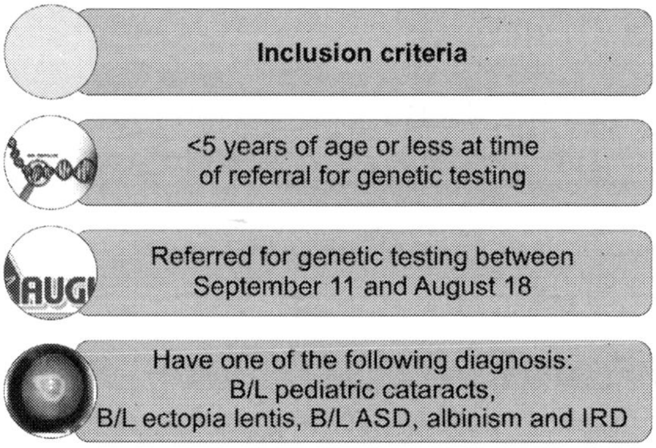

(ASD: anterior segment dysgenesis; IRD: inherited retinal disease)

FIG. 1: Inclusion criteria.

Key Message

⊙ *Like other medical interventions, diagnostic genetic tests should be meticulously evaluated before their introduction into routine practice. Genetic testing helps to identify an etiological diagnosis in majority of preschool children with IEDs. This prevented further unnecessary testing and provided the prospect for anticipatory guidance in significant subsets of patients.*

ARTICLE 17

Genetic testing for Parkinson disease: current practice, knowledge, and attitudes among US and Canadian movement disorders specialists

Alcalay RN, Kehoe C, Shorr E, Battista R, Hall A, Simuni T, et al. Genetic testing for Parkinson disease: current practice, knowledge, and attitudes among US and Canadian movement disorders specialists.
Genet Med. 2020;22:574-80.

Abstract*

Purpose: In view of the upcoming precision medicine-designed clinical trials for GBA and LRRK2 for disease modification in Parkinson disease (PD), there is a need to promote the practice of genetic testing in movement disorders specialists. Here, we assess the current practice, knowledge, and barriers to genetic testing for PD, among clinicians.

Methods: A questionnaire-based survey was conducted at 146 Parkinson Study Group (PSG) sites in the United States (n = 131) and Canada (n = 15) to assess the knowledge and attitudes about genetic testing for PD among movement disorders specialists.

Results: Out of the 178 (47.6%) PSG clinicians who completed the questionnaire, 41% did not refer any PD patients for genetic testing in the last year and >80% reported <11 patients over the same period. Lack of insurance coverage/cost to the patient and lack of perceived utility emerged as the two most common reasons for the reluctance for genetic testing. On a scale of 0–100, the mean level of comfort in respondents' own ability to genetically counsel PD patients on GBA and LRRK2 was 52 (SD = 28). About 38% of the clinicians could not answer all the questions about the inheritance and penetrance of GBA and LRRK2 variants correctly.

Conclusion: The awareness level among movement disorders specialists about genetic counseling and testing in PD is not satisfactory and there is an urgent need to improve this. *Redrafted abstract

> *"Genetics is about how much information is stored and transmitted between generations."*
>
> **—John Maynard Smith**

COMMENT

The understanding of the genetics of Parkinson disease (PD) has escalated in recent years, sanctioning a shift from observational studies, unfolding genotype–phenotype correlations, to interventional ones. Numerous clinical trials that will incorporate participants who are carriers of selected genetic variants are commencing worldwide. Of all genes linked to increased PD risk, those encoding glucocerebrosidase (*GBA*, OMIM 606463) and leucine-rich repeat kinase-2 (*LRRK2*, OMIM 609007) pathogenic variants are presently the most actively beleaguered for clinical development, in early phase (I and II) interventional studies. In preparation for upcoming precision medicine-designed clinical trials for *GBA* and *LRRK2*, we evaluated movement disorders specialists' contemporary practice, knowledge, attitudes, and impediments to genetic testing in PD.

An anonymous questionnaire was sent to movement malady specialists at 146 Parkinson Study Group (PSG) sites in the United States (n = 131) and Canada (n = 15) to gauge their knowledge and attitudes about genetic testing for PD.

One hundred seventy eight (47.6%) PSG clinicians completed the questionnaire. Forty-one percent of clinicians had not referred any PD patients for genetic evaluation in the last year and >80% testified referring fewer than 11 patients over the same period. Most common reasons for not referring for genetic testing encompassed lack of insurance coverage/cost to the patient and lack of distinguished utility. On a scale of 0–100, the mean level of comfort in respondents' own ability to genetically counsel PD patients on *GBA* and *LRRK2* was 52 (SD = 28) (**Fig. 1**). Sixty percent of clinicians correctly answered all questions regarding the inheritance and penetrance of *GBA* and *LRRK2* variants.

Continued

Continued

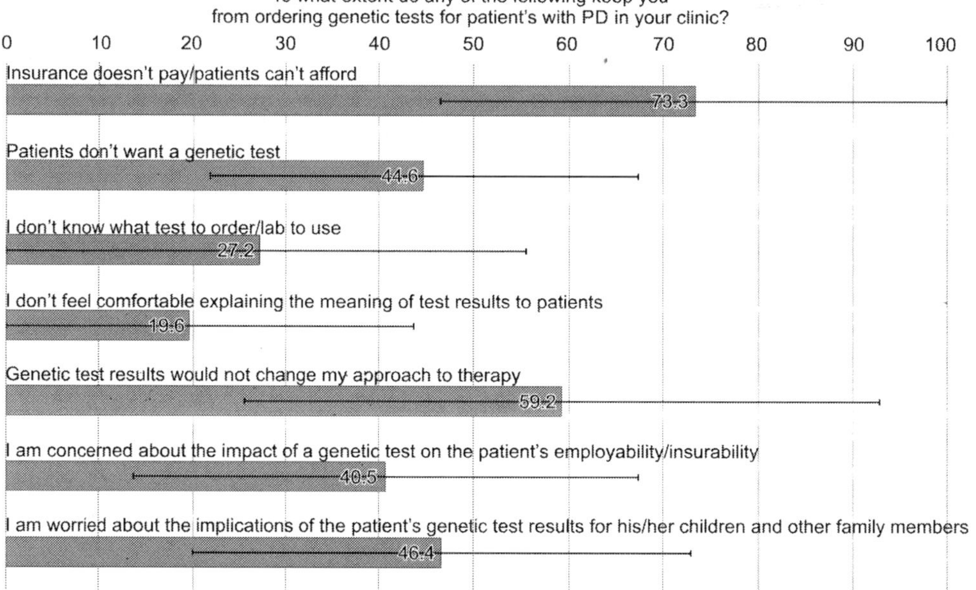

FIG. 1: Responses to the question: "To what extent do any of the following keep you from ordering genetic tests for patients with Parkinson disease (PD) in your clinic?" Participants scored each option on a scale from 0 to 100. Orange bars denote the mean grade for each response, and horizontal black lines represent the standard deviation. All respondents answered each question independently.

Key Message

⊙ *Despite over 20 years ever since the first PD gene was reported and a growing number of newly identified variants, the results of this anonymous survey of PD clinicians clearly validate that referral to PD-focused genetic counseling and testing is not a common practice in 2019. At present, genetic testing in PD is not standard of care, but may be expedient in certain cases for prognosis estimation and referral to clinical trials. Since referral to genetic testing is not a common practice, in most cases, neither patients nor their clinicians are mindful of the patients' pathogenic variant status. There is an exigent need to increase knowledge and ease practical barriers to genetic counseling and testing in PD.*

ARTICLE 18

The epigenetic regulation of HsMar1, a human DNA transposon

Renault S, Genty M, Gabori A, Boisneau C, Esnault C, de Bernonville TD, et al. The epigenetic regulation of HsMar1, a human DNA transposon.
BMC Genet. 2019;20:17.

Abstract

Background: Both classes of transposable elements (DNA and RNA) are tightly regulated at the transcriptional level leading to the inactivation of transposition via epigenetic mechanisms. Due to the high copies number of these elements, the hypothesis has emerged that their regulation can coordinate a regulatory network of genes. Herein, we investigated whether transposition regulation of *HsMar1*, a human DNA transposon, differs in presence or absence of endogenous *HsMar1* copies. In the case where *HsMar1* transposition is regulated, the number of repetitive DNA sequences issued by *HsMar1* and distributed in the human genome makes *HsMar1* a good candidate to regulate neighboring gene expression by epigenetic mechanisms.

Results: A recombinant active *HsMar1* copy was inserted in HeLa (human) and CHO (hamster) cells and its genomic excision monitored. We show that *HsMar1* excision is blocked in HeLa cells, whereas CHO cells are competent to promote *HsMar1* excision. We demonstrate that de novo *HsMar1* insertions in HeLa cells (human) undergo rapid silencing by cytosine methylation and apposition of H3K9me3 marks, whereas de novo *HsMar1* insertions in CHO cells (hamster) are not repressed and enriched in H3K4me3 modifications. The overall analysis of *HsMar1* endogenous copies in HeLa cells indicates that neither full-length endogenous inactive copies nor their inverted terminal repeats seem to be specifically silenced, and are, in contrast, devoid of epigenetic marks. Finally, the *SETMAR* gene, derived from *HsMar1*, presents H3K4me3 modifications as expected for a human housekeeping gene.

Conclusion: Our work highlights that de novo and old *HsMar1* are not similarly regulated by epigenetic mechanisms. Old *HsMar1* are generally detected as lacking epigenetic marks, irrespective their localization relative to the genes. Considering the putative existence of a network associating *HsMar1* old copies and *SETMAR*, two nonmutually exclusive hypotheses are proposed: Active and inactive *HsMar1* copies are not similarly regulated or/and regulations concern only few loci (and few genes) that cannot be detected at the whole genome level.

"The rate of increase in the fitness of any organism at any time is equal to its genetic variance in fitness at that time."

—Ronald A Fisher

COMMENT

Transposable elements (TEs) are nomadic genetic elements signifying a prevalent part of eukaryotic genomes, including human. They are known to spectacle significant genetic consequences, promoting innumerable types of mutation such as disrupting genes (upon neo-insertions) or prompting recombination between homologous sequences at divergent loci. Ahead of these foreseeable consequences in view of TEs mobility and/or amplification, other more bewildering effects relying on TEs occurrence were illustrated during the two last decades. First, TEs possess their own regulatory sequences, and then could alter the normal expression array of neighboring genes. It has also been shown that amplification of various TEs family can offer new gene regulatory networks. Finally, exaptation of several TEs is believed to drive various genetic modernisms.

Both classes of TEs (DNA and RNA) are stringently regulated at the transcriptional level leading to the inactivation of transposition via epigenetic methods. Due to the high copies number of these elements, the hypothesis has emerged that their regulation can harmonize a regulatory network of genes. Herein, it was investigated whether, transposition regulation of *HsMar1*, a human DNA transposon, contrasts in presence or absence of endogenous *HsMar1* copies.

To track the transposition of a complete and active *HsMar1* element, a tool was designed. An excision cassette was composed of an active *HsMar1* copy inserted in opposite orientation between the CMV promoter (pCMV) and the GFP-coding sequence, thus preventing the expression of GFP. LoxP sequences were added at both *HsMar1* ends. Upon *HsMar1* excision (provided in *trans* by HSMAR-RA, the reconstructed active *HsMar1* transposase or by CRE expression), pCMV allows the expression of GFP in recombinant cells. The assay was designed in order to block GFP expression in absence of *HsMar1* excision. GFP has his own start codon allowing its expression, if *HsMar1* was removed between the pCMV and the ORF of GFP. The construct also contains a selection marker (the puromycin resistance gene), the whole being enframed by PiggyBac ends.

The excision cassette was introduced in HeLa and CHO genomes using PiggyBac transposition. Each recombinant line contained at least one copy of the excision cassette (**Figs. 1A** to **D**).

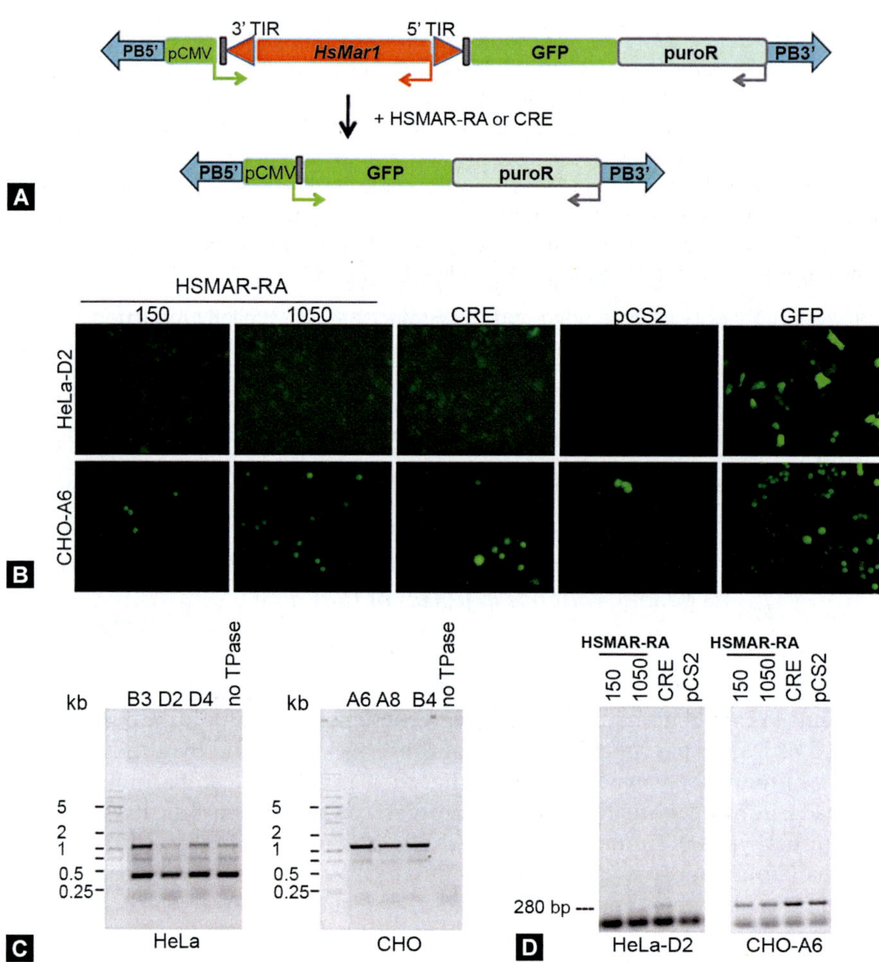

FIGS. 1A TO D: *HsMar1* excision in two genetic backgrounds: Human (HeLa cells) and non-human (CHO cells).

Key Message

⦿ *It is highlighted here that de novo and old HsMar1 are not equally regulated by epigenetic mechanisms. Old HsMar1 are generally detected as lacking epigenetic marks, irrespective their localization relative to the genes. Ruminating on the presumed existence of a network associating HsMar1 old copies and SETMAR, two non-mutually exclusive hypotheses are proposed—active and inactive HsMar1 copies are not similarly delimited or/and regulations concern only few loci (and few genes) that cannot be perceived at the whole genome level.*

ARTICLE 19

20-year follow-up of statins in children with familial hypercholesterolemia

Luirink IK, Wiegman A, Kusters DM, Hof MH, Groothoff JW, de Groot E, et al. 20-year follow-up of statins in children with familial hypercholesterolemia.
N Engl J Med. 2019;381:1547-56.

Abstract*

Background: The statin therapy in children with familial hypercholesterolemia is known to reduce the risk of cardiovascular diseases but most of the studies have focused on its short-term efficacy. We conducted a 20-year follow-up study for evaluation of effects of statins on this population in relation to cardiovascular events.

Methods: A study was conducted on 214 patients that included participants of a previously conducted placebo-controlled trial for evaluation of the 2-year efficacy and safety of pravastatin in familial hypercholesterolemia, and their 95 unaffected siblings. A questionnaire-based survey and blood investigations, along with measurement of carotid intima–media thickness, were done. The data obtained was then compared with that of their 156 parents affected with cardiovascular disease.

Results: Of the original cohort, 184 of 214 patients with familial hypercholesterolemia (86%) and 77 of 95 siblings (81%) were seen in follow-up; among the 214 patients, data on cardiovascular events and on death from cardiovascular causes were available for 203 (95%) and 214 (100%), respectively. A decrease of 32% from the baseline level was observed in the mean low-density lipoproteins cholesterol (LDL-C) level (from 6.13 to 4.16 mmol/L); 20% of the patients (37) achieved the treatment goals (LDL-C 100 mg/dL). Mean progression of carotid intima-media thickness over the entire follow-up period was 0.0056 mm/year in patients with familial hypercholesterolemia and 0.0057 mm/year in siblings (mean difference adjusted for sex: −0.0001 mm/year; 95% confidence interval −0.0010 to 0.0008). The patients with familial hypercholesterolemia had a lower cumulative incidence of cardiovascular events and death from cardiovascular causes at 39 years of age as compared to their affected parents (1% vs. 26% and 0% vs. 7%, respectively).

Conclusion: Our study showed that statin therapy in children with familial hypercholesterolemia slows down the progression of carotid intima–media thickness and also reduces the risk of cardiovascular disease in adulthood. (Funded by the AMC Foundation) *Redrafted abstract

"Not knowing when the dawn will come, I open every door."

—**Emily Dickinson**

COMMENT

Familial hypercholesterolemia is a common autosomal-dominant condition of lipoprotein metabolism. It is caused by mutations in genes encoding key proteins involved in the low-density lipoprotein (LDL) receptor endocytic and salvaging pathways. As a result of which, severely elevated plasma levels of LDL cholesterol (LDL-C) increase from birth onward in patients with familial hypercholesterolemia, and these patients are at high risk for untimely cardiovascular disease.

Statins are the preferred pharmacologic therapy for familial hypercholesterolemia. Since, the first functional and morphologic transformations of the arterial wall occur in childhood, there is universal conformity that treatment should start at a young age. The European Atherosclerosis Society (EAS) consensus panel and the current American College of Cardiology–American Heart Association guidelines for familial hypercholesterolemia encourage initiation of statins from 8 years to 10 years of age, respectively.

In the current study, we aimed to discourse differential progression in both subclinical atherosclerosis and clinical cardiovascular disease in patients with familial hypercholesterolemia who started statin treatment in childhood, and to parallel the outcomes with those in both patients with untreated familial hypercholesterolemia and healthy persons.

All 214 children with familial hypercholest-erolemia who had undergone randomization from 1997 through 1999 in a double-blind, single-center, placebo-controlled trial, which gauged the 2-year efficacy and safety of pravastatin, were eligible for the current study. The amassed incidence of cardiovascular events and of death from cardiovascular causes at 39 years of age was lower among the patients with familial hypercholesterolemia than among their affected parents (1% vs. 26% and 0% vs. 7%, respectively) (**Fig. 1**).

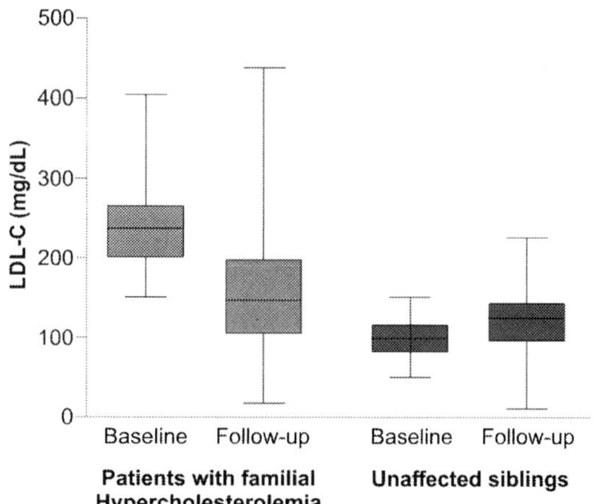

FIG. 1: Low-density lipoprotein cholesterol (LDL-C) levels of patients with familial hypercholesterolemia and their unaffected siblings at baseline and at follow-up.

Key Message

⊙ *In this analysis, initiation of statin therapy throughout childhood in patients with familial hyper-cholesterolemia slackened the progression of carotid intima–media thickness and reduced the risk of cardiovascular disease in adulthood.*

ARTICLE 20

C-type natriuretic peptide analogue therapy in children with achondroplasia

savarirayan R, Irving M, Bacino CA, Bostwick B, Charrow J, Cormier-Daire V, et al. C-type natriuretic peptide analogue therapy in children with achondroplasia.
N Engl J Med. 2019;381:25-35.

Abstract*

Background: Inhibition of endochondral ossification is the basic pathology underlying achondroplasia, a genetic disorder. This results in disproportionate short stature and may lead to serious complications. Here, we evaluate the dose-dependent efficacy and safety of Vosoritide, a biologic analog of C-type natriuretic peptide and a potent stimulator of endochondral ossification, for treatment of achondroplasia.

Methods: A multinational, phase 2, dose-finding study and extension study was conducted on children (5–14 years of age) with achondroplasia. The safety profile of vosoritide was evaluated by enrolling a total of 35 children in four sequential cohorts. They received vosoritide as follows: Once-daily subcutaneous dose of 2.5 µg/kg body weight (8 patients in cohort 1), 7.5 µg/kg (8 patients in cohort 2), 15.0 µg/kg (10 patients in cohort 3), or 30.0 μg/kg (9 patients in cohort 4). After 6 months, the dose in cohort 1 was increased to 7.5 μg/kg and then to 15.0 μg/kg, and in cohort 2, the dose was increased to 15.0 μg/kg. No change in dose was made for cohort 3 and 4. Almost 24-month dose-finding study was completed at the cutoff date, and 30 patients were enrolled for an ongoing long-term extension study. About 42 months was the median duration of follow-up for both studies.

Results: All the 35 patients enrolled showed adverse events during the treatment periods, while 4 of them had serious adverse events (11%). During the first 6 months of treatment, cohort 3 showed a dose-dependent increase in the annualized growth velocity. Also, a sustained increase in the annualized growth velocity was observed at doses of 15.0 and 30.0 μg/kg for up to 42 months of follow-up.

Conclusion: In our study, once-daily subcutaneous administration of vosoritide in children with achondroplasia was associated with mild side effects. Also, we could observe a sustained increase in the annualized growth velocity for up to 42 months. (Funded by BioMarin Pharmaceutical; ClinicalTrials.gov numbers, NCT01603095, NCT02055157, and NCT02724228.) *Redrafted abstract

> *"There is only corner of the universe you can be certain of improving, and that's your own self."*
>
> —**Aldous Huxley**

COMMENT

Achondroplasia is the most common form of disparate short stature, with a prevalence of 1 in 25,000 live births. The condition is instigated by an autosomal-dominant mutation in the fibroblast growth factor receptor 3 gene (*FGFR3*) that constitutively actuates the mitogen-activated protein kinase (MAPK)–extracellular signal-regulated kinase pathway in chondrocytes, which inhibit endochondral ossification. Achondroplasia is associated with a condition-specific profile of developmental milestones, functional restraints affecting quality of life, and chronic pain, all of which lead to psychosocial challenges. Mortality is increased from birth to 4 years of age and in the fourth and fifth decades of life.

C-type natriuretic peptide, encoded by *NPPC*, and its receptor, natriuretic peptide receptor 2 (NPR2), are puissant stimulators of endochondral ossification. Once-daily subcutaneous administration of vosoritide (recombinant C-type natriuretic peptide analog) promotes long-bone growth in juvenile, skeletally normal mice, and monkeys and corrects the dwarfism phenotype in mice with achondroplasia. On the basis of favorable preclinical findings, the current phase 2 dose-finding study and the still-ongoing extension study were conducted to evaluate the use of vosoritide in children with achondroplasia.

In a multinational, phase 2, dose-finding study and extension study, we evaluated the safety and side effect profile of vosoritide in children (5–14 years of age) with achondroplasia. At the time of data cutoff, the 24-month dose-finding study had been completed, and 30 patients had been enrolled in an ongoing long-term extension study; the median duration of follow-up amidst both studies was 42 months.

In the course of the treatment interludes in the dose-finding and extension studies, adverse events occurred in 35 of 35 patients (100%), and serious adverse events occurred in 4 of 35 patients (11%). Therapy was discontinued in 6 patients (in 1 because of an adverse episode). During the foremost 6 months of treatment, a dose-dependent increase in the annualized growth velocity was discerned with vosoritide up to a dose of 15.0 μg/kg, and a sustained increase in the annualized growth velocity was observed at doses of 15.0 and 30.0 μg/kg for up to 42 months (**Figs. 1A** and **B**).

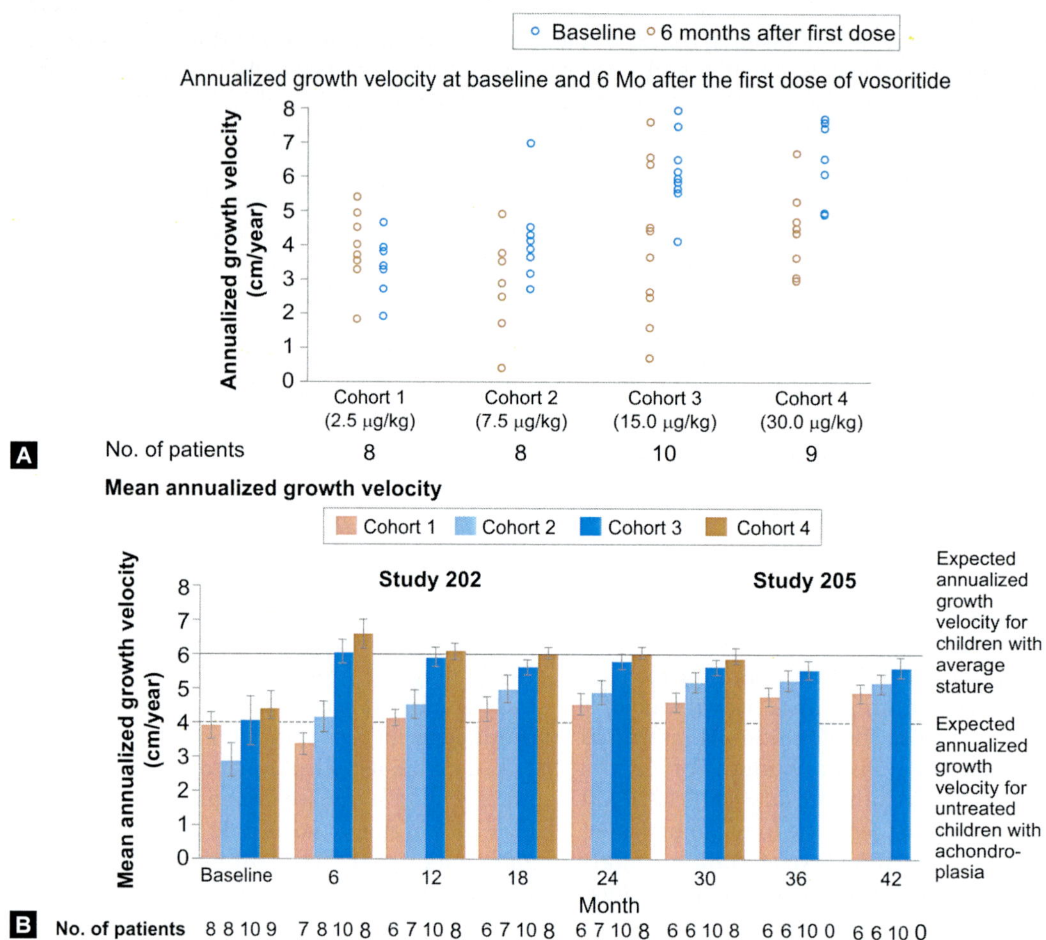

FIGS. 1A AND B: Annualized growth velocity at baseline and during the treatment period.

Key Message

- *In children with achondroplasia, once-daily subcutaneous administration of vosoritide was coupled with a side effect profile that appeared mostly mild. Treatment ensued a sustained increase in the annualized growth velocity for up to 42 months.*

ARTICLE 21

Ambient particulate air pollution and daily mortality in 652 cities

Liu C, Chen R, Sera F, Vicedo-Cabrera AM, Guo Y, Tong S, et al. Ambient particulate air pollution and daily mortality in 652 cities.
N Engl J Med. 2019;381:705-15.

Abstract*

Background: Differences in model specification and publication bias has prevented the systematic evaluation of time-series studies of air pollution. Here, we evaluate the associations of inhalable particulate matter (PM_{10}) (aerodynamic diameter of $\leq$10 μm) and fine $PM_{2.5}$ (aerodynamic diameter $\leq$2.5 μm) with daily all-cause, cardiovascular, and respiratory mortality across multiple countries or regions.

Methods: We collected daily data on mortality and air pollution from 652 cities in 24 countries or regions. Overdispersed generalized additive models with random effects meta-analysis were used to investigate the associations. To test the robustness of the associations, we used two pollutant models and pooling of the concentration–response curves from each city was done to estimate this association at a global level.

Results: Our study showed a 0.44% increase in daily all-cause mortality with an increase of 10 μg /m^3 in the 2-day moving average of PM_{10} concentration. Further, this was also associated with increase of 0.36% (95% CI 0.30–0.43) in daily cardiovascular mortality, and 0.47% (95% CI 0.35–0.58) in daily respiratory mortality. For same change in $PM_{2.5}$ concentration, the increase was 0.68% (95% CI 0.59–0.77), 0.55% (95% CI 0.45–0.66), and 0.74% (95% CI 0.53–0.95), respectively. Adjustment for gaseous pollutants did not affect the associations, which were stronger in locations with lower annual mean PM concentrations and higher annual mean temperatures. A consistent increase in daily mortality with increasing PM concentration was observed in the pooled concentration–response curves that showed steeper slopes at lower PM concentrations.

Conclusion: Short-term exposures to PM_{10} and $PM_{2.5}$ were independently associated with daily all-cause, cardiovascular, and respiratory mortality in >600 cities across the globe. This study also provides an evidence of link between mortality and PM concentration, as already established in regional and local studies. (Funded by the National Natural Science Foundation of China and others) *Redrafted abstract

> *"Environmental pollution is not only humanity's treason to humanity but also a treason to all other living creatures on earth!"*
>
> **— Mehmet Murat ildan**

COMMENT

The undesirable health effects of short-term exposure to ambient air pollution are quite well documented. Particulate matter (PM), especially, provokes public health concerns because of its widespread human exposure to this pollutant as well as its toxicity. PM, which incorporates inhalable particles with an aerodynamic diameter of 10 μm or less (PM_{10}) and fine particles with an aerodynamic diameter of 2.5 μm or less ($PM_{2.5}$), is emitted from combustion sources or formed through atmospheric chemical transformation. Given the extensive evidence regarding their effects of health, the daily and annual mean concentrations of PM_{10} and $PM_{2.5}$ are regulated according to the World Health Organization (WHO) Air Quality Guidelines and standards in major countries.

The associations of inhalable PM with an aerodynamic diameter of 10 μm or less (PM_{10}) and fine PM were evaluated with daily all-cause, cardiovascular, and respiratory mortality across numerous countries. Daily data on air pollution and mortality were collected from 652 cities in 24 countries (**Fig. 1**). Over dispersed generalized additive models were used with random effects meta-analysis to investigate the correlations. Two-pollutant models were fitted to test the vigor of the associations. Concentration–response curves from each city were pooled to allow global estimates to be derived.

The final evaluation included 59.6 million deaths from any cause or nonexternal causes, 20.1 million deaths from cardiovascular diseases, and 5.6 million deaths from respiratory diseases. Associations were stronger in places with lower annual mean PM concentrations and higher annual mean temperatures. The pooled concentration–response curves bared an unswerving increase in daily mortality with increasing PM concentration, with steeper slopes at lower PM concentrations.

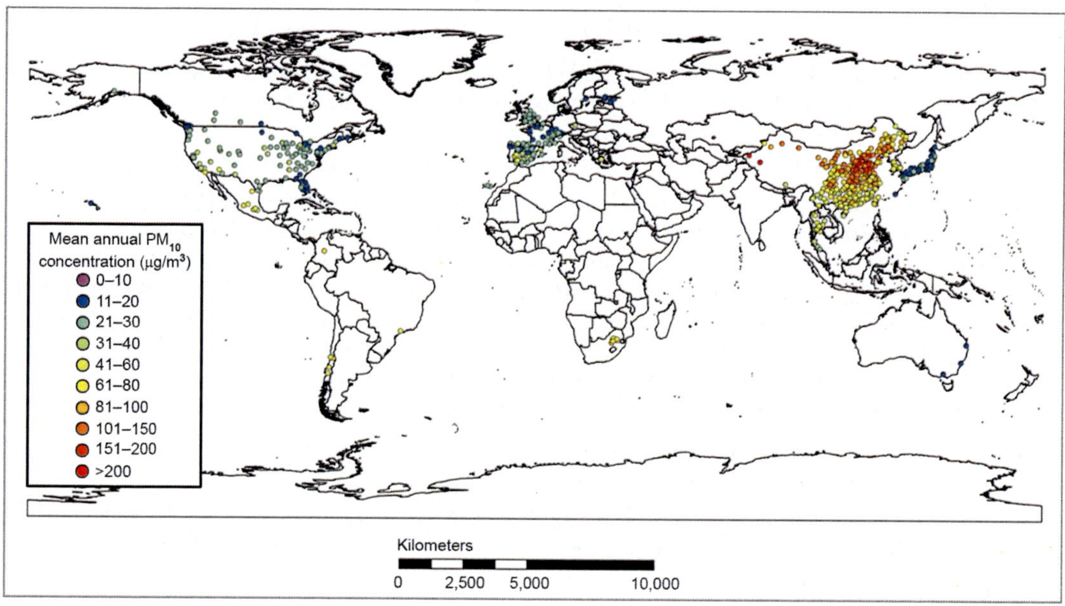

FIG. 1: Distribution of the cities with data on PM$_{10}$.

Key Message

⊙ *Independent associations concerning short-term exposure to PM$_{10}$ and PM$_{2.5}$ and daily all-cause, cardiovascular, and respiratory mortality in >600 cities across the globe were seen. These data buttress the evidence of a link between PM concentration and mortality ascertained in regional and local studies.*

Section 7: Nephrology and Hypertension

Section Editor: Vivekanand Jha

Associate Editors: Gopesh K Modi, Joyita Bharati

ARTICLE 1

Effects of nicotinamide and lanthanum carbonate on serum phosphate and fibroblast growth factor-23 in CKD: the COMBINE trial

Ix JH, Isakova T, Larive B, Raphael KL, Raj DS, Cheung AK, et al. Effects of nicotinamide and lanthanum carbonate on serum phosphate and fibroblast growth factor-23 in CKD: the COMBINE trial.
J Am Soc Nephrol. 2019;30:1096-108.

Abstract*

Management of hyperphosphatemia and high fibroblast growth factor 23 (FGF 23) levels remains a treatment target in advanced chronic kidney disease (CKD). To enhance the effect of intestinal phosphate binder, lanthanum carbonate (LC), a randomized trial was conducted to see the additive benefit of nicotinamide (NAM). Around 205 patients with estimated glomerular filtration rate (eGFR) between 20 and 45 mL/min/1.73 m^2 (mean 32 mL/min/1.73 m^2) with mean baseline serum phosphate of 3.7 mg/dL and median FGR 99 pg/mL (10 and 99 percentile: 59, 205) were randomized in a 2 × 2 study design randomized double blind placebo-controlled trial into four groups: (1) NAM plus LC, (2) NAM plus LC placebo, (3) LC plus NAM placebo, or (4) double placebo for 12 months. However, after 12 months, neither the serum phosphate nor the FGF 23 levels reduced in any study group. *Redrafted abstract

"Reductionism and real life—It does not always add up."

COMMENT

Cardiovascular disease burden in chronic kidney disease (CKD) patients is the biggest reason for their morbidity and mortality. CKD and its associated variables impose a cardiovascular risk factor burden that outweighs the conventional cardiovascular risk factors. Hyperphosphatemia is ubiquitous in CKD and the levels have been associated with cardiovascular outcome and vascular calcification in a large number of studies. The risk starts building up even with modest elevation of serum phosphate levels. Fibroblast growth factor 23 (FGF 23) levels start rising to counter the serum phosphate elevation by augmenting urinary phosphate excretion. The downside is the association of high FGF levels with left ventricular hypertrophy and increased risk of heart failure.

Intestinal phosphate binders work by reducing the availability of absorbable phosphate in gut. Just as it happens in biology, as a consequence of phosphate binders the sodium phosphate active cotransporter 2b (Npt2b) on the intestinal epithelial cells gets upregulated. The natural next step would then be to block Npt2b. High dose nicotinamide (NAM) does just that. There are studies that show reduction in serum phosphate levels with NAM in patients with end stage kidney disease. The background for this trial is thus set on pragmatic application of phosphate absorption dynamics. Of course, it must be reiterated that even lowering serum phosphate is not synonymous with reduction in hard endpoints of health benefits in CKD.

The CKD Optimal Management with Binders and Nicotinamide (COMBINE) thus tests the efficacy of these two agents in moderate CKD individually or as a synergistic/additive combination. Unfortunately, over the course of 1 year, it fails in both the objectives of lowering serum phosphate or FGF 23 levels in either scenario of lanthanum carbonate (LC) or NAM alone or in combination. The duration of 12 months is enough to demonstrate not only the efficacy but also the ability to ensure compliance and tolerability over some length of time.

The study population was representative of typical kidney clinic patient profile: Mean age 69 years, 38% women, mean estimated glomerular filtration rate (eGFR) 32 mL/min/1.73 m^2 and mean serum phosphate 3.7 mg/dL. Although the mean body mass index (BMI) over 30 may not represent all populations. The results did not change even on subgroup analysis on patients with serum phosphate >4 mg/dL at baseline. The investigators had measured 24 hours urinary phosphate excretion as a surrogate for net reduction in intestinal phosphate absorption. As expected, LC did achieve this goal of reduced phosphate absorption. NAM on the other hand did not change urinary phosphate excretion implying that it was ineffective in reducing intestinal phosphate absorption. It also did not exert additive effect on reducing intestinal phosphate absorption with LC.

What makes these agents to further lose favor is >40% participants in N-L arm and almost a third in either N or L arm discontinued the drug due to gastrointestinal side effects and pill burden. While a large drop out will drive the results to null hypothesis and the usual argument would be to go on searching with another strategy for a benefit. In reductionist approach this is can be justified but the final endpoint is the overall benefit to a patient. Then synthesis of all that we have unearthed should be put in real life context where the proportion of noncompliant patients might be even more and is likely to nullify any small benefit if it were actually present. Besides, outside a trial, another burden on patient will be cost per added medication. And, even if some reduction is serum phosphate or FGF 23 is obtained, it will have to walk the mile for actual health benefit. The current evidence should inspire alternative or novel approaches rather than trying to press for more juice from what has hitherto been unrewarding in a nicely done trial.

Key Messages

- *Clinical nephrology has been seeking interventions to reduce serum phosphate and FGF 23 in CKD.*
- *Intestinal phosphate binders such as lanthanum carbonate (LC) have been partly successful in this endeavor.*
- *Blocking additional pathway for phosphate absorption with nicotinamide (NAM) in an additive manner was tried in CKD patients. The strategy did not yield any benefit over a period of 12 months.*

ARTICLE 2

Intravenous iron in patients undergoing maintenance hemodialysis

Macdougall IC, White C, Anker SD, Bhandari S, Farrington K, PIVOTAL Investigators Committees, et al. Intravenous iron in patients undergoing maintenance hemodialysis.
N Engl J Med. 2019;380:447-58.

Abstract

The PIVOTAL multicenter, open-label trial with a noninferiority design tested the safety and efficacy of high dose intravenous (IV) iron therapy in patients undergoing hemodialysis in the UK. A total of 2,141 adult patients in their first year on hemodialysis were randomized in 1:1 ratio to either a reactive strategy of relatively small doses of IV iron (0–400 mg monthly) when ferritin was <200 ng/mL or TSAT was <20% or a proactive strategy of a 600 mg iron load in month 1 followed by 400 mg monthly when ferritin was <700 ng/mL and TSAT was <40%.

The primary trial endpoint was the composite of nonfatal myocardial infarction, nonfatal stroke, hospitalization for heart failure, or death, assessed in a time-to-first-event analysis. Secondary endpoints included death, infection rate, and dose of an erythropoiesis-stimulating agent (ESA). Noninferiority would be met if the upper boundary of the 95% confidence interval for the hazard ratio for the primary endpoint did not cross 1.25 (**Fig. 1**).

A total of 1,093 patients were randomized to the proactive group and 1,048 to the reactive group. The patients in the proactive group received a median monthly iron dose of 264 mg—a mean of 3.8 g of iron in the first year, then an average of 200 mg per month from 12 months onward. The patients in the reactive group were never iron loaded, yet still required a median of 145 mg (mean of 1.8 g of iron during the first year then 165 mg per month).

A total of 320 patients (29.3%) in the high-dose group had a primary endpoint event, as compared with 338 (32.3%) in the low-dose group. The hazard ratio of 0.85 (95% CI 0.73–1.00) was statistically significant for superiority (p = 0.04), suggesting that the proactive approach reduced the rate of major cardiovascular events.

Proactive iron loading led to more rapid improvement of anemia and reduced transfusions in the first year, with hemoglobin averaging 11.2 g/dL versus 10.6 g/dL at 3 months, and 0.3 g/dL higher in the proactive group at 9 months. The median monthly ESA dose was 29,757 IU in the high-dose group and 38,805 IU in the low-dose group. This translated to ~7,000 and ~9,000 units/week for the proactive and reactive groups, respectively. Infections were not increased with high-dose IV iron.

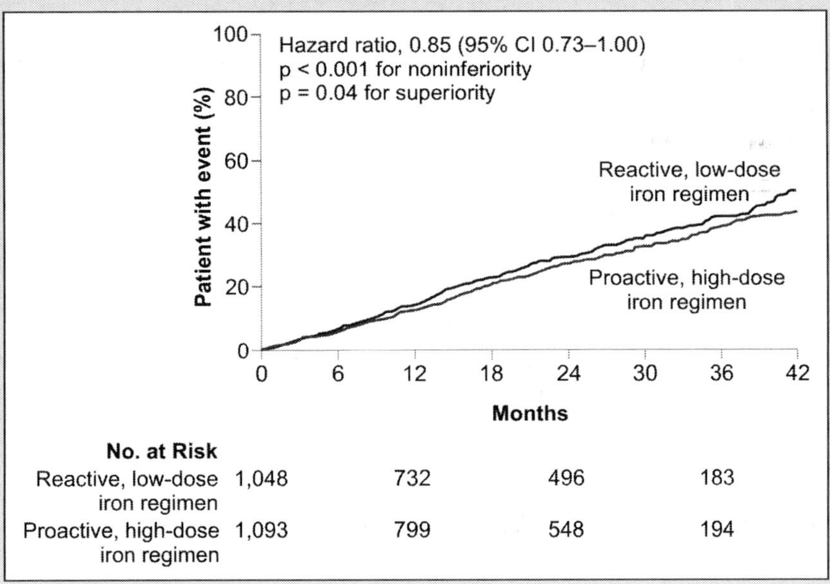

FIG. 1: Shows the comparison between the two treatment arms on the primary end point (death from any cause).

"Ironic – more is not less with IV iron for anemia of kidney disease."

COMMENT

Anemia is ubiquitous among patients on dialysis. The management is centered on erythropoiesis-stimulating agents (ESAs), but the critical role of iron has been long recognized. There are several reasons behind the iron deficiency of chronic kidney disease (CKD)—insufficient iron intake and uptake from the gut, occult or overt blood loss from the gastrointestinal (GI) tract, menorrhagia, hemodialysis-associated blood loss, and frequent blood sampling for diagnostic purposes. Elevated hepcidin hampers GI iron absorption and blocks iron release from hepatocytes and macrophages.

Consensus on the correct dose of iron has been plagued by worries about iron toxicity (infection, iron overload). The increased risk of deaths in patients on hemodialysis in the 1998 Normal Hematocrit Trial was correlated the dose of IV iron in a post-hoc analysis.

The recommendations prior to PIVOTAL suggested maintaining ferritin levels >200 ng/mL and avoiding intravenous (IV) iron when ferritin exceeds 500 ng/mL. Studies have shown that IV iron can raise hemoglobin levels and transferrin saturation and lower ESA dose requirements, even in highly inflamed patients on dialysis with serum ferritin levels of 500–1,200 ng/mL. However, this approach had not been tested in large, long-term studies.

These findings again emphasize the need for randomized controlled trials (RCTs), since PIVOTAL clearly shows that proactive IV iron administration reduces cardiovascular events and deaths, need for transfusions and ESA doses but does not increase infections in patients on hemodialysis. These findings are exact opposite of prior observational studies and post-hoc analyses that had identified higher risks of death, major adverse cardiovascular events, CKD progression, or infection in patients who had been treated with prolonged, high-dose IV iron.

PIVOTAL findings comprehensively allay the concerns raised about the dangers of IV iron, support eliminating the ferritin limit, and provide reassurance that maintaining high iron stores is beneficial in patients on hemodialysis.

These results also validate the findings of the 2007 DRIVE trial, which showed that IV iron compared with no iron raised hemoglobin levels, lowered ESA doses by about 25% and reduced treatment costs. A post-hoc analysis of this trial reported that IV iron did not increase infection rates and reduced serious adverse events.

Some cautionary flags about generalizability have been raised—the trial was done only in UK units, used only iron sucrose, and followed a particular dosing schedule (more frequent smaller doses may be even better tolerated), had a relatively short follow-up time (2.1 years). Studies that extend the proactive approach to diverse populations, other iron formulations, determine the long-term safety would be valuable.

Is there no upper limit to how much iron we can give? This trial does not answer that question. Hemochromatosis is associated with much higher ferritin levels and TSATs >70%. An observational study of 58,058 hemodialysis patients set a threshold dose of 400 mg/month above which IV iron tended to be associated with higher mortality.

Key Messages

- *High dose IV iron provides cardiovascular benefits and reduces ESA requirement in patients on dialysis.*
- *A more thorough refutation of the hypothesis that generous IV iron use will harm patients on dialysis is hard to imagine.*

ARTICLE 3

Atrasentan and renal events in patients with type 2 diabetes and chronic kidney disease (SONAR): a double-blind, randomized, placebo-controlled trial

Heerspink HJ, Parving HH, Andress DL, Bakris G, Correa-Rotter R, SONAR Committees Investigators, et al. Atrasentan and renal events in patients with type 2 diabetes and chronic kidney disease (SONAR): a double-blind, randomized, placebo-controlled trial.

Lancet. 2019;393:1937-47.

Abstract

The SONAR trial reported the result of long-term treatment with the selective endothelin-A (ETA) receptor antagonist atrasentan (0.75 mg daily), a selective ETA receptor antagonist in patients with type 2 diabetes mellitus (T2DM) and chronic kidney disease (CKD). This randomized, double-blind placebo-controlled trial was conducted at 689 sites in 41 countries. It followed an enrichment design to select patients more likely to respond and less likely to develop fluid retention. Patients had to have a baseline brain natriuretic peptide (BNP) <200 pg/mL, no history of heart failure or severe peripheral edema. Then they entered an enrichment period that selected patients for albuminuria response plus lack of substantial fluid retention (an increase in bodyweight ≥3 kg and a BNP increase to ≥300 pg/mL) once on atrasentan.

Out of a total of 11,087 screened patients, 5,117 entered the enrichment period and 2,648 successfully completed run-in. Of these, 1,325 were assigned to atrasentan and 1,323 to placebo. The primary outcome events were sustained (>30 day) doubling of serum creatinine and end-stage kidney disease (ESKD) (estimated glomerular filtration rate <15 mL/min/1.73 m^2 sustained for ≥90 days, chronic dialysis for >90 days, kidney transplantation, or death from kidney failure). The trial was event-driven and was terminated prematurely by the sponsor when it was predicted that the prespecified number of events would not be reached at a median follow-up of 2.2 years. Around 79 (6.0%) of 1,325 participants in the atrasentan group and 105 (7·9%) of 1,323 in the placebo group had a primary composite renal endpoint event [hazard ratio (HR) 0.65 (95% CI 0.49–0.88); p = 0.0047]. There was no significant interaction between responder and nonresponder status, suggesting that results were similar overall. The difference was significant for doubling of serum creatinine [HR 0.61 (95% CI 0.43–0.87)] but not for end-stage renal disease (ESRD) [HR 0.73 (95% CI 0.53–1.01)]. No significant beneficial effects of atrasentan were detected on risks of hospital admission for heart failure [HR 1.33 (95% CI 0.85–2.07); p = 0.208] or all-cause mortality [HR 1.09 (95% CI 0.75–1.59); p = 0.65]. Effects on the primary outcome were maintained across subgroups, including by sex, age, albuminuria or glycemia, and kidney function. Serious adverse events, including fluid retention and anemia, occurred more frequently in the atrasentan group than in the placebo group. The authors concluded that atrasentan reduced the risk of renal events in patients with diabetes and CKD who were selected to optimize efficacy and safety, and supported its role in protecting renal function in patients with T2DM at high risk of developing end-stage kidney disease (ESKD) (**Fig. 1**).

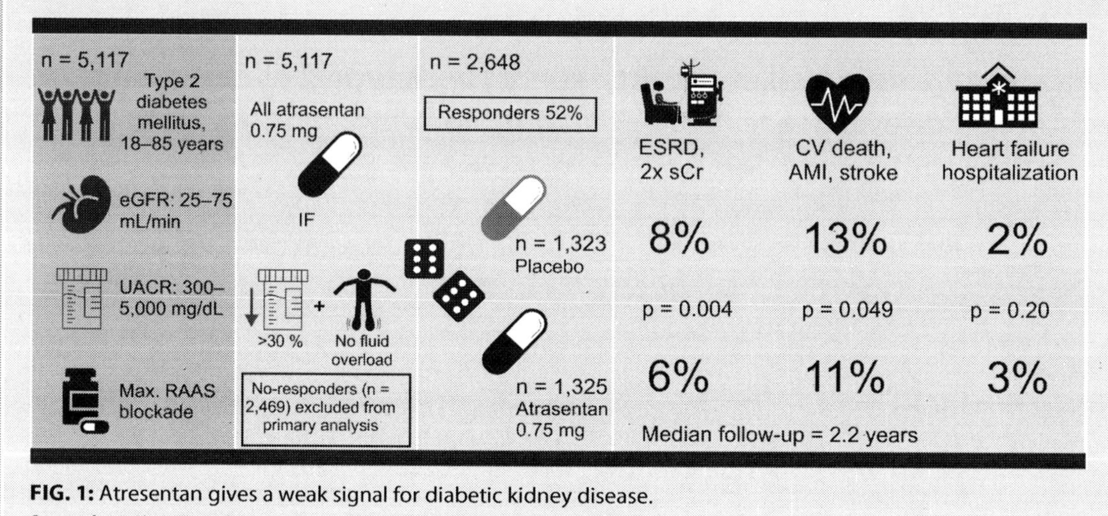

FIG. 1: Atresentan gives a weak signal for diabetic kidney disease.
Source: http://www.nephjc.com/news/2019/6/11/sonar-the-visual-abstract

"So near and yet so far: Why a successful intervention will not reach clinical practice?"

COMMENT

Endothelin-1, a vasoactive peptide with cytokine-like properties, produces complex and opposing actions within the vasculature and contributes to the pathogenesis of diabetic kidney disease (DKD). There are at least four known receptors—ETA, ETB1, ETB2, and ETC. Endothelin-A (ETA) receptor activation mediates sodium retention, fibrosis and inflammation, whereas ETB receptor activation facilitates sodium excretion via activation of the nitric oxide synthase in the collecting duct and inhibition of epithelial sodium channel activity as well as protection against the actions of ETA receptor activation on fibrosis and inflammation. Atrasentan, a selective ETA receptor antagonist, was initially studied for the potential treatment of cancer.

Strong rationale exists that selective ETA receptor antagonists could reduce or slow the progression of kidney injury and disease. Early successes with ETA antagonists in decreasing albuminuria in DKD patients, however, were marred by volume overload. The randomized controlled trial (RCT) examining avosentan for nephroprotection had to be terminated early due to increased heart failure rates.

To get over this issue, SONAR used a clever design that preselected patients most likely to benefit and less prone to the most common adverse of atrasentan. This personalized approach facilitated demonstration of a positive outcome for the primary endpoint (progression of DKD), but compromises the external validity of the results and implementation of such an enrichment strategy in routine busy clinical practice. Notably, atrasentan did not provide a cardiovascular advantage.

Even though SONAR has demonstrated that atrasentan preserves renal function in addition to decreasing albuminuria, this agent is unlikely to be widely used. The most important confounders are CREDENCE findings, because the field has shifted toward a new benchmark of renin–angiotensin system (RAS) blockade plus sodium-glucose cotransporter-2 (SGLT-2) inhibitor.

These are interesting hypotheses that need to be examined in new clinical trials. At this time, it has been speculated that AbbVie may not be interested in further exploring this potentially life-saving drug. An important factor in the calculus is the short remaining patent life for most of these compounds.

> ### Key Messages
>
> ⊙ *Atrasentan favorably influences the course of certain patients with DKD but is difficult to use in routine clinical practice.*
>
> ⊙ *Can simultaneous use of atrasentan and SGLT-2 inhibitor on top of RAS blockade provide further nephroprotection and reduce the residual risk? Could this combination offset any potential deleterious effect of atrasentan on heart failure?*

ARTICLE 4

Canagliflozin and renal outcomes in type 2 diabetes and nephropathy

Perkovic V, Jardine MJ, Neal B, Bompoint S, Heerspink HJ, Charytan DM, CREDENCE Trial Investigators, et al. Canagliflozin and renal outcomes in type 2 diabetes and nephropathy.
N Engl J Med. 2019;380:2295-306.

Abstract*

The CREDENCE double blind randomized trial assigned 4,401 type 2 diabetes mellitus (T2DM) patients with diabetes and albuminuric kidney disease to receive canagliflozin, an oral sodium-glucose cotransporter-2 (SGLT-2) inhibitor at 100 mg/day or placebo and followed them for a median of 2.62 years. Patients needed to have kidney disease—as defined by estimated glomerular filtration rate (eGFR) 30–90 mL/min/1.73 m^2 and UACR 300–5,000 mg/g, and be on treatment with angiotensin converting enzyme (ACE) blockade. Treatment was maintained until patients started kidney replacement therapy. The primary endpoint was a composite of end-stage kidney disease (ESKD), doubling of serum creatinine or death from renal or cardiovascular cause. The trial was event-driven, and terminated early because of the evidence of benefit in a prespecified interim analysis.

Canagliflozin decreased the combined primary endpoint by 30% [hazard ratio (HR) 0.70; 95% confidence interval (CI) 0.59–0.82; p = 0.00001] and the secondary endpoints – both renal (ESKD, doubling of serum creatinine or renal death) [HR 0.66 (95% CI 0.53–0.81; p < 0.001)] as well as cardiovascular (death or hospitalization for heart failure) [HR 0.69 (95% CI 0.57–0.83; p ≤ 0.001)]. The risk of ESKD was reduced by 32% (p = 0.002).

Canagliflozin was safe, in fact, serious adverse events significantly less frequent in the treatment arm than for placebo HR 0.87 (95% CI 0.79–0.97). Some adverse effects that raised concerns in prior canagliflozin trials such as amputation and fracture were not increased in frequency. The HR for diabetic ketoacidosis was increased, but the absolute risk was low: Only 11 out of 2,200 patients developed this event.

The data suggest that for every 1,000 patients treated for 2.5 years, canagliflozin would prevent the composite primary outcome of ESKD, doubling of the serum creatinine level, or renal or cardiovascular death; prevent 22 hospitalizations for heart failure and 25 composite events of cardiovascular death, myocardial infarction, or stroke. *Redrafted abstract

"Changing paradigm in treatment of diabetic kidney disease: CREDENCE opens the door."

COMMENT

Diabetic kidney disease (DKD) is a devastating complication of diabetes that increases the risk of kidney failure that needs kidney replacement therapy and an increased risk of premature death, mainly due to cardiovascular disease. According to Global Burden of Disease data, DKD was the cause of >425,000 deaths in 2017, increased by 37% in the last decade, and accounted for 35% of deaths from chronic kidney disease (CKD) worldwide. Type 2 diabetes mellitus (T2DM) was responsible for >80% of these DKD deaths.

Renin–angiotensin system (RAS) blockade is the standard of care for patients with proteinuric DKD for protection from development of kidney failure. However, it is worth pointing out that neither the IDNT (irbesartan), nor the RENAAL (losartan) trials showed any benefit on a secondary cardiovascular outcome of cardiovascular death, myocardial infarction, unstable angina, heart failure resulting in hospitalization, stroke, peripheral revascularization or limb amputation. Further, the kidney risk protection was incomplete – with a residual risk of 6–8/100 patient-years for individual endpoints and 11/100 patient-years for the combined endpoint of doubling of serum creatinine or end-stage kidney disease (ESKD). This means that the search for an agent that could provide further protection is very much ongoing.

Canagliflozin belongs to a class of molecules that inhibit the enzyme sodium-glucose cotransporter-2 (SGLT-2) cotransporter involved in 90% of glucose reabsorption in the proximal renal tubule. This reduces the renal threshold of glucose from 180 to 40–120 mg/dL, leading to loss of glucose in urine excretion and lower blood glucose levels. On the basis of this property, SGLT-2 inhibitors were tested and approved as a new class of hypoglycemic agents.

Secondary outcome results of the cardio-vascular outcomes trials of SGLT-2 inhibitors—the EMPA-REG OUTCOME (Empagliflozin Cardiovascular Outcome Event Trial in Type 2 Diabetes Mellitus Patients), CANVAS Program (CANagliflozin cardioVascular Assessment Study), and the DECLARE-TIMI (Dapagliflozin Effect on Cardiovascular Events–Thrombolysis in Myocardial Infarction) study showed strong signal of renoprotection. Making a clear conclusion regarding kidney-related benefits was not possible, however, since most of the participants enrolled these studies had normal kidney function.

Still, the guidelines recommendations were modified to suggest considering SGLT-2 inhibitor to lower serum glucose for albuminuric DKD patients with relatively preserved renal function based, but stopped short of recommending SGLT-2 inhibitors to treat DKD.

These findings naturally prompted setting up of trials to investigate the effect of these molecules on DKD. CREDENCE is the first RCT of any SGLT-2 inhibitors in which the whole study population had DKD and the primary endpoint was renal. The study findings are unequivocal, and provide solid evidence for a new therapeutic indication for canagliflozin to treat DKD. The addition of canagliflozin, and possibly other SGLT-2 inhibitors with proven renoprotection, to the armamentarium of drugs that delay kidney function decline DKD has been widely hailed and is leading to rapid change in clinical practice guidelines worldwide.

The CREDENCE sets a new standard of care treatment of DKD. The combination of canagliflozin and RAS blockade achieved a very low residual kidney risk. The agent was effective at estimated glomerular filtration rate (eGFR) below the current limits of 60 mL/min/1.73 m^2 for initiation and 45 mL/min/1.73 m^2 for maintenance. Since the drug was not stopped until patients initiated renal replacement therapy (RRT), there should be no limits for canagliflozin prescription based on eGFR. The eGFR was 30–44 mL/min/1.73 m^2 in 31% of the patients and 45–60 mL/min/1.73 m^2 in 29%. This helps expanding the indication for treatment of DKD beyond the current eGFR limits that canagliflozin should not be initiated when eGFR is <60 mL/min/1.73 m^2.

Interestingly, the hypoglycemic effect of canagliflozin in CREDENCE was mild—the mean difference in glycosylated hemoglobin (HbA1c) between the treatment and placebo groups was 0.25% over the study period and only 0.11% at the

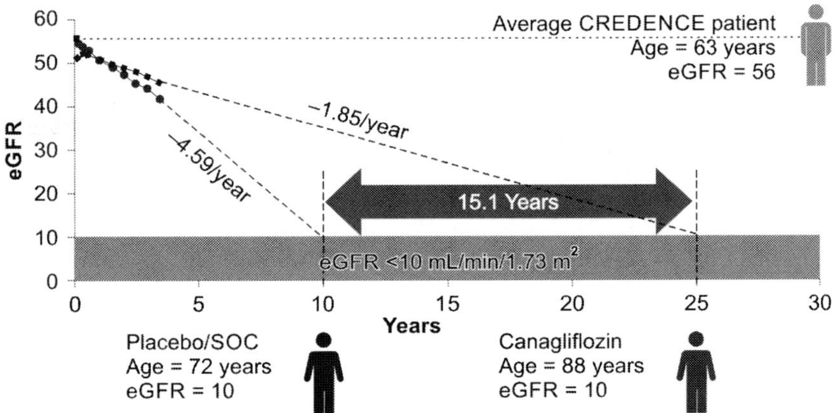

FIG. 1: The projected effects of SGLT-2 inhibitors on. eGFR based on CREDENCE data.

end of the study. Despite this moderate effect on HbA1c, end-stage renal disease (ESRD) events were reduced by 32% (**Fig. 1**). These findings imply that renal protection can be expected following treatment with canagliflozin irrespective of the HbA1c levels. This is a vital finding, since the hypoglycemic effect of SGLT-2 inhibitors is likely to come down as GFR declines.

The sum of these observations is from being primarily an antidiabetic agent, SGLT-2 inhibitors can be used primarily to treat DKD, independent from any antidiabetic effect.

The question that follows then is—will SGLT-2 inhibition help patients with other types of kidney disease as well? This hypothesis is being examined in the EMPA-KIDNEY (The Study of Heart and Kidney Protection with Empagliflozin; NCT03594110) and DAPA-CKD (A Study to Evaluate the Effect of Dapagliflozin on Renal Outcomes and Cardiovascular Mortality in Patients with Chronic Kidney Disease; NCT03036150).

So what is the mechanism of nephroprotection independent of the antidiabetic effects of these agents? The most widely accepted hypothesis is the impact on glomerular hyperfiltration related to tubuloglomerular feedback inducing afferent arteriole vasoconstriction. This complements the efferent arteriole vasodilation by RAS blockade and further lowers intraglomerular pressure, glomerular hyperfiltration and albuminuria. Eventually, circulating angiotensin II and atrial natriuretic peptide levels decrease, inflammation comes down and intrarenal oxygenation increases. Other mechanisms include lowering body weight, blood pressure, uric acid, plasma volume and proximal tubular cell glucotoxicity, oxidative stress, inflammation and oxygen consumption and increasing natriuresis, hemoglobin levels and insulin sensitivity.

Key Message

⊚ *Sodium-glucose cotransporter-2 inhibitors reduce the risks for CVD and CKD progression in patients with type 2 diabetes mellitus and glucose lowering is a side effect.*

ARTICLE 5

A phase 3 trial of difelikefalin in hemodialysis patients with pruritus

Fishbane S, Jamal A, Munera C, Wen W, Menzaghi F, KALM-1 Trial Investigators. A phase 3 trial of difelikefalin in hemodialysis patients with pruritus.
N Engl J Med. 2020;382:222-32.

Abstract*

Treatment of uremic pruritus was attempted by targeting the activity of peripheral neurons and immune cells residing in skin. Difelikefalin is a selective agonist of kappa opioid receptors with potential antipruritic activity. The efficacy of intravenous difelikefalin (0.5 µg/kg bodyweight thrice a week) in reducing pruritus was assessed in a cohort of patients on regular hemodialysis in a double-blind, placebo-controlled, phase 3 trial. The primary outcome was an improvement in 24-hour Worst Itching Intensity Numerical Rating Scale (WI-NRS; score range 0–10 with higher score implying severe itching). The secondary outcomes were changes in quality of life impact of itching. Around 378 patients were randomized and 51.9% (82 of 158) in the difelikefalin group were benefitted as measured by at least a 3-point WI-NRS score change compared to 30.9% (51 of 165) in the placebo arm. Diarrhea, dizziness, and vomiting were more common in the treatment arm. *Redrafted abstract

"Doping the uremic itch/pruritus."

COMMENT

Uremic pruritus is a major symptom in chronic kidney disease (CKD) patients. Its prevalence and intensity increases in hemodialysis patients. It is frustrating for the patients and healthcare providers because of its impact of quality of life, sleep and lack of effective treatments. Being a nonlife-threatening issue in the midst of a life-threatening disease condition, the symptom has perhaps remained orphan. For years the treatment has been a hit and trial with a variety of local and systemic agents essentially comprising emollients, moisturizers, phototherapy, and antihistamines with added attempts using gabapentin, pregabalin and steroids.

The sensation of pruritus is mediated by chemokines secreted by the immune cells in skin and by the stimulation of the nerve endings that carry the signal to brain in response to a variety of stimuli. Peripherally distributed kappa opioid receptors are part of that orchestra of signals. Difelikefalin activates these very receptors on neurons and immune cells. It does not cross blood brain barrier thereby minimizing chances of neurological adverse effects.

This drug was studied part of KALM-1 trial at 56 sites in the United States. The pruritus and associated effects were studied with various scales. Concomitant antipruritic medications that were already running in almost 40% of patients were continued. The Worst Itching Intensity Numerical Rating Scale (WI-NRS) score of 4 or above indicates moderate-to-severe itching. A 3-point reduction was considered a significant primary outcome measure. Additionally, itch related quality of life was measured with two instruments: (1) 5-D itch scale (score range 5–25; degree, duration, direction, disability and distribution of itch), and (2) Skindex-20 multidimensional questionnaire (score 0–60; effect of itching of disease, mood and emotional distress, and social functioning). The mean (SD) baseline WI-NRS score was 7.1 (1.4) and 7.3 (1.6) in both the groups. The changes at the end of 12-week period are shown in the **Table 1**. It is obvious that difelikefalin led to an improvement in all scales that were measured. Interestingly, even the placebo arm experienced improvement in the score indicating some benefit of the existent pruritus treatments. More likely, it points to the

TABLE 1: Itching related scores and efficacy of difelikefalin uremic pruritus.

Scale	Difelikefalin (n = 189)	Placebo (n = 189)	p value
>3-point reduction in WI-NRS score	82/158	51/165	<0.001
≥4-point improvement in 5D scale*	–5.0 (0.3)	–3.7 (0.3)	<0.001
Change in Skindex-10 score*	–17.2 (1.3)	–12 (1.2)	<0.001

*Least square mean change.
(WI-NRS: Worst Itching Intensity Numerical Rating Scale)

complex nature of this symptom both in terms of pathophysiology and its natural course. The investigators looked for the possibility of physical dependence to the drug with the Short Opioid Withdrawal Scale (ShOWS) and Objective Opioid Withdrawal Scale (OOWS) and there was no evidence of physical dependence with difelikefalin in line with its inactivity at mu or delta opioid receptors.

The clinically meaningful benefit with this agent definitely warrants doing long-term studies and extending it to predialysis CKD patients as well.

Key Messages

- Uremic pruritus is a disabling condition and affects quality of life significantly.
- The options for treatment of uremic pruritus have been very restricted and have not seen any new development for quite some time.
- Difelikefalin, a kappa opioid receptor agonist has shown promise in this randomized trial and thus promises to be a new treatment for this condition.

ARTICLE 6

Effects of sodium bicarbonate in CKD stages 3 and 4: a randomized, placebo-controlled, multicenter clinical trial

Melamed ML, Horwitz EJ, Dobre MA, Abramowitz MK, Zhang L, Lo Y, et al. Effects of sodium bicarbonate in CKD stages 3 and 4: a randomized, placebo-controlled, multicenter clinical trial.
Am J Kidney Dis. 2020;75:225-34.

Abstract

Neutralization of metabolic acidosis has been advocated for helping with progression of chronic kidney disease (CKD), associated mineral and bone disorder and muscle dysfunction. Around 149 patients with CKD stage 3 and 4 [mean estimated glomerular filtration rate (eGFR) 24 mL/min/1.73 m^2] participated in a three center, randomized, placebo-controlled clinical trial to evaluate the effects of administering sodium bicarbonate (0.4 mEq/kg of body weight). The primary outcome measures were changes in muscle function testing and bone mineral density. Muscle biopsies were also performed to look for subcellular and biochemical changes. The mean (SD) age, eGFR and baseline serum bicarbonate for the study cohort were 61 (12.6) years, 36.3 (11.2) mL/min/1.73 m^2 and 24 (2.20) mEq/L. The mean follow-up was 1.35 (0.75 years). The serum bicarbonate remained significantly higher than baseline in the intervention arm compared to placebo on repeated measurements across the study period with the highest value being at 2-month assessment at 26.4 (2.2) mEq/L. The results did not show any difference in functional muscle strength testing or bone mineral density between the groups. There was significant albeit small reduction in serum potassium in the study arm by 0.1 mEq/L. The intervention thus did not benefit either of the primary endpoints in stage 3 and 4 CKD patients.

"A pinch of soda for muscle and bone health in chronic kidney disease."

COMMENT

Metabolic acidosis is the hallmark of chronic kidney disease (CKD) and worsens with progressive loss of glomerular filtration rate (GFR). Experimental data suggests this can amplify kidney damage and hasten the progression of CKD. Similar evidence exists that metabolic acidosis can accelerate bone resorption and impede new bone formation. It is also linked to metabolic bone disease. There is uncontrolled evidence to support alkali supplementation for improving muscle strength. This study tried to address these questions in a randomized placebo-controlled trial. It evaluated a comprehensive set of measures to ensure picking up any benefit that might be present. These included sit-to-stand test that measures the time for 10 successive sit to stand maneuvers from a straight back chair. Handgrip strength measurement and bone mineral density using dual-energy X-ray absorptiometry (DEXA) scan besides routine biochemistry and estimated GFR (eGFR) change over time. Muscle biopsies were obtained in a subset of patients and were analyzed for gene expression studies, protein composition changes to examine for catabolism and inflammatory markers in muscle.

It is disappointing to find no benefit whatsoever of sodium bicarbonate supplementation in the CKD stage 3 and 4 on muscle strength, muscle composition or bone mineral density and GFR loss. The sound physiological basis of the study could not fructify into a cheap and safe treatment modality. These findings are contradictory to observations in general population and even some unblinded smaller studies in CKD wherein alkali supplementation improved functional status, reduced muscle catabolism and even reduced loss of GFR with time. But this narrative is not uncommon wherein randomized placebo-controlled trials throw up results contrary to what has been reasonably accepted or assumed.

While this study finds no benefit of sodium bicarbonate supplementation, it is still difficult to accept that correction of metabolic acidosis will have no benefits in CKD. In this study the participants had normal serum bicarbonate at enrollment. It is likely the benefits are restricted to people with low serum bicarbonate at inception. It is also plausible that patients with normal bicarbonate need a detailed acid base analysis to enrich the at-risk population or they need higher doses of alkali or higher serum bicarbonate level target.

This study thus very elegantly establishes futility of sodium bicarbonate in CKD stage 3 and 4 with normal bicarbonate at usual doses and leaves the room open to newer strategies for addressing the acid base consequences of CKD.

Key Messages

⊙ *Metabolic acidosis is always seen in CKD and its treatment has potential to help muscle function, bone health and overall mortality.*

⊙ *Sodium bicarbonate supplementation in moderate CKD with normal serum bicarbonate does not add any benefit to above parameters.*

ARTICLE 7

Patiromer versus placebo to enable spironolactone use in patients with resistant hypertension and chronic kidney disease (AMBER): a phase 2, randomized, double-blind, placebo-controlled trial

Agarwal R, Rossignol P, Romero A, Garza D, Mayo MR, Warren S, et al. Patiromer versus placebo to enable spironolactone use in patients with resistant hypertension and chronic kidney disease (AMBER): A phase 2, randomized, double-blind, placebo-controlled trial.
Lancet. 2019;394:1540-50.

Abstract

The AMBER trial evaluated the feasibility and safety of combining a novel potassium binder patiromer with spironolactone in patients with resistant hypertension with chronic kidney disease (CKD) [estimated glomerular filtration rate (eGFR) between 25 and 45 mL/min/1.73 m^2]. The primary outcome was the proportion of patients who continued to remain on spironolactone at week 12 with patiromer added to offset the risk of hyperkalemia. The study screened 547 subjects from 62 centers in Europe and USA. Of these, 295 patients who had resistant hypertension and steady state serum potassium between 4.3 and 5.1 mEq/L were randomized to patiromer (8.4 g once a day) or placebo in addition to open label spironolactone. At the end of 12-week study period, a significantly higher proportion of patients in the patiromer arm continued on spironolactone 86% versus 66% (between-group difference 19.5%; 95% CI 10.0–29.0; p < 0.0001) compared to placebo indicating that patiromer ameliorated hyperkalemia risks with spironolactone and thereby allowing better hypertension management in this population of patients.

"Overcoming the potassium barrier for treating resistant hypertension in chronic kidney disease."

COMMENT

Resistant hypertension is challenge in medical practice. Defined as uncontrolled blood pressure while on three or more classes of antihypertensive medications, it is prevalent in almost 10% of all hypertensive subjects. The burden of resistant hypertension is many folds higher in chronic kidney disease (CKD) patients and it multiplies risks of cardiovascular disease and the tendency to progression to end stage kidney disease.

Chronic kidney disease patients face many impediments in hypertension management. These include a limitation of sodium excretion and the risk of hyperkalemia that becomes especially important with drugs acting through renin–angiotensin–aldosterone pathway (RAAS). Spironolactone is an aldosterone antagonist and a potassium sparing diuretic. It has an established place in the management of resistant hypertension and heart failure. One of its major side effects is hyperkalemia which gets pronounced in CKD patients. As mentioned earlier these patients are preferably treated with angiotensin converting enzyme (ACE) inhibitors or angiotensin II receptor blocker (ARB).

Patiromer is newer oral nonabsorbable potassium binding polymer with better tolerability and efficacy profile compared to conventional potassium binding resins such as calcium or sodium polystyrene sulfonate. Its potassium lowering ability and better tolerability was exploited to facilitate the addition of spironolactone to a triple drug antihypertensive regime in CKD patients [estimated glomerular filtration rate (eGFR) between 25 and 45 mL/min/1.73 m^2 and serum potassium 4.3 and 5.1 mEq/L] while mitigating the risk of hyperkalemia. While the primary outcome was proportion of subjects who continued on spironolactone, a couple of secondary outcomes measures were also examined. The patients who were on ACE inhibitors or ARB continued these agents. The study design is notable for its rigor on screening protocols and run in period to ensure steady state potassium levels and automated office blood pressure readings. Patients were also given automated monitors for home blood pressure monitoring. The drug compliance was monitored by serum levels of patiromer metabolites.

The key results showed that 23% of patients on placebo had to discontinue spironolactone due to hyperkalemia as against only 7% subjects in the patiromer group. Both groups achieved a substantial fall in systolic blood pressure of 10.8–11.7 mm Hg. The compliance was over 90% and the adverse events similar between both groups. Mean eGFR reduced in both groups by 1.4–2.1 mL/min/1.73 m^2 and this was reversed after discontinuation of study drugs. Almost 20% patients had a 30% decrease in eGFR and no patient developed reduced low magnesium levels.

The study does enrich the armamentarium for treating resistant hypertension in CKD allowing the use of spironolactone in combination with patiromer. Aldosterone blockade will also confer advantages that go beyond blood pressure control. The rigorous methodology and this being the first randomized controlled trial (RCT) of its kind is a value addition to the practice of nephrology. But some considerations still remain. The effect of most antihypertensive medications often gets altered with longer follow-up. The risk of potassium rise remains ever present in the natural history of CKD and thus experience will have to build up in clinical practice. The pill burden is always a concern in this population and this might create serious consequences if patients develop hyperkalemia due to noncompliance with patiromer.

Nevertheless, this elegant robust study creates a road map that can be used in specific patients with good monitoring for improving CKD, hypertension and cardiovascular disease outcomes.

Key Messages

- *Patiromer is a newer potassium binding polymer for reducing potassium absorption in gut and thus it can be used for preventing and/or treating hyperkalemia.*
- *Spironolactone is recommended for treatment of resistant hypertension.*
- *Patiromer facilitated the use of spironolactone in CKD patients with resistant hypertension by keeping the risk of hyperkalemia at bay.*

ARTICLE 8

Prediction system for risk of allograft loss in patients receiving kidney transplants: international derivation and validation study

Loupy A, Aubert O, Orandi BJ, Naesens M, Bouatou Y, Raynaud M, et al. Prediction system for risk of allograft loss in patients receiving kidney transplants: international derivation and validation study.
BMJ. 2019;366:l4923.

Abstract*

This international cohort study endeavored to develop and validate a method for prediction of long-term kidney allograft failure after kidney transplantation. Data from 4,000 consecutive kidney transplants performed at four French centers between 2005 and 2014 was collected prospectively and 32 prognostic factors that can impact kidney allograft survival were modeled. The output of this model comprising eight significant functional, histological, and immunological variables was integrated into a risk prediction score called iBox. The score was validated in another cohort of 3,557 transplants done at six centers in Europe and

USA and it was further tested in three randomized controlled trials (RCTs) in transplant immunosuppression. The primary outcome was allograft failure defined as return to dialysis or pre-emptive retransplant. Among the 7,557 kidney transplant recipients included, 1,067 (14.1%) allografts failed after a median post-transplant follow-up time of 7.12 (interquartile range 3.51–8.77) years. The iBox score showed accurate calibration and discrimination (C index 0.81, 95% confidence interval 0.79–0.83). The performance of the iBox was also confirmed in the validation cohorts from Europe (C index 0.81, 0.78–0.84) and the US (0.80, 0.76–0.84). iBox stood the test of the prospective RCTs as well.

The performance of iBox risk prediction score makes it the most accurate and integrative prediction tool for kidney transplant outcomes. *Redrafted abstract

"Doctor, how long will my transplanted kidney last?"

COMMENT

Science in a big measure is an effort in predictions. And medical science in particular is always striving for predicting outcomes of diseases and benefits of treatment interventions. The accuracy of prediction assumes a vital position in planning interventions and policy. In this age of patient reported outcomes, predictions are of substantial interest for the patients who invest resources and face the consequences of their decisions about various treatments and interventions.

Predicting the longevity of the transplanted kidney or conversely predicting the long-term kidney allograft failure is a key measure for transplant biologists, physicians, policy makers, clinical researchers, patients and their donors.

A lacuna has always existed in accurately predicting the survival of kidney allografts. And with steadily improving biological understanding, ensuing technologies and treatments, such a measure is needed to assess the utility of any intervention or advancement rather sooner than having to wait for decades for the natural history to unfold.

This group of investigators has assorted important prognostic variables into a risk prediction score (iBox). This initiative is remarkable for the incorporation of large number of transplant patients' data in the development of the prediction score. The variables used to create the iBox were selected after a univariate regression involving recipient's demographics; transplant characteristics such as donor age, donor hypertension and diabetes, ischemia time, use of thymoglobulin induction; immunological parameters such as human leukocyte antigen (HLA) mismatch, donor specific antibodies based on single antigen bead assays; functional parameters—estimated glomerular filtration rate (eGFR), proteinuria and allograft histopathology data. Of note histopathology data on the graft was available for almost all the transplants in the derivation cohort. The analyses also allowed creation of a simplified iBox model that was based on eGFR, proteinuria and circulating donor specific antibodies. Expectedly, this was inferior to the full model in terms of prediction capability.

In total, 1,067 (14%) grafts were lost from the total of 7,557 transplants. Not only did the integrated iBox model performed very well in the derivation cohort, it showed good discrimination performance in the external validation cohort with C statistic of 0.81 in Europe and 0.80 in the US. The performance was replicated in context of three large randomized controlled trials (RCTs) in transplant immunosuppression with C index of 0.87, 0.82–0.92. Conventionally, models are considered useful for informing about decisions when C statistic is >0.70 and at values >0.8, it is a strong decision-making tool.

This prediction model performed better than all existing scoring systems. Another advantage of iBox is its application for prediction of graft outcome at any time point after transplant. Most existent scoring systems inform about allograft survival at the time of transplant. Hence they are deployed for organ allocation and making a long-distance projection which is subject to being subverted by events on follow-up. iBox scoring can be reliably carried out at any time point after transplant and thus it becomes a useful tool for long-term management of transplant patients.

While iBox is a significant milestone, it is important to highlight we can expect even better prediction models as we incorporate information from evolving biomarkers, genomics and proteomics data into models that are driven by deep learning paradigms. And, it is equally evident that benefits of all such future models including iBox, that harness data produced by high end expensive diagnostics, may not percolate to the large majority of end-stage renal disease (ESRD) subjects who reside in low- and middle-income nations. Nevertheless, the availability of a reliable and useful tool is big step forward.

Key Messages

- ⊛ *A new prediction tool for estimating the life of kidney allograft has been developed. It is called iBox.*
- ⊛ *This integrates all important variables and performs across the transplant centers and across the journey from day of transplant to anytime during its course.*
- ⊛ *As of date iBox is the best prediction for kidney allograft failure risk.*

ARTICLE 9

Long-term safety and efficacy of veverimer in patients with metabolic acidosis in chronic kidney disease: a multicenter, randomized, blinded, placebo-controlled, 40-week extension

Wesson DE, Mathur V, Tangri N, Stasiv Y, Parsell D, Li E, et al. Long-term safety and efficacy of veverimer in patients with metabolic acidosis in chronic kidney disease: a multicenter, randomized, blinded, placebo-controlled, 40-week extension. *Lancet. 2019;394:396-406.*

Abstract

Metabolic acid is ubiquitous in chronic kidney disease (CKD) and is associated with adverse outcomes. Veverimer, is a new molecule developed to treat metabolic acidosis. It is a nonabsorbed, counterion-free, polymeric drug that selectively binds and removes hydrochloric acid from the gastrointestinal lumen. In this a multicenter, randomized, blinded, placebo-controlled, 40-week extension of a 12-week parent study, patients with CKD (eGFR 20–40 mL/min/1.73 m^2) and metabolic acidosis (serum bicarbonate 12–20 mmol/L), were assigned to veverimer (6 g/day) or placebo. The primary objective was safety assessment for the period of study. The study also assessed the trends of serum bicarbonate concentration and physical functioning. The study included 196 patients (114 veverimer and 82 placebo). By the end of the study, fewer patients on veverimer discontinued treatment prematurely (3% vs. 10%, respectively). The incidence of adverse events was not only similar to placebo but tended be lesser in veverimer arm. The effect of serum bicarbonate was substantive. Around 63% patients on veverimer had a sustained increase in serum bicarbonate (≥4 mEq/L or normalization) at the end of study compared to 38% in placebo group, p = 0.0015). Simultaneously, veverimer resulted in significantly improved patient-reported physical functioning [Kidney Disease and Quality of Life–Physical Function Domain (KDQoL-PFD)] versus placebo and significantly better time to do the repeat chair stand test. The study launches a new drug for treatment of metabolic acid in CKD without the pitfalls of sodium bicarbonate.

"Veverimer: True offspring of elegant physiology."

COMMENT

Chronic kidney disease (CKD) patients uniformly develop metabolic acidosis as glomerular filtration rate (GFR) falls. There have been reports of association of chronic acidosis with faster decline in GFR, bone loss, catabolism and perhaps even higher mortality. The treatment options for metabolic acidosis have relied upon oral sodium bicarbonate supplementation and dietary interventions to reduce ingested acid load. Dietary manipulation by increasing fruit and vegetable has its own limitations and sodium bicarbonate has not yet stood the test of well-designed blinded randomized trials. Besides that, sodium bicarbonate can potentially lead to sodium load and consequent risk of worsening hypertension and hypervolemia. This makes it unsuitable for patients who need to be on strict salt intake restriction.

Veverimer is a novel, nonabsorbed polymer that is designed to treat metabolic acidosis by binding hydrochloric acid in the gastrointestinal tract and removing it from the body through excretion in the feces, thereby decreasing the total amount of acid in the body and increasing serum bicarbonate (**Fig. 1**). Veverimer is specifically designed to bind with high selectivity and remove hydrochloric acid. Its design does not deliver sodium or other counterions, potentially allowing for chronic treatment of metabolic acidosis in patients with CKD and common comorbidities such as hypertension, cardiovascular disease, heart failure or edema.

The novelty of this drug was initially tested in a 12-week study and this same cohort of patients was involved in this 40-week extension to assess its safety as primary outcome measure. Unlike the other study by Melamed et al. in this publication, the participants had baseline bicarbonate between 12 and 20 and not 24 mEq/L. The study also examined the durability of the impact on serum bicarbonate concentration and if that lead to better physical performance. The target bicarbonate concentration to titrate the dose of veverimer was 22–29 mEq/L. The mean (SD) baseline bicarbonate value was 17.2 (1.4) and 17.1 (1.5) in the active and placebo arms. With respect to primary outcome the dosing compliance, defined as >80% doses being taken, was 100% for veverimer. And it was

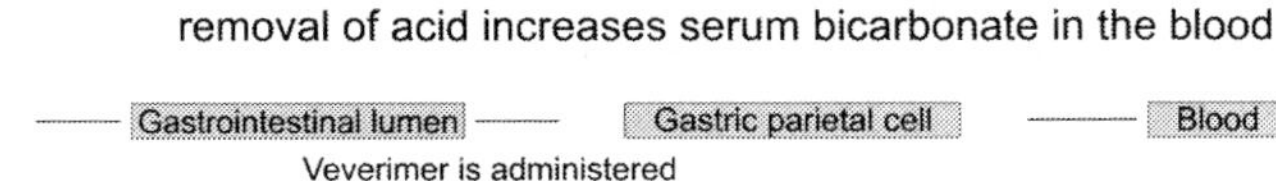

Veverimer binds and removes acid in the GI tract
removal of acid increases serum bicarbonate in the blood

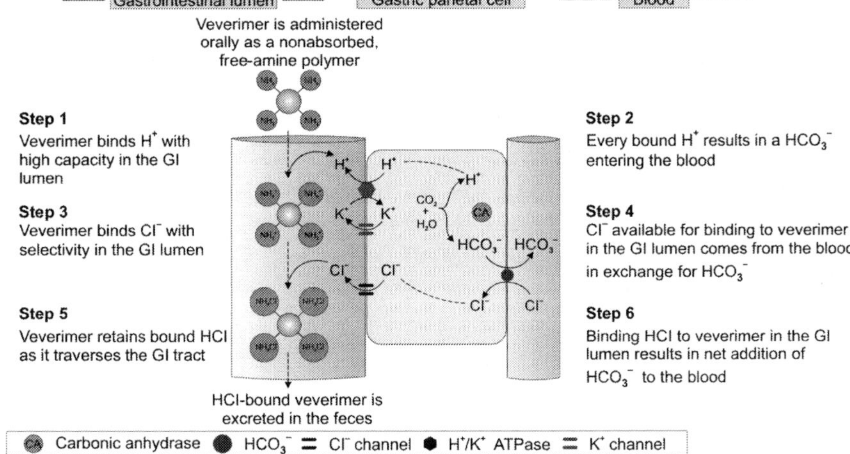

FIG. 1: Working of veverimer: It selectively binds to hydrochloric acid in gut leading to delivery of bicarbonate in blood stream.

Source: https://www.tricida.com/veverimer/.

well tolerated with a safety profile that matched the placebo to the extent more patients on placebo discontinued treatment prematurely (10% vs. 3%). There were no apparent adverse effects on electrolytes and lipid profile. The good news is that veverimer arm reported significant improvement in physical functioning on the KDQoL-PFD which quantifies the degree of limitation in performing daily activities such as climbing stairs and walking (p < 0.0001).

The mean change in the placebo-subtracted treatment effect in the KDQoL-PFD was 12.1 points which is far more than the threshold or 3–5 point change for it to be considered as clinically meaningful. And the range of activities that was positively influenced is actually important for activities of daily living. In fact, this degree of improvement in physical functioning outperforms many standard interventions such as anemia correction with erythropoiesis stimulating agents.

Even though it was not part of the primary outcome analysis, the veverimer arm also experienced a significant reduction in composite clinical endpoint of death, renal replacement therapy or a 50% decline in estimated GFR (eGFR) (p = 0.0224).

What has not been addressed in the study is the impact of proton pump inhibitors or H2 receptor antagonists which reduce gastric acid production in context of veverimer function and efficacy.

This study has many exciting results. A new drug finds its place in therapeutics and its role might extend to non-CKD metabolic acidosis treatment as well. Its elegance lies in delivering a treatment from principles of basic physiology. Further, treatment of metabolic acidosis with veverimer was associated with significantly improved hard clinical endpoints. The only caution would be to wait for the replication of results in similar, larger and longer-term studies designed to test improved hard clinical outcomes.

Key Messages

- ◉ *Veverimer is a novel compound: Nonabsorbed, counterion-free, polymeric drug that selectively binds to hydrochloric acid in gut leading to delivery of bicarbonate in blood stream.*
- ◉ *This trial shows good results with veverimer treatment in CKD with low bicarbonate levels.*
- ◉ *The benefits extend from improved serum bicarbonate levels, better physical functioning and perhaps decrease in progression of CKD.*

ARTICLE 10

Automatic measurement of kidney and liver volumes from MR images of patients affected by autosomal dominant polycystic kidney disease

van Gastel MD, Edwards ME, Torres VE, Erickson BJ, Gansevoort RT, Kline TL. Automatic measurement of kidney and liver volumes from MR images of patients affected by autosomal dominant polycystic kidney disease. *J Am Soc Nephrol. 2019;30:1514-22.*

Abstract*

Autosomal dominant polycystic kidney disease (ADPKD) leads to the formation and incessant growth of cysts in kidneys and also in liver. Hitherto, the measurement of total kidney volume (TKV) and total liver volumes (TLV) riddled with cysts was done by manual tracing and subsequent computations. A deep learning protocol with automated segmentation method for TKV and TLV was developed and validated. The development of the deep learning network involved 440 magnetic resonance images from ADPKD patients—80% for training and 20% for validation. It was further tested on images from 100 patients. The model's performance also assessed for longitudinal follow-up on 45 of these 100 patients. Measurement of TKV and TLV by the manual method was considered the gold standard. TKV and TLV measured by the automated approach correlated highly with manually traced TKV and TLV (intraclass correlation coefficients, 0.998 and 0.996, respectively), with low bias and high precision (<0.1% ± 2.7% for TKV and −1.6% ± 3.1% for TLV); this was comparable with inter-reader variability of manual tracing. For longitudinal analysis, bias and precision were, 0.1% ± 3.2% for TKV and 1.4 ± 2.9% for TLV growth. The technique of automated TKV and TLV driven by deep learning networks was successfully developed and validated. *Redrafted abstract

"Machine learning to measure polycystic kidney and liver volumes."

COMMENT

The incessant development of cysts in kidneys and liver is the hallmark of autosomal dominant polycystic kidney disease (ADPKD). Total kidney volume (TKV) is now akin to a biomarker to predict future chronic kidney disease (CKD) and its progression to end-stage renal disease (ESRD) in patients with ADPKD. It also serves as an outcome measure to assess the impact of interventions aimed at preventing or retarding the progression of disease. The current standard treatment for ADPKD includes vasopressin antagonist tolvaptan and TKV is one of the key parameters that guides its use. Similarly, treatments are emerging for liver cysts and total liver volume (TLV) will provide a similar benchmark for assessment of benefits. To be able to measure small growth differences with low variability, manual planimetry was used in clinical trials investigating treatment effect on kidney growth. With manual tracing, these volumes are calculated from a set of contiguous images by summing the products of the slice thickness and the slice area measurements within the kidney or liver boundaries. Obviously, the method is labor intensive and costs time. This restricts its use in trial settings and not routine clinical care. The automation of this process is the product of a collaborative effort of Developing Intervention Strategies to Halt Progression of Autosomal Dominant Polycystic Kidney Disease (DIPAK) Consortium at The Netherlands and the Human Imaging Core of Mayo Clinic PKD center, USA. MRIs were done at baseline and after 120–132 weeks as part of the DIPAK study and the DICOM image data transferred to Mayo Clinic. Semantic segmentation of liver and kidney images was done by convolutional neural network architecture developed by the Mayo Clinic investigators. The performance was compared to the TKV and TLV calculated by manual tracing method both in terms of absolute percentage differences in values, interclass correlation coefficient and Bland Altman analyses. The results showed that automated method was as good as manual method. The variation between automated method and manual approach was as much as it is observed between two trained persons. The automated method was at par with manual tracings for detecting small changes in TKV over time. In fact, the reclassification of TKV dependent risk categories with automated measurement was only 2% compared to manual reference method.

The glomerular filtration rate (GFR) in ADPKD remains normal for a substantial period of time while the cysts continue to develop and grow. TKV measurement can identify and prognosticate patients when they are technically "subclinical" thereby extending the window of opportunity to help these patients. The automated method capitalizes on the power of artificial learning as it evolves into deep learning and neural networks where in the system or computer finds its own rules and methods based on its experience, i.e., data volumes, dimensions and depth to deliver the output. Automated measurement of TKV takes only few seconds compared to 60–120 minutes for manual tracing measurement. There is one more bottleneck automation overcomes. The images can be transferred across the globe like they were done in this study making this technique available to wider group of users. And with its capacity to mine into millions of scans over time the deep learning model will surely outsmart the best of trained personnel and the issues of learning curve in training people. Machine learning will reinvent the way we practice medicine and live our lives. The disruption is already in motion.

Key Messages

- *Total kidney volume (TKV) is an important prognostic variable in ADPKD.*
- *TKV measurement by MRI is required for treatment decisions and it is a surrogate for designing clinical trials in ADPKD.*
- *The power machine learning and neural networks has been utilized to make this process automated with excellent precision and reproducibility. This will make it available to clinicians at large.*

ARTICLE 11

Renal denervation in isolated systolic hypertension using different catheter techniques and technologies

Fengler K, Rommel KP, Lapusca R, Blazek S, Besler C, Hartung P, et al. Renal denervation in isolated systolic hypertension using different catheter techniques and technologies.
Hypertension. 2019;74:341-8.

Abstract*

The study reports findings of a post-hoc analysis of the RADIOSOUND-HTN (A Three-arm Randomized Trial of Different Renal Denervation Devices and Techniques in Patients with Resistant Hypertension) trial assessing the impact of adjustment for baseline blood pressure values on efficacy of renal denervation (RDN), with special emphasis on isolated systolic hypertension (ISH).

The RADIOSOUND-HTN was a randomized clinical trial (RCT) that examined three different RDN techniques for patients with resistant hypertension (office SBP >160 mm Hg or DBP >90 mm Hg despite ≥3 classes of antihypertensive drugs including a diuretic – radiofrequency ablation (RFA) of the main renal artery (n = 39); radiofrequency ablation of the main renal artery, branches, and accessories (n = 39); and ultrasound-based main renal artery ablation (n = 42). Symplicity spyral catheter and paradise ultrasound catheter were used for RFA and ultrasound ablation, respectively. Among 120 study participants across the 3 arms, ISH and combined systolic-diastolic hypertension were equally distributed (61 and 59 participants, respectively). Blood pressure reduction at 3 months was more pronounced in patients with combined hypertension than in patients with ISH (13.3 ± 11.7 vs. 5.9 ± 11.8 mm Hg, respectively, p = 0.001). This difference was significant for RFA of the renal main arteries and ultrasound-based ablation of the main renal artery treatment but did not reach significance in the RFA of the main and branch arteries group.

Patients with ISH were older (67.9 ± 9.3 vs. 58.7 ± 8.6 years) and had lower 24-hour systolic (146.0 ± 9.7 vs. 153.7 ± 12.7 mm Hg) and diastolic (73.8 ± 6.1 vs. 93.6 ± 8.9 mm Hg) blood pressure. After adjustment for baseline blood pressure and age, the initially observed difference in blood pressure reduction between participants with combined hypertension and ISH [10.6 (7.2–13.9) vs. 8.1 (4.9–11.2) mm Hg, respectively] was no longer statistically significant (p = 0.34). Further adjustment for other baseline parameters (renal function, smoking, diabetes mellitus, and use of vasodilators) revealed no difference in blood pressure reduction between the two populations. The authors conclude that the value of ISH as predictor for successful RDN might have been overestimated.

In the main study report the daytime ambulatory systolic blood pressure (SBP) (primary endpoint) was reduced more at 3 months in the ultrasound group than in the group with RF ablation of the main renal artery, the SBP reduction was not significantly different between the ultrasound ablation group and the group with main renal artery plus side branch ablation. The results of this study suggested that ultrasound ablation may create lesions with greater depth in the main renal arteries so that treatment of renal artery branches and accessory arteries with ultrasound may not be necessary. *Redrafted abstract

"Renal denervation—a cat with nine lives."

COMMENT

Over 1 billion people worldwide have hypertension and >9 million annual deaths are attributed to complications of hypertension (HTN) such as myocardial infarction, stroke, and kidney failure. Even though there are several effective antihypertensive agents, successful management of high blood pressure remains challenging, and therefore, an important global priority.

A bit of history is in order. Before effective antihypertensive drugs became available, patients with severe HTN were treated with surgical splanchnicectomy to interrupt sympathetic nerves in the lower thoracic and lumbar regions. This treatment did lower BP and reduce mortality but carried high perioperative morbidity and had severe side effects. Overactivity of renal sympathetic efferent nerves can decrease renal blood flow, decrease urinary excretion of salt and water, and increase renin release from the kidney whereas the sympathetic sensory afferents increase systemic sympathetic activity through a central action.

Renal denervation (RDN), a more sophisticated method of altering sympathetic tone, was introduced about a decade ago with the hope that it will improve management of patients with drug-resistant hypertension. Surgical RDN had been shown to reduce BP in several animal models of HTN. This minimally invasive procedure based on sound hypothesis, created a lot of enthusiasm and seems to be effective in uncontrolled studies, but fell at the hurdle when examined in a randomized, sham-controlled trial – the Renal Denervation in Patients with Uncontrolled Hypertension (SIMPLICITY-HTN-3) study. Neither the office nor the 24-hour ambulatory systolic BPs were lower in the group that received the intervention when compared with sham treatment.

After a few twists and turns that led to modifications in the denervation technique, in particular inclusion of more distal and branch renal artery radiofrequency ablation, it seems that RDN is back on track, supported by findings of four sham-controlled trials. Extending the ablation to distal segment of the main renal artery or the arterial branches result in significantly greater reductions in both renal norepinephrine (NE) levels and axon density than conventional treatment of just the main renal artery.

Ultrasound-driven catheter-based circumferential ablation has also been developed—it uses a piezoelectric crystal on the end of the catheter centered in the renal artery by inflation of a water-cooled balloon.

Identification of patients most likely to benefit from RDN remains an important and clinically relevant issue. It is notable that patients with isolated systolic hypertension (ISH) have been excluded from recent sham control studies, because they are considered to be poor responders. SYMPLICITY HTN-3 and the Global SIMPLICITY showed that blood pressure reduction was greater in patients with combined hypertension than in patients with ISH. The pathophysiology of ISH, related to arterial stiffness makes it more difficult for control to be achieved, leaving these patients with higher risk for cardiovascular events. In an RDN study, responders had a lower pulse wave velocity, and patients with higher pulse wave velocity had more often ISH (**Fig. 1**).

However, exclusion of patients with ISH would render RDN inappropriate for the vast majority of patients over the age of 50 years. According to the US NHANES 80% of patients over 50 years of age has ISH. Further, they represent 67% of all untreated and 80% of all inadequately or partially treated participants. The current analysis suggests

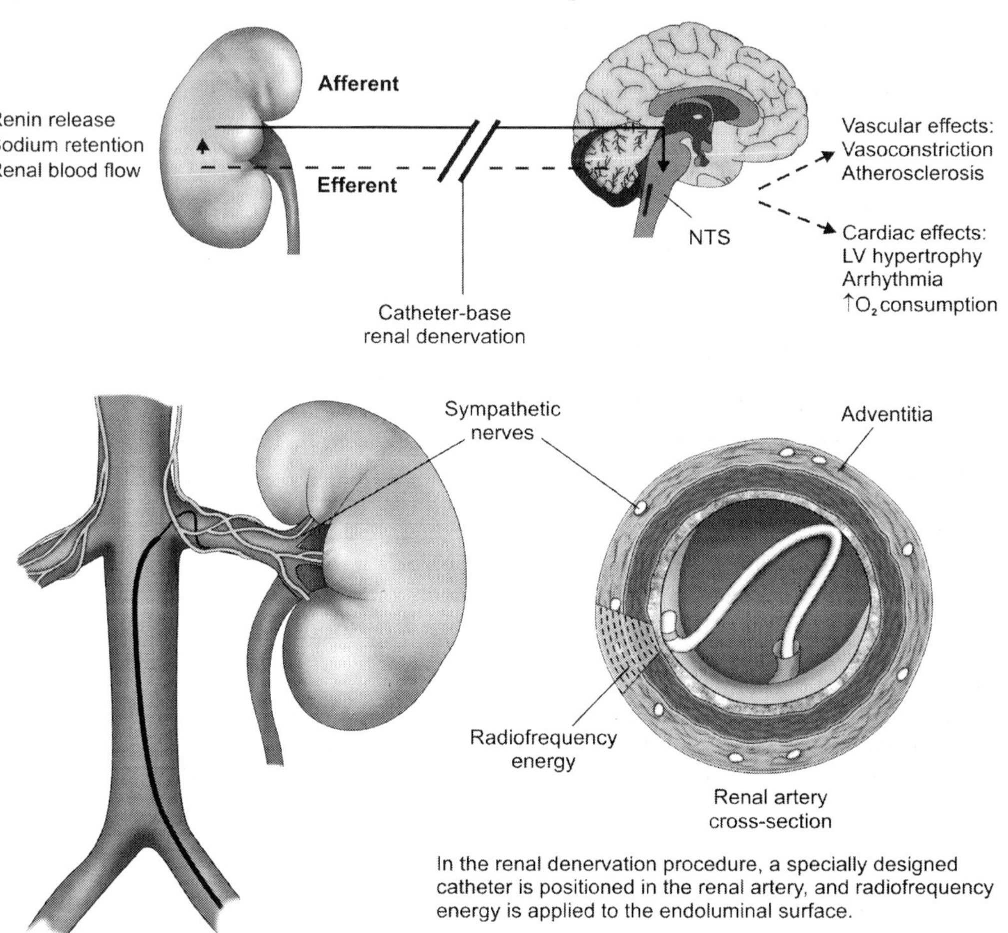

$\uparrow O_2$ consumption

In the renal denervation procedure, a specially designed catheter is positioned in the renal artery, and radiofrequency energy is applied to the endoluminal surface.

FIG. 1: The putative mechanism of action of renal denervation.

Source: https://consultqd.clevelandclinic.org/taking-aim-at-resistant-hypertension/

we need to rethink that assumption. A separate trial is needed perhaps in patients with ISH.

This post-hoc analysis has some important limitations—starting from its post-hoc nature which makes the study findings hypothesis-generating that needs to be tested in future randomized controlled trials. The study was not sham-controlled, the study population consisted of patients with resistant hypertension solely and excluded those over the age of 75 years, reducing the generalizability of the findings. The latter are expected to have primarily ISH, and information about the efficacy of RDN in this ever increasing age group is urgently needed.

Key Message

⊙ *Renal denervation is back on track, but needs to address the needs of the largest and most rapidly growing hypertensive population—the elderly with isolated systolic hypertension.*

ARTICLE 12

Rituximab or cyclosporine in the treatment of membranous nephropathy

Fervenza FC, Appel GB, Barbour SJ, Rovin BH, Lafayette RA, MENTOR Investigators, et al. Rituximab or cyclosporine in the treatment of membranous nephropathy.
N Engl J Med. 2019;381:36-46.

Abstract*

In this prospective, randomized trial, Fervenza et al. asked the question whether the anti CD-20 monoclonal antibody rituximab is noninferior to treatment with cyclosporine for inducing and maintaining remission of proteinuria in patients with this membranous nephropathy (MN).

They enrolled patients with nephrotic syndrome (proteinuria >5 g/24 h) and preserved kidney function (eGFR >40 mL/min/1.73 m^2) despite 3 months of angiotensin converting enzyme (ACE) blockade. The assigned treatments were two doses of rituximab 1,000 mg each, administered 14 days apart; repeated at 6 months in case of partial response or oral cyclosporine 3.5 mg/kg of body weight per day for 12 months. The primary outcome was a composite of complete or partial remission of proteinuria at 24 months.

A total of 130 patients were enrolled – 65 in either arm. At 24 months, 39 patients (60%) in the rituximab group and 13 (20%) in the cyclosporine group were in remission (risk difference 40%; 95% CI 25 to 55; p < 0.001 for both noninferiority and superiority). In particular, there was a large difference between the rituximab group and the cyclosporine group regarding the percentage of patients with complete remission (35% vs. none). Among antiphospholipase A 2 receptor (PLA2R) positive patients, the decline in antibody titer was faster and of greater magnitude and duration in the rituximab group. Serious adverse events occurred in 17% in the rituximab group and 31% in the cyclosporine group (p = 0.06). Progressive loss of renal function was slower with rituximab than with cyclosporine over the whole trial period, probably owing to the chronic nephrotoxic effects associated with cyclosporine (**Fig. 1**).

The authors concluded that rituximab was superior to cyclosporine in maintaining proteinuria remission up to 24 months. *Redrafted abstract

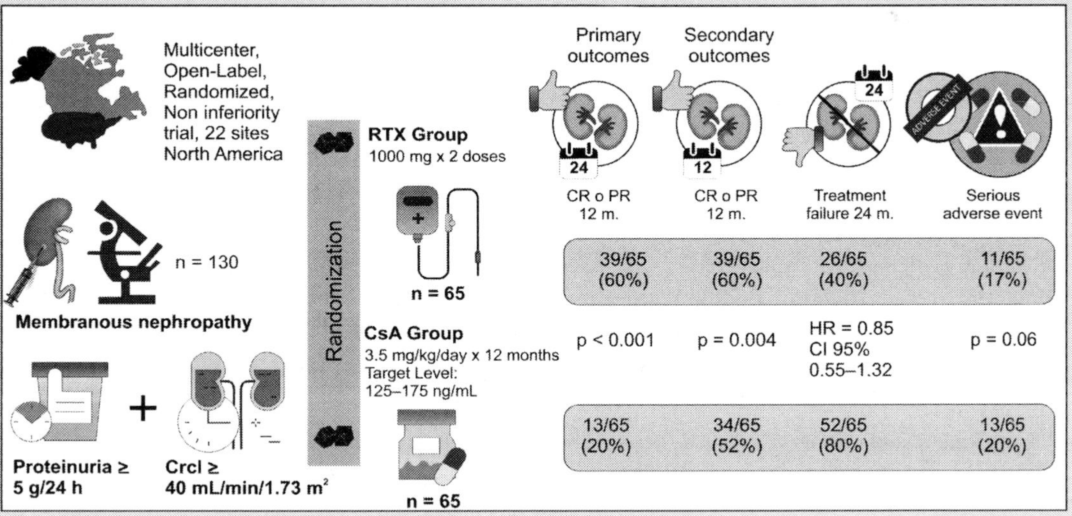

FIG. 1: An overview of MENTOR comparing rituximab with cyclosporine.
Courtsey: Christhian Munoz @CristhianMuM.
Source: https://twitter.com/CristhianMuM/status/1195807665819127814

"Rituximab for membranous nephropathy—avoiding the real question."

COMMENT

Membranous nephropathy (MN) develops as a result of an autoimmune process that leads to IgG deposition in the subepithelial space of glomerular capillaries and is the leading cause of nephrotic syndrome in adults worldwide. According to some reports, the incidence of this condition is growing. About one-third of the patients progress to develop kidney failure. Another third have persistent proteinuria and are at an elevated risk of cardiovascular disease and infection. Identification of patients at high risk of progression is an important goal since all of the current treatments that aim to interfere with the pathogenetic pathways carry significant toxicity.

A combination of alkylating agents and steroids has been shown be effective inducing clinical remission and prevent development of kidney failure in patients with membranous nephropathy in at least three long-term randomized controlled trials (RCTs). Since this combination is associated with short and long term risks (not shown in these RCTs), alternative treatment options have been explored. Calcineurin inhibitors, mainly cyclosporine, are used as primary therapy in North America, without definite evidence of benefit, however.

The results of this trial are consistent with the current western world-centric notion that rituximab should replace cyclosporine, the most frequently used immunosuppressive drug for the treatment of primary MN.

However, demonstration that rituximab is better than cyclosporine in inducing remissions in MN leaves the glass with treatment options for these patients still half-full. The authors were clever in their choice of cyclosporine as the comparator agent. The results must be examined in light of the existing compelling clinical trial data show that a combination of alkylating agents (chlorambucil/cyclophosphamide) and steroids are the most effective regimen for long-term dialysis free kidney survival in primary MN and hence should be the preferred comparator treatment arm for any new agent.

The world is inexorably moving toward an antibody-based therapy. Will anti-CD20 antibodies become the treatment of choice for all patients with membranous nephropathy? At this time it does not look likely. Rituximab therapy may fail in upto one-third of patients or cause complications. Fully humanized anti-CD20 antibodies, such as ofatumumab, may become viable alternatives to reduce the complication risk. Other agents in development that might be helpful include anti-CD38 antibodies, such as daratumumab and isatuximab that target plasma cells or engineering of T cells with chimeric antigen receptor technology.

Let's examine the place of the humble alkylating agent-based regimens. Concerns have been raised about the risk of adverse events, hence development of safer and effective drugs is considered desirable. New drugs (almost all of which are biologicals) are certain to be expensive and likely unaffordable for patients in developing countries, thus widening the therapeutic apartheid. We should also test strategies aimed at improving the safety profile of the (cheap) alkylating-agent based regimen, such as eliminating the methylprednisolone bolus, reducing the dose of alkylating agents and using antibody (PLA2R, THSD7A) level monitoring and stopping treatment early in those who show rapid immunological response.

Key Messages

- *Rituximab is superior to cyclosporine in inducing remission of proteinuria.*
- *We need an RCT of rituximab with the current standard of care—the alkylating-agent based regimen.*

ARTICLE 13

Efficacy and safety of mycophenolate mofetil versus levamisole in frequently relapsing nephrotic syndrome: an open-label randomized controlled trial

Sinha A, Puraswani M, Kalaivani M, Goyal P, Hari P, Bagga A. Efficacy and safety of mycophenolate mofetil versus levamisole in frequently relapsing nephrotic syndrome: An open-label randomized controlled trial.
Kidney Int. 2019;95:210-8.

Abstract

Background: Mycophenolate mofetil (MMF) and levamisole are commonly used in treating children with frequently relapsing and steroid dependent nephrotic syndrome. Whereas MMF is an expensive drug, levamisole is cheap and would cater to majority in developing countries. Comparative studies are lacking.

Method: Prospective, randomized, open-label, parallel group trial comparing efficacy of 12 months of MMF with 12 months of levamisole to decrease frequency of relapses in children aged 6–18 years with frequently relapsing (FR) or steroid dependent (SD) nephrotic syndrome (NS). Prior therapy with immunosuppressive therapy, other than alternate day steroids (<1 mg/kg/day) and cyclophosphamide (<6 months of study entry), was an exclusion criteria. Randomization was stratified for steroid dependence. Patients entered the study during relapse and steroids were tapered and stopped by 3 months of entry. Secondary outcomes included treatment failure, sustained remission, and frequent relapses. Treatment failure was defined as occurrence of steroid resistance, steroid toxicity, 2 or more serious adverse events attributed to relapses, and specific and unacceptable drug-associated adverse effects.

Results: About 149 children were randomized 1:1 into MMF (76) and levamisole (73) groups. Steroid dependence was seen in 28% at randomization and 21% had received prior (>6 m back) cyclophosphamide therapy. The incidence of relapses was 1.34 relapses per person-year and did not vary between the two groups (mean difference: –0.29; 95% CI: –0.65 to 0.08 relapses/person-year; p = 0.12) and therapy with MMF was associated with a relative relapse rate of 0.93 (95% CI: 0.71–1.21; p = 0.58) as compared to levamisole. About 15% of patients in both the groups had frequent relapses requiring alternate immunosuppression. About 50% had infrequent relapses and 20–30% had sustained remission until the last median follow-up of 43 months. Median time to first relapse was >6 months—median 8.8 (MMF) and 6.8 (levamisole), respectively.

Conclusion: Mycophenolate mofetil was not superior to levamisole in reducing the frequency of relapses in children between 6 and 18 years of age with FR or SD nephrotic syndrome.

"Levamisole as good as mycophenolate mofetil: Why buy a cow when milk is cheap?"

COMMENT

Comparative studies on therapy of frequently relapsing (FR) or steroid dependent (SD) nephrotic syndrome are the basis for use of immunosuppressive therapy for steroid-sparing and remission maintenance effects. Both mycophenolate mofetil (MMF) and levamisole are steroid-sparing agents used in children with moderately severe FR and SD nephrotic syndrome. Levamisole was recently shown to be more effective than placebo in children on alternate day steroids for FR nephrotic syndrome (FRNS). While MMF was found to be inferior to calcineurin inhibitors in treating FRNS, it has been shown to be effective in maintaining remission in children with FRNS in observational studies. In this randomized parallel group study comparing MMF with levamisole in predominantly FRNS children, MMF was not superior to levamisole in reducing frequency of relapse and cumulative steroid exposure. The incidence of relapses was 1.34 relapses per person-year and did not vary between the two groups (mean difference: –0.29; 95% CI –0.65 to 0.08 relapses/person-year; p = 0.12) and therapy with MMF was associated with a relative relapse rate of 0.93 (95% CI 0.71–1.21; p = 0.58) as compared to levamisole. Compared to the preceding year, relapse rates were decreased significantly after MMF and levamisole therapy. There were no differences in the secondary outcome of frequency of relapses and treatment failure among the two groups (**Figs. 1A** and **B**). On exploratory analysis using multivariable Cox regression, disease severity, i.e., steroid dependence was shown to be predictive of risk (hazards) of relapse as compared to frequent relapsers, independent of age, sex, number of relapses in the preceding year, or intervention (MMF or levamisole). Time to first relapse was longer in the MMF group than levamisole group in this subgroup of SD nephrotic syndrome. However, the risk (hazards) for frequent relapses and treatment failure were similar between the two groups. Also, there were no predictors for frequent relapses or treatment failure. MMF was used at 750–1,000 mg/m^2 and

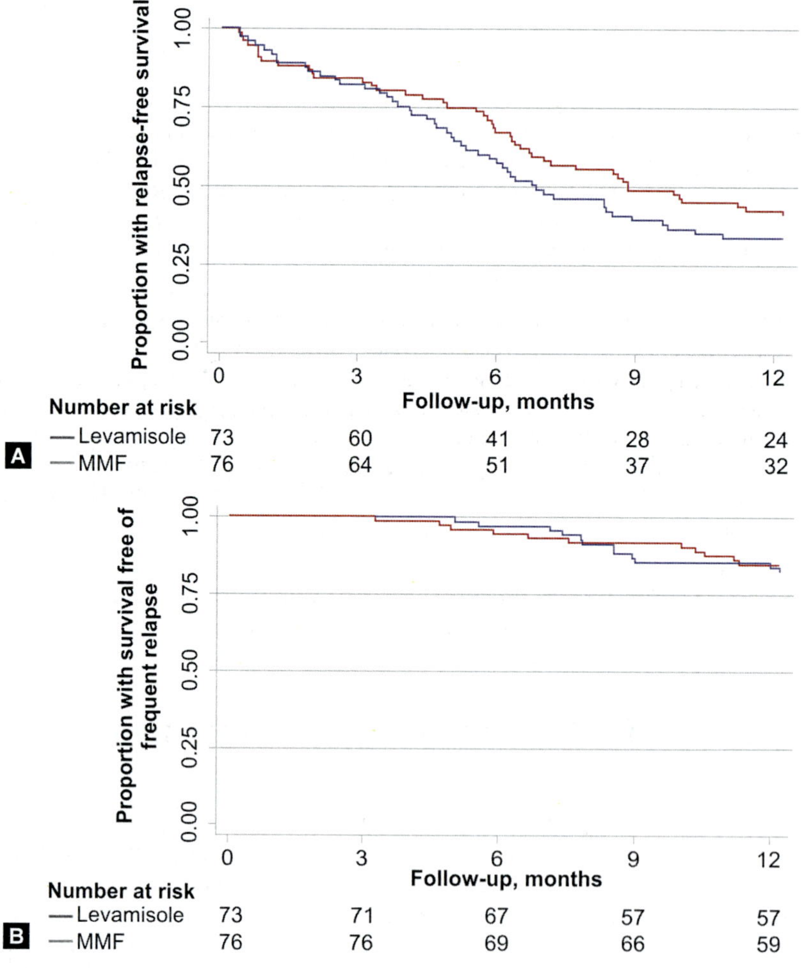

(MMF: mycophenolate mofetil)

FIGS. 1A AND B: Kaplan–Meier survival estimates. (A) Time to first relapse, and (B) time to frequent relapses in patients treated with levamisole (blue line) or mycophenolate mofetil (MMF; red line). The median time to first relapse was similar for patients treated with MMF and levamisole (8.8 vs. 6.8 months; log rank p = 0.25). At 12 months, 15.5% of patients administered MMF and 17.7% of patients receiving levamisole showed frequent relapses (p = 0.72).

blood levels were not measured. Lesser proportion of patients in sustained remission in MMF group in this study compared to previous trials was hypothesized to be due to use of a lower dose of MMF than used generally (1,000–1,200 mg/m^2). This could also be the reason for nonsuperiority of MMF over levamisole in this study. Both MMF and levamisole were found to be safe.

Key Messages

- *In a group of children with FRNS (predominantly), MMF and levamisole were similar in efficacy (frequency of relapses) and safety.*
- *Randomized trials using MMF at appropriate dose (1,000–1,200 mg/m^2) in a cohort of only FR or only SD nephrotic syndrome (or both but stratified at study entry) would provide more insight into the most appropriate therapy in them.*

ARTICLE 14

Long term tapering versus standard prednisolone treatment for first episode of childhood nephrotic syndrome: phase III randomized controlled trial and economic evaluation

Webb NJ, Woolley RL, Lambe T, Frew E, Brettell EA, PREDNOS Collaborative Group, et al. Long term tapering versus standard prednisolone treatment for first episode of childhood nephrotic syndrome: phase III randomized controlled trial and economic evaluation.
BMJ. 2019;365:l1800

Abstract*

Objective: This study aimed to evaluate whether prolonging initial prednisolone treatment from 8 to 16 weeks among children who have idiopathic steroid-sensitive nephrotic syndrome results in improvement in the pattern of disease relapse.

Methods: This was a double blinded, parallel group, phase III randomized placebo-controlled trial including children between 1 and 14 years of age across 125 UK hospitals with first episode of steroid sensitive nephrotic syndrome. Children were randomized to receive an extended 16-week course of prednisolone or a standard 8 week course of prednisolone. A minimization algorithm ensured balanced treatment allocation by ethnicity (South Asian, white, or other) and age (5 years or less, 6 years or more). The primary outcome measure was time to first relapse over a minimum follow-up of 24 months. Secondary outcome measures were relapse rate, incidence of frequently relapsing nephrotic syndrome and steroid-dependent nephrotic syndrome, use of alternative immunosuppressive treatment, rates of adverse events, behavioral change, quality adjusted life years, and cost-effectiveness from a healthcare perspective.

Results: Time to first relapse (hazard ratio 0.87; 95% confidence interval 0.65–1.17; log rank p = 0.28) and incidence of frequently relapsing nephrotic syndrome [extended course 60/114 (53%) vs. standard course 55/109 (50%); p = 0.75] did not differ between the 16 week versus 8 week prednisolone therapy groups. There were no statistically significant differences in serious adverse event rates or adverse event rates, with the exception of behavior, which was poorer in the standard course group. However, scores on the Achenbach child behavior checklist did not differ. Extended course treatment was associated with a mean increase in generic quality of life and cost savings.

Conclusions: In UK children with steroid-sensitive nephrotic syndrome, there was no improvement in clinical outcomes when extension of the initial course of prednisolone treatment was done from 8 to 16 weeks. Though, evidence was found of a short-term health economic benefit via decreased use of resource and enhanced quality of life. *Redrafted abstract

"Duration of steroid therapy in childhood nephrotic syndrome: What is the best bet?"

COMMENT

The standard treatment of children with steroid sensitive nephrotic syndrome (SSNS) is typically based on International Study of Kidney Disease in Children (ISKDC) recommendation— prednisolone 60 mg/m^2 daily for 4 weeks followed by 40 mg/m^2 prednisolone for subsequent 4 weeks, making a total of 8 weeks of therapy. About 50% of these children develop a frequent relapsing (FR) or steroid dependent (SD) course sooner or later in the future. While some clinical predictors of FR/SD course such as younger age at onset of nephrotic syndrome, increased time to enter remission at the first episode, are largely nonmodifiable, treatment duration (8 weeks vs. <8 weeks) has been proved to be a crucial modifiable predictor of future course. From the Cochrane review of different corticosteroid regimen for children with SSNS published in 2015, it appears that older and recent studies had contradictory findings. While older studies (with significant risk of bias) stated benefit of extended therapy (>8 weeks) in terms of risk of FR course, recent studies (lesser risk of bias) stated otherwise. Moreover, adverse effects were not uniformly reported. Therefore, the PREDNOS trial, randomized controlled trial, looking at 237 children across multiple centers in the UK has straightened out the evidence for treatment duration of first episode of SSNS. The standard treatment arm received the usual ISKDC regimen for 8 weeks and the extended treatment arm received 60 mg/m^2 prednisolone for 4 weeks, followed by gradual tapering by 10 mg/m^2 every 2 weeks for a total of 12 weeks. Of the total 237 patients recruited, 223 were left for intention to treat analysis. Randomization was done in a 1:1 ratio and allocation was balanced by ethnicity (South Asian, white, others) and age (5 years or less and 6 years or more). The cumulative dose of prednisolone after completion of the trial was not statistically different in the two arms. The primary outcome, time to first relapse, was similar in the two arms (139 days in extended arm vs. 87 days in standard arm) (**Fig. 1**). About 80% of children in both the groups developed relapses in the 2-year follow-up. None of the secondary outcomes such as proportion developing FR/SD course, number of relapses and number requiring alternative immunosuppression, were different. The extended course was found to be slightly more cost-effective than the standard course as there were lesser unplanned visits and medications and small increase in quality of life. There were no significant differences between the two arms in terms of drug-related serious adverse events, blood pressure control, growth, cataract, and quantitative behavioral data. Hence, the trial concludes that 8 weeks of prednisolone therapy remains the most appropriate duration to treat first episode SSNS in children, until further evidence suggests otherwise.

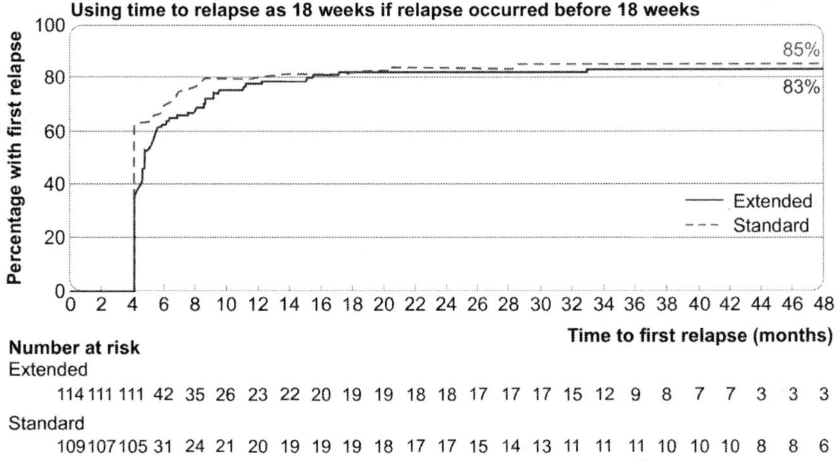

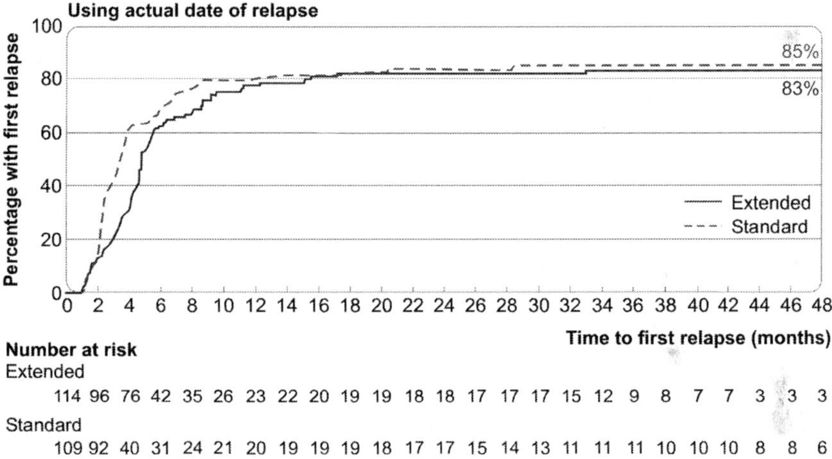

FIG. 1: Time to first relapse in participants receiving extended or standard course of prednisolone treatment.

Key Messages

- *Extending the duration of prednisolone therapy beyond 8 weeks is not helpful to delay first relapse in children with first episode SSNS.*
- *Extended duration of prednisolone might be useful as a cost-effective measure for using healthcare resources.*

ARTICLE 15

Effects of hemodiafiltration versus conventional hemodialysis in children with ESKD: the HDF, heart and height study

Shroff R, Smith C, Ranchin B, Bayazit AK, Stefanidis CJ, Askiti V, et al. Effects of hemodiafiltration versus conventional hemodialysis in children with ESKD: The HDF, Heart and Height Study
J Am Soc Nephrol. 2019;30:678-91.

Abstract*

Background: Hemodiafiltration (HDF) is associated with better middle molecule clearance and survival benefits in adults. Children on dialysis have poor cardiovascular health owing to chronic inflammatory milieu, repeated hemodynamic stress, and secondary hyperparathyroidism. Outcomes of HDF in children have not been reported previously.

Methods: Prospective nonrandomized observational study comparing conventional hemodialysis (HD) with online postdilution HDF in incident and/or prevalent children on dialysis (between 5 and 20 years of age). The primary outcomes were change in carotid intima-media thickness (cIMT) and height over 1-year follow-up.

Results: Of 190 children screened, 133 were studied: 78 in the HD group and 55 in HDF group. cIMT scores increased in the study time-period in the HD group and remained static in HDF group. Height standard deviation (SD) scores increased slightly in the HDF group as compared to HD group. There was better serum beta-2 microglobulin clearance in the HDF group and levels remained static despite no residual kidney function. Blood pressure SD scores remained static in HDF group, whereas, they increased in the HD group. Patient-reported outcomes, mainly dialysis recovery time, were better in HDF group than HD group.

Conclusion: In incident and prevalent children on dialysis, HDF provided better subclinical cardiovascular measures and better growth as compared to HD. Randomized trials would confirm the findings. *Redrafted abstract

*"Hemodiafiltration benefits **Heart** and **Height** in children—the 3"H" stand together."*

COMMENT

A total of 133 children from 10 countries (Europe and North America) between 5 and 20 years on two dialysis modalities, post-dilution online hemodiafiltration (HDF) and conventional hemodialysis (HD), were examined prospectively for cardiovascular and growth outcomes. This was a nonrandomized prospective comparative observational study and therefore, selection and allocation biases would be expected inherently. Propensity-score matching, was done to overcome confounding factors. Most patients did not have significant residual kidney function. The primary endpoints included change in carotid intima-media thickness (cIMT) standard deviation (SD) scores and change in height SD scores at 1-year follow-up. Secondary endpoints included 24-hour ambulatory blood pressure monitoring, health-related quality of life, pulse-wave velocity, left ventricular mass index (LVMI), biochemical measures. The median convection volume achieved in the HDF group was 13.2 L/m^2, within the target range of 12–15 L/m^2. cIMT increased by +0.41 SD score in the HD group, whereas, it decreased by 0.07 SD scores in the HDF group (**Figs. 1A** to **C**). Change in height SD score remained static in HD group, whereas, height SD score increased slightly in HDF group. Both these outcomes were inversely related to serum beta-2 microglobulin levels. However, the possible interaction of height scores with pubertal status was not looked at, and most children were >10 years of age. The HD group had higher annualized mean arterial pressure (MAP) SD scores compared to HDF group. Also, the HD group had a trend toward higher LVMI change than the HDF group. Serum beta-2 microglobulin levels

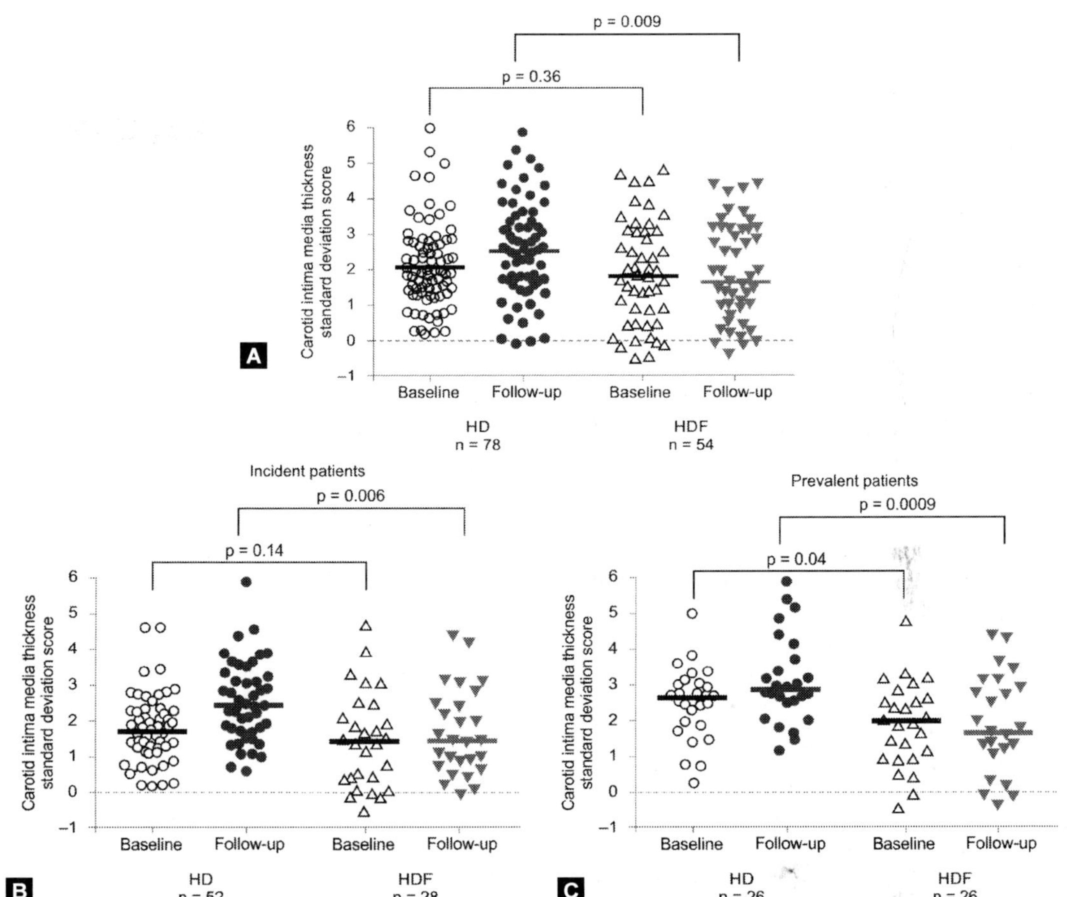

(cIMT: carotid intima media thickness; HD: hemodialysis; HDF: hemodiafiltration; SD: standard deviation)

FIGS. 1A TO C: At 12 months the cIMT SD score increased in the HD group and remained static in the HDF group. (A) cIMT SD scores at baseline and 12 months for HD and HDF cohorts are shown. cIMT increases significantly from 0 to 12 months in the HD cohort (p = 0.02) but remains static in HDF (p = 0.89), with a significant difference between groups at 12 months (p = 0.009). (B and C) cIMT SD score at baseline and 12 months in incident and prevalent patients on HD and HDF. Data are shown as median and interquartile range.

decreased over the 12 months period in the HDF group, however, C-reactive protein levels (lower than HD group) remained static in this group. HDF group also had decreased PTH levels at 12 months compared to HD group, although serum calcium, phosphate, and 25-hydroxy vitamin D were similar in both groups. The positive change in cIMT in HDF reflected better fluid removal and middle molecule clearance (inflammatory markers and possibly, FGF23). Of note, the post dialysis recovery time was shorter in HDF group (few minutes or less in 70% of patients) as compared to HD (hours). Other patient-reported outcomes such as dizziness, headache, school attendance were also lesser in the HDF group. The laboratory

benefits of HDF in this study appear to be mostly because target convective volumes were achieved. Most patients (~70%) had dialysate sodium set at <138 mmol/L and diffusive gain of sodium and excess interdialytic weight gain was unlikely. However, intradialytic BP variation was not studied and in the absence of a randomized design, better hemodynamic tolerability in HDF could be merely reflecting patient-related characteristics. Growth hormone resistance is prevalent in children on HD. Removal of insulin-like growth factor-1 (IGF-1) binding proteins (middle molecules) by HDF might have contributed to better growth in this group, short of data on interaction between pubertal status and height.

Key Messages

- *HDF is associated with better subclinical cardiovascular measures and growth than HD in children on dialysis.*
- *Randomized trials looking at long-term survival benefits in addition to hemodynamic and middle-molecule clearance would be required to confirm the superiority of HDF.*

ARTICLE 16

Primary vesicoureteral reflux; what have we learnt from the recently published randomized, controlled trials?

Garin EH. Primary vesicoureteral reflux; what have we learnt from the recently published randomized, controlled trials? *Pediatr Nephrol. 2019;34:1513-9.*

Abstract*

Recently conducted randomized trials in children with primary vesicoureteral reflux (VUR) have paved the way for a relook at the pathophysiology and link between VUR and urinary tract infection (UTI). Nondilating VUR has been convincingly shown to be innocuous as most resolve spontaneously with time. Therefore, extensively investigating and treating a child with the first febrile UTI seems an overstated approach. However, at the same time the evidence on dilating VUR causing long-term renal damage still needs to be explored. Similarly children with frequent symptomatic UTIs also need to be well-represented in larger clinical trials to understand the benefits of long-term antibiotic prophylaxis. This review has summarized the evidence base for medical treatment and clinical relevance of primary VUR in children. *Redrafted abstract

"Primary vesicoureteral reflux in the children: Randomized trials provoke reassessment of the approach to management."

COMMENT

Vesicoureteral reflux (VUR) is the reflux (backflow) of urine from the vesicle (bladder) to the ureter with or without extension into the pelvicalyceal system. The prevalence of VUR varies with frequency of testing for it, i.e., with voiding cystourethrogram (VCUG). It also depends on the indication for testing for it, i.e., antenatal hydronephrosis or symptomatic urinary tract infection (UTI). Further, mild-to-moderate VUR resolves spontaneously over time, and therefore, the prevalence decreases with age.

Following questions are answered in this review.

1. Does VUR predispose to UTI? Although theoretical plausibility of VUR predisposing to UTI has been imbibed among physicians since antiquity, recent high quality evidence does not support it.

2. Does VUR predispose to acute pyelonephritis or renal scars? Focal defects in renal scans obtained at the time of infection were taken as representing acute pyelonephritis in previous observational studies. Increased use of renal scans showed focal scars in about 60% of those with higher grades of VUR. However, it is not evident that these scars resulted from acquired

UTIs or they were congenitally present. While it is clear that nondilating VUR does not predispose to acute pyelonephritis and renal scars, better quality studies evaluating its presence in dilating VUR (grade III and above) are needed to arrive at a conclusion.

3. Does antibiotic prophylaxis prevent UTI in those with VUR? There are conflicting observations made by randomized trials largely owing to lack of homogeneity of studies in terms of grades of VUR, age and sex of children and control group included. The RIVUR trial showed that recurrent UTI was lesser (13%) in those on antibiotic prophylaxis compared to 24% in the placebo group over 2 years of follow-up. Of note, the significant difference in the UTI rates were shown only in children younger than 2 years and with grade I–II VUR, not higher grades. A recent meta-analysis concluded that antibiotic prophylaxis prevents recurrent UTI even in those with high VUR grades. As of now, caution needs to be exercised in prescribing long-term antibiotic prophylaxis and aggressive monitoring should be done for detecting resolution of high grade VUR.

4. Does antibiotic prophylaxis decrease recurrence rate UTI? The PRIVENT study reported long-term antibiotic prophylaxis to reduce the recurrence rates of UTI in children with symptomatic UTI, with or without VUR. At the same time, pooled data from 3 other randomized trials did not show protective role of antibiotics in reducing recurrent UTI rates.

5. Does antibiotic prophylaxis decrease risk of acute pyelonephritis? Limited evidence suggests that antibiotic prophylaxis does not decrease acute pyelonephritis.

6. Does antibiotic prophylaxis decrease renal scars? None of the randomized trials have shown effectiveness of antibiotic prophylaxis in reducing renal scars, a secondary outcome in all trials. What is needed to be addressed in future studies? To identify the subset of patients with VUR who are at the highest risk of long-term renal damage. This would, of course, include the group with grade IV–V VUR and those with frequent symptomatic UTIs (including acute pyelonephritis). Further interventions need to be studied better in this subgroup if it is at risk of future renal damage. A brief summary of current recommendations for antibiotic prophylaxis in children with VUR is shown in **Table 1**.

TABLE 1: Management approach for primary vesicoureteral reflux (VUR) and febrile urinary tract infection (UTI).

VUR grade	Management
Grade I	No antibiotic prophylaxis
Grade II	No antibiotic prophylaxis
Grade III	No antibiotic prophylaxis
Grade IV	Uncertain, lack of conclusive evidence on antibiotic prophylaxis
Grade V	Uncertain, lack of conclusive evidence on antibiotic prophylaxis
First febrile UTI	Ultrasonography of kidneys, ureter and bladder; if abnormal, VCUG and decide; if normal, treat the episode
Recurrent febrile UTI	Antibiotic prophylaxis to reduce rates; Evaluate for bladder bowel dysfunction

(VCUG: voiding cystourethrogram)

Key Messages

- *Nondilating VUR (grade I–III) do not lead to increased risk of recurrent UTI, acute pyelonephritis, or renal damage, therefore, does not warrant prolonged antibiotic prophylaxis and frequent aggressive investigations.*
- *Future studies addressing interventions in the subset with dilating VUR and those with frequent symptomatic UTIs are required.*

ARTICLE 17

Acute kidney injury

Ronco C, Bellomo R, Kellum JA. Acute kidney injury.
Lancet. 2019;394:1949-64.

Abstract

Acute kidney injury (AKI) is a part of a syndrome in the context of clinical status of patients; not a single disease. While it is conventionally defined based on serum creatinine and urine output criteria, neither of these markers have sufficient diagnostic accuracy. Novel biomarkers are increasingly used in the research context as many lack specificity to be used in clinical practice. Specific care-bundles with respect to clinical context should be used in managing AKI. Prevention of AKI would depend on knowledge of and robust monitoring of risk factors of AKI in an individual patient. Management strategies for fluid imbalance and acid base disorders are better supported by high-quality evidence. Renal replacement therapy is usually started at the onset of complications which do not respond to conservative management.

"Acute Kidney Injury: Deceptively simple."

COMMENT

Acute kidney injury (AKI) is defined as increased serum creatinine over hours to days, decreased urine output, or both. It is a part of various syndromes such as sepsis, cardiorenal, hepatorenal, urinary tract obstruction, etc. The approach to management of a patient with AKI is based on the syndrome specification. Surrogate markers, such as kidney size (on imaging) and trend of serum creatinine during follow-up, are used to infer rapidity of kidney injury often. Serum creatinine is not sensitive to diagnose AKI as about 50% of glomerular filtration rate (GFR) must be lost before a detectable change in serum creatinine can be noted. Similarly, urine output is neither sensitive nor specific to diagnose AKI. Hypovolemia could cause oliguria without real kidney injury, and in cases of acute interstitial nephritis, urine output might be preserved or more. Although acute tubular necrosis (ATN) is a widely used term to denote pathology of most AKI, tubular necrosis is uncommonly observed on kidney biopsies. Milder forms of injury such as tubular cell simplification, mitosis and cell sloughing are sensitive and specific pathological correlates of AKI. Despite being milder forms of ATN, these lesions can lead to decreased GFR through activation of tubuloglomerular feedback.

While use of novel AKI biomarkers gained momentum recently, these are now only used in research as they lack specificity (**Table 1**). Among all these markers, urinary tissue inhibitor of metalloproteinases 2 (TIMP-2) and insulin-like growth factor binding protein 7 (IGFBP7) are kidney stress markers which aid in predicting AKI (as per standard criteria) and are US FDA approved as first diagnostic test for AKI. These tests should ideally be used in critically ill patients or those with defined exposure to kidney insult, so that their value in clinical decision making remains precise. Risk factors for AKI include poor renal functional reserve, such as advanced age and preexisting chronic kidney disease (CKD). The pathophysiology of AKI varies with the clinical context of the patient. Prevention of AKI is based on identifying risk factors and triggers of AKI. Biomarker-driven implementation of specific bundles for AKI care are shown to reduce rates of AKI. While restrictive fluid therapy is not favored in the context of major abdominal surgery (RELIEF trial), standard fluid therapy does not result in reduced AKI in septic patients. Hydration with isotonic saline remains the cornerstone for preventing contrast-associated AKI. There is no single criterion to decide renal

TABLE 1: Characteristics of acute kidney injury biomarkers.

	Sample type	Class	Appearance or peak after injury*	Functional role in the kidney
Tissue inhibitor of metalloproteinase-2; insulin-like growth factor binding protein 7	Urine	Stress	Immediately after cardiopulmonary bypass, peaks at 6–24 h	Cell-cycle arrest: Can induce cell-cycle arrest—thought to be a protective mechanism*
Neutrophil gelatinase associated lipocalin	Urine or plasma	Damage	<4 h after cardio-pulmonary bypass, peaks at 4–6 h	Iron trafficking: Binds to iron siderophore complexes in renal tubular epithelial cells; tubular epithelial genesis: Forms an iron-siderophore complex (holo-neutrophil gelatinase associated lipocalin), which is secreted by the ureteric bud, and can induce the genesis of tubular epihtelium; anti-inflammatory and anti-apoptotic
Kidney injury marker-1	Urine	Damage	12–24 h; peaks at 2–3 days	Renal recovery and tubular regeneration: Clearance of apoptotic bodies; anti-inflammatory effect
Liver-type fatty acid binding protein	Urine	Damage	Unknown	Fatty acid uptake and intracellular transport: mobilises lipid peroxides from cytoplasm of tubular epithelial cells to tubular lumen; *L-FABP* gene expression is increased by peroxisome proliferator activated receptor -α hypoxaemia
Cystatin C	Serum or urine	Function	NA	None, filtration marker; cystatin C is normally taken up by renal tubular epithelial cells; as such its appearance in the urine indicates tubular dysfunction
Pro-enkephalin	Serum	Function	NA	None, filtration marker

* Available evidence for the time from injury to detection of the marker. Filtration markers have a variable relationship to injury so specific times are not possible to establish.

(NA: not applicable)

replacement therapy (RRT) in patients with AKI. Most units practice RRT timing based on emergent indications. Continuous RRT (CRRT) is used for hemodynamically unstable patients as a standard in the developed world; in developing countries, it is based on local availability. A trial of discontinuation of RRT is given upon spontaneous diuresis (>500 mL/day) typically. AKI may represent a continuum which ends in CKD in some patients owing to maladaptive repair.

Key Messages

⊙ *AKI is not a single disease, rather a syndrome specific to clinical context of a patient.*

⊙ *Specific care bundle in relation to clinical contexts help in preventing and managing AKI.*

⊙ *Renal replacement therapy is typically started when complications of AKI start to develop.*

ARTICLE 18

Roxadustat treatment for anemia in patients undergoing long-term dialysis

Chen N, Hao C, Liu BC, Lin H, Wang C, Xing C, et al. Roxadustat treatment for anemia in patients undergoing long-term dialysis.
N Engl J Med. 2019;381:1011-22.

Abstract*

This trial, conducted in China, examined the safety and efficacy of the new hypoxia-inducible factor prolyl hydroxylase inhibitor roxadustat by comparing it with standard therapy (epoetin alfa) for the treatment of anemia in patients undergoing dialysis.

A total of 305 patients who had been on treatment with epoetin alfa for at least 6 weeks were randomly assigned in a 2:1 ratio to either continue epoetin alfa three times per week or receive roxadustat for 26 weeks. The trial had a noninferiority design with the lower boundary of the two-sided 95% confidence interval (CI) for the difference between two groups set at 1.0 g/dL. The target hemoglobin value was 10–12 g/dL.

A total of 204 received roxadustat and 101 were in the epoetin alfa group, and 162 and 94, respectively completed the 26-week treatment period. Statistical noninferiority was established (difference, 0.2 ± 1.2 g/dL; 95% CI –0.02 to 0.5). Roxadustat led to a numerically greater change in hemoglobin level from baseline to weeks 23–27 (0.7 ± 1.1 vs. 0.5 ± 1.0 g/dL), increased the transferrin level (difference, 0.43 g/L; 95% CI 0.32–0.53), maintained the serum iron level (difference, 25 µg/dL; 95% CI 17–33), attenuated decreases in the transferrin saturation (difference, 4.2%; 95% CI 1.5–6.9), led to greater decrease in total and low-density lipoprotein cholesterol (LDL-C) at week 27 (difference, –22 mg/dL; 95% CI –29 to –16 and –18 mg/dL; 95% CI –23 to –13 respectively), and greater a mean reduction in hepcidin of (30.2 ng/mL 95% CI –64.8 to –13.6 vs. 2.3 ng/mL, 95% CI –51.6 to 6.2). Hyperkalemia and upper respiratory infection occurred at a higher frequency in the roxadustat group, and hypertension occurred at a higher frequency in the epoetin alfa group. *Redrafted abstract

"Anemia of kidney disease—There is a pill for that."

COMMENT

Anemia, caused by reduced production of erythropoietin by the kidneys, is widely recognized as a major complication of kidney failure that has a major impact on health and happiness. Until erythropoietin came along, a high proportion of dialysis patients required blood transfusions that led to complications such as viral infections, iron overload and immunological sensitization.

All this changed in 1989 when recombinant erythropoietin therapy was first approved—these agents were able to increase hemoglobin levels resulting in vastly improved quality of life and decreased cardiac hypertrophy and mortality. Ever since that time, erythropoiesis-stimulating agents (ESAa) (along with oral and intravenous iron) have been the used the world over to correct anemia at all stages of chronic kidney disease

(CKD). The belief in positive effects of ESAs was so high that the FDA expanded the label for epoietin alfa to include positive effects on health, sex life, well-being, life satisfaction and happiness. ESA therapy carries a number of disadvantages, including the need for parenteral administration, need to be accompanied by intravenous iron supplementation, and pure red cell aplasia in a minority.

More serious issue became apparent when studies asked the question: would full reversal of anemia further improve outcomes? Multiple studies showed, at best, no improvement in outcome and, at worst, increased risks of stroke and death. The Correction of Anemia with Epoetin Alfa in Chronic Kidney Disease (CHOIR) study showed a higher risk of a composite endpoint that included death and cardiovascular events, and the Trial to Reduce Cardiovascular Events with Aranesp Therapy (TREAT) showed a higher risk of stroke. The findings of these studies, along with that of the Cardiovascular Risk Reduction by Early Anemia Treatment with Epoetin Beta (CREATE) study that did not show any benefit on reduction of the risk of any of the primary cardiovascular outcomes led to lowering of the goals regarding hemoglobin level in patients on dialysis to a range of 9–11 g/dL, and those not on dialysis were recommended to be treated only for reduction in the risk of transfusions or to treat symptomatic anemia.

Discovery of these new class of small molecule orally active hypoxia-inducible factor prolyl hydroxylase inhibitors (PHIs) promise to change this paradigm. These agents prevent the degradation of hypoxia-inducible factor (HIF) by the oxygen-sensing prolyl hydroxylase domain (PHD) enzymes. HIF binds to the hypoxia responsive element and promotes transcription of *EPO* gene.

In addition to increasing erythropoietin levels, these agents have a number of additional effects. These include positive effects on inflammation, iron handling, and reduction of hepcidin level. The latter finding was noted in this trial. Reduced hepcidin levels allow better utilization of existing iron stores and facilitate oral iron absorption, potentially avoiding the use of high doses of intravenous iron. Further, patients receiving HIF PHIs have lower serum levels of erythropoietin than those receiving erythropoietin, which will help from protection of putative "EPO toxicity" (**Fig. 1**). There was no difference in the hemoglobin rise among patients with elevated or normal C-reactive protein levels, suggesting the potential utility of roxadustat for patients who have a high inflammatory state. The lowering of total cholesterol, low-density lipoprotein cholesterol, and triglycerides was another beneficial side-effect, related to effect on acetyl coenzyme A and 3-hydroxy-3-methylglutaryl coenzyme A (HMG-CoA) reductase.

This trial showed a higher risk of hyperkalemia, a finding that has not been not reported in trials of other HIF PHIs, so hyperkalemia may be an off-target effect of roxadustat rather than a class effect.

The major limitations of this trial is the relatively small sample size (compared to CHOIR and TREAT), and short follow-up. Adverse events may yet appear when larger, longer trials are completed. ESAs act specifically on the erythropoietin receptor, which is selectively expressed in red blood cell precursors. However, the HIF pathway exists in all cells and regulates the expression of hundreds of genes. Thus, PHD inhibitors can have other on-target effects. The extent and the nature of these effects will depend on the pharmacokinetic parameters, dosing

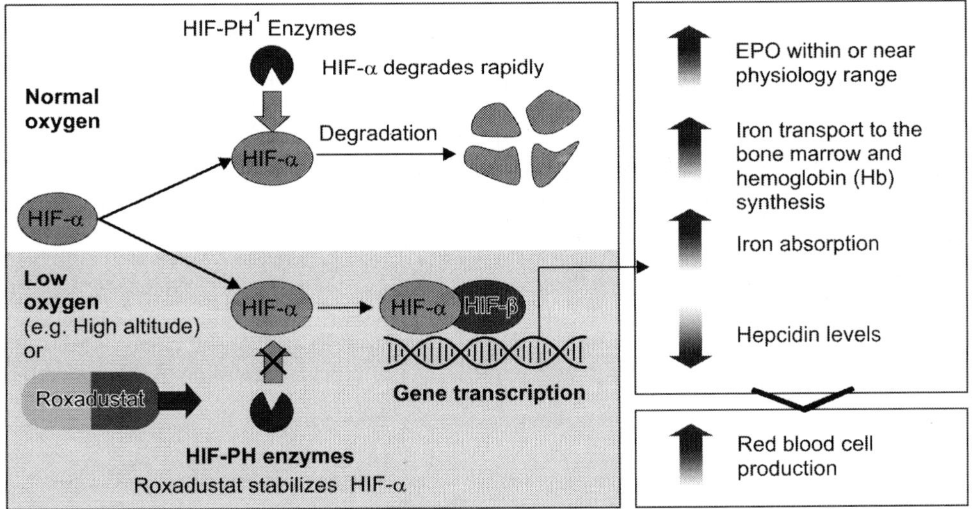

FIG. 1: Mechanism of action of PHI-HIF inhibitors.
Source: https://www.sec.gov/Archives/edgar/data/921299/000156459016013728/fgen-10k_20151231.htm

schedules and the activity of the chosen inhibitor against the three different PHD enzymes. It is hypothesized that intermittent, partial inhibition of PHD enzymes in the remaining renal tissue and/or the liver is sufficient to increase erythropoietin levels and ameliorate renal anemia.

This trial provides reasonable cause to think again that anemia of CKD might be reversed fully and safely, attributing the previously shown lack of benefit from normalization of the hemoglobin level to adverse effects from high doses and blood levels of erythropoietin.

Key Message

- *This trial has enabled us to ask: Can roxadustat therapy normalize the hemoglobin level in patients with anemia and allow them to reap the benefit of improved oxygen delivery without the increased risks associated with normalization of the hemoglobin level by erythropoietin-stimulating agents?*

ARTICLE 19

A clinically applicable approach to continuous prediction of future acute kidney injury

Tomašev N, Glorot X, Rae JW, Zielinski M, Askham H, Saraiva A, et al. A clinically applicable approach to continuous prediction of future acute kidney injury.
Nature. 2019;572:116-9.

Abstract

In this article, the authors describe the findings of collaborative work conducted with machine-learning researchers from DeepMind, a Google subsidiary. They asked the question: Can an artificial intelligence driven computational model predict the likelihood of developing acute kidney injury (AKI) in the near future.

Researchers used data from the US Veterans Affairs (VA) clinical database of 703,782 adult patients across 172 inpatient and 1,062 outpatient sites. Each patient contributed multiple data points in the 72-hour period preceding the AKI event, giving a total of >6 billion clinical-event entries. They used a method called ablation analysis to determine the factors linked to the risk of developing AKI and used "recurrent neural network", a machine-learning algorithm and created a time-updated prognostic model (**Fig. 1**).

The area under the receiver operator characteristic curve of their model was 0.92 for prediction of AKI within the next 48 hours, which means that the patient who would develop AKI in the next 48 hours will have the higher score 92% of the time. This performance is better than previous models that have used novel serum and urine biomarkers to predict AKI. The model predicted 55.8% of all AKI episodes, and 90.2% of those that required subsequent dialysis. However, it would generate 2 false alerts for every true alert. About 57% of the false alerts occurred in patients with pre-existing CKD, 24% related to an AKI episode that appeared to have resolved.

The model correctly identified substantial future increases in seven auxiliary biochemical tests in 88.5% of cases. It also provided information about factors most salient to the computation of risk prediction.

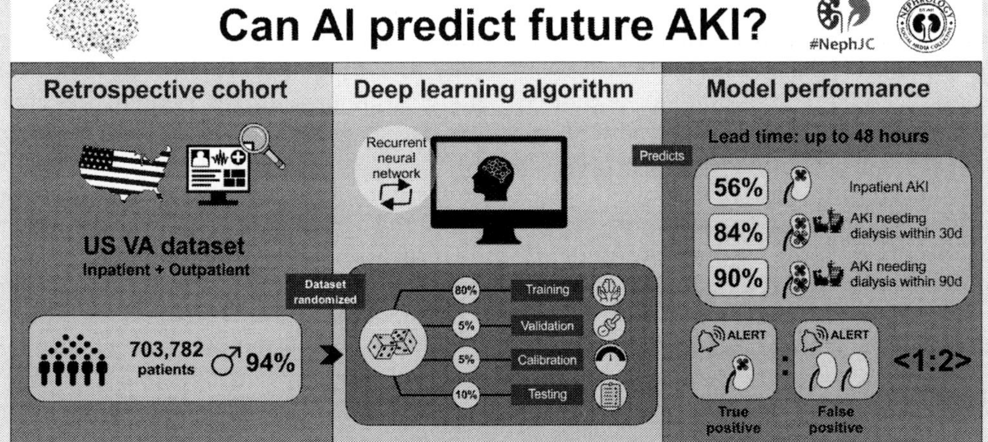

FIG. 1: A visual abstract by Dr Harish Seethapathy describing the prediction of in-hospital AKI using deep learning.

Source: http://www.nephjc.com/news/2019/9/24/artificial-intelligence-and-aki-the-visual-abstract

"Artificial intelligence comes to nephrology."

COMMENT

Acute kidney injury (AKI) is a major clinical problem and has been called a humanitarian issue by the International Society of Nephrology. In 2013, it was estimated that every year 13 million people develop AKI around the world, of whom 1.7 million die. A large proportion of AKI develops in hospitalized patients, especially those with multiple morbidities, after surgery or other interventions and those receiving multiple drugs. About 10–25% of all hospital admissions are complicated by AKI. Cate of AKI carries high cost (> US$ 100 billion worldwide) and increases the duration of hospital stay. Prevention of AKI has been emphasized as an important public health goal.

The widescale adoption of electronic health record (EHR) technology has led to an unprecedented accumulation of medical data. Attempts to use data to develop automated alerts based on simple algorithms have been developed but have been plagued by low sensitivity. The findings presented in this study are exciting and indicate that it might be possible to use deep learning approaches to guide the prevention of clinically important events such as AKI.

It is important to consider the price of these alerts – according to the authors there would be two false predictions for every 1 positive prediction and about 3% of hospitalized patients would alert on a daily basis. While these are early days, performance of such models can be made to vary by determining cut points that generate an alert threshold for taking action. It is important to consider what action should follow the alert. For the authors, the action is "trigger a daily clinical assessment", which has few downsides and a false alert carries little penalty. Different cut points may be needed that prompts for interventions that carry risk (such as empirical volume resuscitation).

Routine use of such models presents in real-world practice might present challenges. The study used 620,000 variables as inputs collected in the Veterans Affairs (VA) system database. Many of these features may not be captured by the EHRs in other health systems. Further, any one of these inputs can "break", for example when systems are upgraded, leading to degradation or even failure of the predictive algorithm. Finally, these algorithms need real-time computing power which is not available everywhere. The authors used deidentified data in DeepMind lab. In real-world, institutions may not want potentially sensitive patient information going to third parties and want to perform these calculations on site.

A solution could be development of models that maximize predictive power with fewer inputs. In contrast to the predictive power of 0.92 given by the recurrent neural network model, the authors also reported that a simple logistic regression with the same inputs that yielded an area under the curve of 0.86, which is still very impressive and emphasizes the value of data. Some experts in machine learning have raised the need of identifying the differential contribution of time-variant versus time-invariant features to the overall prediction. In other words, are individuals alerting because they are at high risk from the moment they enter the hospital (based on an elevated baseline Scr, the presence of diabetes, or other chronic conditions) others because of the dynamic changes that take place during hospitalization.

It raises the very interesting question for nephrologists. Suppose an alert is triggered and a "pre-AKI" consult arrives—what do we do now? According to the authors, the expected action is "clinical assessment", but it may lead to expectation of an "action". At this time, we do not have any therapies to offer. Management of hemodynamics and avoidance of nephrotoxins are the only appropriate responses. However, fluid therapy is not entirely without risk, and the justification to withhold a potentially beneficial but potentially nephrotoxic antibiotic in a patient with currently normal kidney function is not straightforward, given there were 2 false alerts to every true one. Such decisions can only be justified after trials are conducted that randomize pre-AKI alerting to usual care would seem particularly valuable at this point.

The other issue related to the relation between timing of the insult and the clinical manifestations of AKI. A nephrotoxic drug might not cause damage until a cumulative toxicity threshold has been reached, and this may take several doses. Such a lead time creates an opportunity to identify subtle cues. On the other hand, AKI event has already developed in the cases of most patients with sepsis-associated AKI giving little, if any, opportunity for data mining. Similarly, surgery-associated AKI usually manifests in the first 12–24 hours.

An interesting feature was that <7% of records examined by the authors were women, an anomaly related to the VA system that predominantly serves males.

Key Messages

⊙ *Artificial intelligence can help provide clinically usable information.*

⊙ *We need a RCT that randomize pre-AKI alert system to usual care before recommending its routine use.*

ARTICLE 20

Effect of vitamin D and omega-3 fatty acid supplementation on kidney function in patients with type 2 diabetes: a randomized clinical trial

de Boer IH, Zelnick LR, Ruzinski J, Friedenberg G, Duszlak J, Bubes VY, et al. Effect of vitamin D and omega-3 fatty acid supplementation on kidney function in patients with type 2 diabetes: a randomized clinical trial.
JAMA. 2019;322:1899-909.

Abstract*

Background: Chronic kidney disease (CKD) occurs in 40–60% of adults with type 2 diabetes mellitus (T2DM) and is a leading cause of end-stage renal disease. Renin–angiotensin system and inflammatory pathways play role in kidney disease progression.

Methods: Supplementation of vitamin D3 and/or omega-3 fatty acids was tested against placebo to assess their effects on decline of kidney function. Adult men and women with T2DM were randomized into 1 of 4 groups in a 2 × 2 factorial design and followed for 5 years to assess estimated glomerular filtration rate (eGFR) decline. Secondary outcomes were a composite outcome of eGFR decline >40% decline, kidney failure, or death and increase of urine albumin creatinine ratio (uACR), respectively.

Results: Of the 1,312 patients randomized, 934 (71%) completed the study. Adherence to assigned intervention was good. The mean baseline eGFR was 85.8 mL/min/1.75 m^2 and change in eGFR was –12.7 mL/min/1.75 m^2 for the total population. Most patients (70%) were vitamin D replete (serum vitamin D >30 ng/mL) only 16% having serum vitamin D levels <20 ng/mL. There were no differences between the groups in terms of eGFR decline. There were no differences in adverse events between intervention and placebo groups.

Conclusion: Supplementation of vitamin D3 and/or omega-3 fatty acids does not result in slowing of eGFR decline as compared to placebo in adults with T2DM. *Redrafted abstract

"Is vitamin D really 'VITAL' for kidney health?"

COMMENT

Prevention of development and progression of diabetic kidney disease is still an area of intense research. Active vitamin D (1,25-dihydroxyvitamin D) is shown to suppress renin secretion and reduce inflammation in kidney tissues in animal studies. Short-term urine albumin excretion has also been shown to be reduced by active vitamin D in humans. Similarly, omega-3 fatty acid exerts anti-inflammatory effects and so, can probably alter progression of chronic kidney disease (CKD). Observational studies in humans have found association of lower intake of 25-hydroxyvitamin D (vitamin D3) and oily fish with CKD progression. However, the effects of vitamin D3, a safer alternative to active vitamin D, have never been satisfactorily shown in a randomized clinical trial. Vitamin D and Omega-3 Trial to Prevent and Treat Diabetic Kidney Disease (VITAL-DKD), is an ancillary study to VITAL trial which is looking at the effects of these supplements in preventing cancer and cardiovascular diseases. Participants (n = 1,321), adult men >50 years and women >55 years, with a mean estimated glomerular filtration rate (eGFR, 86 mL/min/1.75 m^2) were randomized into 1 of the 4 intervention groups in

a 2 × 2 factorial design. Vitamin D3 (2,000 IU/day) and omega-3 fatty acid (465 mg eicosapentaenoic acid plus 375 mg of docosahexaenoic acid) were administered for 5 years and outcomes (eGFR decline and secondary outcomes) measured at 5 years. A difference in change of eGFR over 5 years of at least 2.3 mL/min/1.75 m^2 between the intervention groups and placebo groups was felt by investigators to reflect clinical relevance. The study population was a relatively healthy population of older adults with DM (of 6–10 years duration) controlled on oral drugs and hypertension (60% on RAS blockade) with only 13% with eGFR <60 mL/min/1.73 m^2 and 9% with urine albumin creatinine ratio (uACR) >30 mg/g. About 30% of the population had insufficient vitamin D levels (20–30 ng/mL) and only 16% had deficient vitamin D levels (<20 ng/mL). Adherence to interventions was seen in 80–90%. Serum levels of vitamin D3 remained different in the intervention and placebo groups until 2 years. The mean change in eGFR over 5 years was –12.7 mL/min/1.73 m^2 in the overall studies population and did not differ between the assigned groups (**Table 1**). No differences were

TABLE 1: Primary outcome: Effects of vitamin D and omega-3 fatty acids on change in estimated glomerular filtration rate (eGFR) from baseline to year 5.

	Active intervention			Placebo			Difference in change from baseline[a]	
	No.	eGFR, mean (95% CI), mL/min/1.73 m^2	eGFR change from baseline, mean (95% CI), mL/min/1.73 m^{2b}	No.	eGFR, mean (95% CI), mL/min/1.73 m^2	eGFR change from baseline, mean (95% CI), mL/min/1.73 m^{2b}	Mean difference (95% CI), mL/min/1.73 m^2	p value[c]
Vitamin D								
Baseline[d]	701	86.3 (84.6–88.0)		607	85.3 (83.7–87.0)			
Year 2	531	80.6 (78.8–82.4)	–5.2 (–6.2 to –4.2)	459	79.3 (77.3–81.2)	–6.1 (–7.1 to –5.1)	0.9 (–0.6 to 2.5)	
Year 5	496	74.3 (72.3–76.2)	–12.3 (–13.4 to –11.2)	438	72.5 (70.6–74.5)	–13.1 (–14.2 to –11.9)	0.9 (–0.7 to 2.5)	0.25
Omega-3 fatty acids								
Baseline[d]	657	85.7 (84.1–87.3)		651	86.0 (84.2–87.8)			
Year 2	499	79.4 (77.6–81.2)	–5.7 (–6.8 to –4.7)	491	80.6 (78.6–82.5)	–5.5 (–6.5 to –4.6)	–0.3 (–1.8 to 1.3)	
Year 5	472	73.7 (71.8–75.6)	–12.2 (–13.3 to –11.1)	462	73.2 (71.1–75.3)	–13.1 (–14.2 to –12.0)	0.9 (–0.7 to 2.6)	0.27

[a] Modeled difference, with positive values indicating higher eGFR at year 5 (slower decline in eGFR from baseline) among participants randomized to the active intervention compared with those randomized to the corresponding placebo intervention. Derived from a linear mixed model that includes adjustment for age, sex, and baseline urine albumin-creatinine ratio and accounts for missing data using multiple imputation.

[b] Change from baseline summarized over all participants using multiple imputation.

[c] Test of the difference in change in eGFR from baseline to year 5.

[d] Four participants were missing baseline eGFR values.

observed between the groups in the secondary composite outcome of eGFR decline of >40%, kidney failure or death. The study was not powered to assess effects of interventions among subgroup with vitamin D3 insufficiency or deficiency who might benefit from it.

Key Messages

⊙ *Vitamin D or omega-3 fatty acid supplementation does not preserve kidney function in relatively healthy patients with type 2 diabetes mellitus.*

⊙ *Further studies on the effects of vitamin D supplementation on kidney function in those with vitamin D deficiency are needed.*

⊙ *The long-term effects of active vitamin D3 (1,25-dihydroxyvitamin D) remains to be evaluated in randomized trials.*

ARTICLE 21

Association of treatment with metformin versus sulfonylurea with major adverse cardiovascular events among patients with diabetes and reduced kidney function

Roumie CL, Chipman J, Min JY, Hackstadt AJ, Hung AM, Greevy RA Jr, et al. Association of treatment with metformin versus sulfonylurea with major adverse cardiovascular events among patients with diabetes and reduced kidney function *JAMA. 2019;322:1-11.*

Abstract*

Objective: To examine the role of metformin or sulfonylurea in preventing major adverse cardiovascular events (MACE) in diabetic patients who developed early kidney dysfunction and continued these therapies.

Methods: A retrospective cohort study of US veterans, with data supplemented by linkage to Medicare, Medicaid, and National Death Index data from 2001 through 2016. Persistent new users of metformin and sulfonylureas who reached a reduced kidney function threshold (estimated glomerular filtration rate <60 mL/min/1.73 m^2 or creatinine ≥1.4 mg/dL for women or ≥1.5 mg/dL for men). Patients were followed up from reduced kidney function threshold until MACE, treatment change, loss to follow-up, death, or study end (December, 2016).

Results: The weighted cohort included 24,679 metformin and 24,799 sulfonylurea users (median age: 70 years) and the median estimated glomerular filtration rate was 55.8 mL/min/1.73 m^2 at study entry (**Fig. 1**). MACE outcomes occurred less frequently in metformin than the sulfonylurea group (23.0 per 1,000 person-years versus 29.2 per 1,000 person-years, respectively). The cause-specific adjusted hazard ratio of mace for metformin was 0.80 (95% CI 0.75–0.86) compared with sulfonylureas.

Conclusions: In diabetic patients with reduced kidney function who persisted with monotherapy, treatment with metformin, in comparison to sulfonylurea, was found to be associated with a risk of MACE. *Redrafted abstract

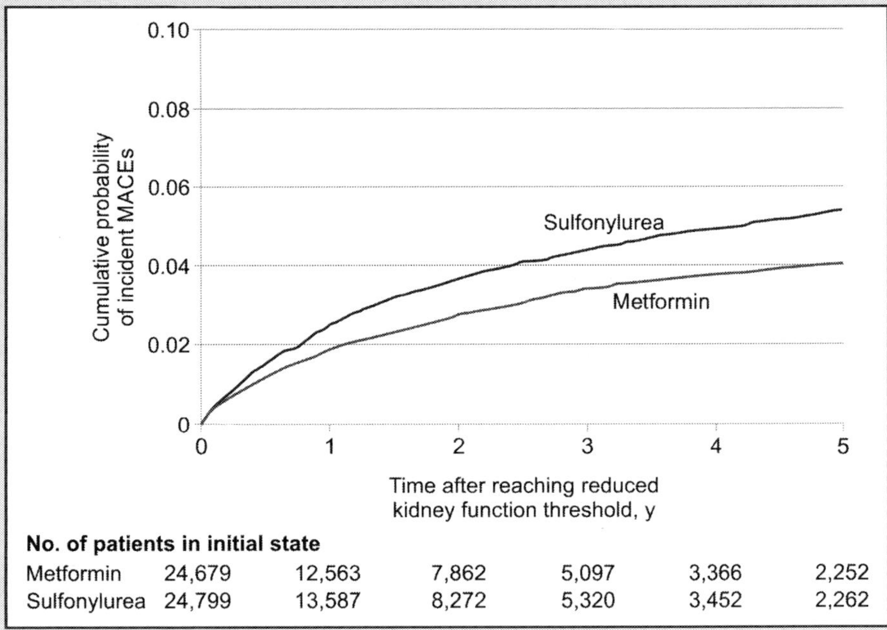

FIG. 1: Competing risk cumulative incidence match-weighted cohort.

"Better reasons for prescribing metformin now?"

COMMENT

Metformin is the first-line drug for type 2 diabetes mellitus (T2DM) as it is beneficial for weight, cheap and relatively nontoxic drug. However, there has been conflicting mandates on the use of metformin in those with reduced kidney function. Although the US FDA had initially issued warnings restricting the use of metformin in those with serum creatinine of ≥1.5 mg/dL, recent modifications by the FDA are in favor of continuing use of metformin in those with mild kidney dysfunction (up to >30 mL/min/1.73 m^2). Apart the UK prospective diabetes study showing cardiovascular benefits of metformin, no large randomized trials have examined this aspect. Observational studies demonstrated safety of metformin in those with mild kidney dysfunction, however, clinical trials showing its efficacy in terms of cardiovascular health are lacking. Among US veterans with T2DM, persistent metformin monotherapy was compared with persistent sulfonylurea monotherapy after the onset of reduced kidney function, i.e., estimated glomerular filtration rate (eGFR) <60 mL/min/1.73 m^2, or serum creatinine of ≥1.5 mg/dL in men or serum creatinine of ≥1.4 mg/dL in women. This was a retrospective study with propensity-matched analysis of 49,478 participants having a mean eGFR of 55.8 mL/min/1.73 m^2 at entry. Participants were followed up for median of 1 year in the metformin group and median of 1.2 years in the sulfonylurea

group for the primary composite outcome of major adverse cardiovascular events (MACE). The cause-specific adjusted hazard ratio for MACE was 0.80 (95% CI 0.75–0.86) in the metformin group as compared to sulfonylurea group, suggesting lower risk of MACE in the metformin group. There were lesser number of patients (3,586 in metformin group and 4,287 in the sulfonylurea group) with second confirmatory reduced eGFR excluding the possibility of an acute reversible kidney injury in some patients. The results were similar, however, statistical significance was not reached. While the findings of this study cannot be generalized to those who start metformin after the onset of reduced kidney function, as of now it seems safe and wise to continue metformin in patients on metformin monotherapy despite onset of mild kidney dysfunction. There is a possibility that the apparent benefits of metformin could be because the comparator sulfonylurea group, had higher risks of cardiovascular complications. However, this seems less likely as sulfonylurea was recently shown to be similar risks of cardiovascular events as linagliptin in the CAROLINA trial. Linagliptin, in turn, is shown to be noninferior to placebo in terms of cardiovascular events. So, it is becoming clearer that both metformin and sulfonylurea are safe and effective in the long-term and can be continued to be used either as monotherapy or add-on therapy.

Key Messages

- *Metformin monotherapy is associated with lower risk of cardiovascular events than sulfonylurea monotherapy in type 2 diabetes mellitus patients with early kidney dysfunction.*
- *The level of kidney dysfunction when metformin should be ideally discontinued needs to be addressed further in randomized trials.*

Section Editor: Gagandeep Singh

Associate Editors: U Meenakshisundaram, Jeyaraj Durai Pandian

ARTICLE 1

Drug repositioning screening identifies etravirine as a potential therapeutic for Friedreich's ataxia

Alfedi G, Luffarelli R, Condò I, Pedini G, Mannucci L, Massaro DS, et al. Drug repositioning screening identifies etravirine as a potential therapeutic for Friedreich's ataxia.
Mov Disord. 2019;34:323-34.

Abstract*

Introduction: Friedreich's ataxia (FRDA), which is an autosomal-recessive cerebellar ataxia, is caused due to mutation of the *frataxin (FXN)* gene; this leads to reduced FXN expression, oxidative stress, and mitochondrial dysfunction. At the present times, there is no treatment for patients of FRDA. As residual FXN levels critically affect disease severity, increasing the FXN levels is the primary aim of specific therapy for FRDA. As this study aimed to develop a new therapy for FRDA, a drug repositioning approach was adopted for recognizing market-available drugs that are able to enhance FXN levels.

Materials and methods: By using a cell-based reporter assay for assessing variation in FXN amount, a high-throughput screening was performed of a library that consisted of 853 US Food and Drug Administration (US FDA)-approved drugs.

Results: In the potentially interesting individuals who were isolated from the screening, attention was focused on etravirine, which is an antiviral drug presently being used as an anti-HIV therapy. It was demonstrated that etravirine can encourage a significant rise in levels of FXN in cells derived from patients of FRDA, by increasing FXN messenger RNA (mRNA) translation. An important finding was that accumulation of FXN in treated patient cell lines was similar to levels of FXN in unaffected carrier cells; this indicates that etravirine could be therapeutically appropriate. Certainly, treatment with etravirine preserves the activity of the iron-sulfur cluster consisting of enzyme aconitase as well as confers resistance to oxidative stress in cells that are derived from patients of FRDA.

Conclusion: Taking into account the excellent safety profile as well as its ability of increasing FXN levels and correcting some of the defects related to the disease, etravirine seems to be a potential candidate for the treatment of FRDA. *Redrafted abstract

"The world we have created is a product of our thinking; it cannot be changed without changing our thinking."

—Albert Einstein

COMMENT

Friedreich's ataxia (FRDA) is an autosomal recessive inherited ataxia which causes progressive degeneration in the nervous system and heart. It has an estimated prevalence of 1 in 50,000 individuals in the white population. Onset is generally around puberty with gait ataxia and incoordination and classical features include dysarthria, areflexia, sensory loss, skeletal abnormalities, and left ventricular hypertrophy. Despite being the most common form of inherited ataxia, FRDA still lacks an adequate approved treatment. Hence, finding a therapy is a paramount medical need.

■ GENETIC BASIS OF FRIEDREICH'S ATAXIA

Friedreich's ataxia is caused by a homozygous hyperexpansion of GAA triplets (from 70 to 1,000) within the first intron of the gene encoding for frataxin (FXN). This mutation reduces transcription of the *FXN* gene attributed to the formation of "sticky" DNA structures and epigenetic modifications, but maintains at least 10–30% of FXN which is essential for survival during embryonic development. Given that reduced amount of FXN is the principal cause of the disease, the main goal of a specific therapy would be to restore physiological FXN levels.

Drug repositioning implies the usage of a drug already in use for another disease/indication for a new indication. The authors of this paper have taken a systematic drug repositioning approach. They screened the US Food and Drug Administration (US FDA)-approved library and isolated 19 compounds among which their attention was focused on etravirine.

Etravirine is an antiretroviral drug used in the lifelong treatment of HIV-infected patients, including children. The authors have shown that it can promote a significant increase in FXN levels in vitro without any toxic effect. It has been shown to promote FXN accumulation in cells derived from FRDA patients, restoring physiological FXN levels. It is proposed that etravirine may function by enhancing the rate of translation of FXN mRNA or by preventing the degradation of FXN protein.

Key Message

⊙ *Treatment of FRDA is often wrought with desperation on the part of the patient's family and the physician because of the lack of any definitive treatment. Etravirine has shown promise in this in vitro study and we can only hope that this drug repositioning leads to a definitive treatment for FRDA.*

ARTICLE 2

Recent advances in idiopathic inflammatory myopathies (IIM)—rapid discoveries of myositis-specific antibodies (MSAS) and myositis-associated antibodies (MAAS)—moving towards 'precision medicine'

Malaviya AN, Bhalla S, Verma S, Kapoor S. Recent Advances in Idiopathic Inflammatory Myopathies (IIM)—Rapid Discoveries of Myositis-specific Antibodies (MSAS) and Myositis-Associated Antibodies (MAAS)—Moving Towards 'Precision Medicine'. *J Assoc Physicians India. 2019;67:68-73.*

Abstract

The progress in the understanding of inflammatory muscle diseases over the past several decades has been slow but steady. The classification given by Bohan and Peter in 1975 was based on clinical features. It served well, but inadequacies were also obvious. The increasing discoveries of autoantibodies in this group of disorders have helped in refining the classification of Bohan and Peter to a large extent. At the present state of knowledge, it is now possible to classify and subclassify this group of diseases using distinct clinical features combined with the type of autoantibodies in well-defined subsets. Not only the subsets help predicting the type of organ involvement and comorbidities but may also help to choose a specific drug for a particular subclass. This approach may lead to the practice of precision medicine for inflammatory myositis.

"Winds of change: Newer advances in inflammatory myopathies."

COMMENT

In the past, inflammatory disease of the striated muscle, depending upon its associated features, has been given different names such as dermatomyositis, polymyositis, amyopathic myositis, and inclusion body myositis. However, in the last few decades this terminology has been changed to the more acceptable, all-encompassing name idiopathic inflammatory myopathies (IIMs). The clinical picture of IIM is highly heterogeneous with variable presentation of painless proximal muscle weakness, typical skin rash, association with other connective-tissue-disease-like clinical features, raised muscle enzymes, and characteristic electromyographic, magnetic resonance imaging (MRI), and histopathological abnormalities.

With so many variables, the clinical presentation of IIM is broad. Over the decades, multiple classification systems have been used to subclassify IIMs with the primary aim of achieving a homogenous pattern of categorizing the subtypes for improvement in specificity of treatment. However, despite the many classification systems, the most recent being the European League Against Rheumatism (EULAR), the difficulties persist. The time-honored system proposed by Bohan and Peter in 1975, based predominantly on clinical features, has remained the most widely accepted and used system till date, but inadequacies have been present.

In 1976, the discovery of the anti-Mi-2 antibody, which was the first "myositis-specific antibody" (MSA), was a practice changing revelation. For the first time, it placed IIMs in the category of systemic inflammatory rheumatic diseases. It also proved that MSAs could help to predict disease subtype, disease course, and prognosis as well as response to a particular treatment. Newer modalities have led to the discovery of many such MSAs which are specific only to IIM, and similar "myositis-associated antibodies" (MAAs) which though seen in IIM are not specific and may be seen in other connective tissue diseases as well. The increasing detection of newer autoantibodies has helped to refine, classify, and subclassify this group of diseases using characteristic clinical features combined with their autoantibodies into well-defined subsets which not only help to predict the type of organ involvement but also play a crucial role in deciding the specific path of treatment. This approach may herald the way to the practice of precision medicine for inflammatory myositis.

Key Messages

- ⊙ *The discovery of myositis-specific and myositis-associated antibodies has revolutionized the approach to inflammatory myopathies.*
- ⊙ *Characteristic clinical features in combination with specific autoantibodies can help to characterize, classify, and prognosticate disease along with deciding treatment regimen.*

ARTICLE 3

Clinical profile of patients with acute intracerebral hemorrhage and ICH score as an outcome predictor on discharge, 30 days and 60 days follow-up

Ojha P, Sardana V, Maheshwari D, Bhushan B, Kamble S. Clinical Profile of Patients with Acute Intracerebral Hemorrhage and ICH Score as an Outcome Predictor on Discharge, 30 Days and 60 Days Follow-up.
J Assoc Physicians India. 2019;67:14-8.

Abstract

Background: Intracerebral hemorrhage (ICH) is one of the most common causes of morbidity and mortality worldwide accounting for 10–15% of all strokes types. ICH score is a validated tool to predict mortality and morbidity at 30-day follow-up period.

Objective: To prospectively evaluate the predictive utility of ICH score in patients presenting with acute ICH on discharge, 30 days and 60 days follow-up period.

Design: Prospective observational study.

Materials and methods: This study was conducted in the Department of Neurology, Government Medical College, Kota, Rajasthan, India from January, 2016 to August, 2016. Total 120 consecutive patients presenting with acute ICH were studied. Data collected included demographics, clinical parameters, cranial computed tomography (CT) findings, and ICH score on presentation. Primary outcome was defined as mortality/ morbidity during hospitalization, on discharge, 30 days and 60 days follow-up. The mRS (modified Rankin score) was used to assess the outcome.

Statistical analysis used: SPSS 19 statistical software. SPSS is known as "Statistical Package for the Social Sciences".

Results: Of the total 120 patients with acute ICH (108 supratentorial and 12 infratentorial) studied, 48 (40%) patients died during hospitalization. Mean age was 66.9 ± 13.5 years. Hydrocephalus, midline shift, and IV extension on presenting CT scan were observed in 20 (16.6%), 44 (36.6%), and 48 (40%) patients, respectively. The independent predictors of increased mortality with statistical significance ($p < 0.001$) were presence of vomiting, seizures, loss of consciousness, lower GCS (≤8), higher ICH score, and ventilator requirement. Statistically, significant ($p \leq 0.001$) radiological features associated with mortality included infratentorial location, presence of hydrocephalus, higher midline shift (58.3% vs. 22.2% OR = 2.6), intraventricular extension of hematoma and a higher baseline hematoma volume. ICH score on admission was significantly ($p < 0.001$) positively correlated with the mRS score on discharge (R = 0.667), 1 month (R = 0.66), and 2 months (R = 0.765) follow-up.

Conclusion: Intracerebral hemorrhage score is a useful tool to predict outcome during hospitalization, on discharge, 1 month and 2 months follow-up. We suggest that ICH score assessment and documentation should become standard procedure in acute care and follow-up of patients with intracerebral hemorrhage.

"Utility of ICH score as an outcome predictor in intracerebral hemorrhage."

COMMENT

Spontaneous intracerebral hemorrhage (ICH) accounts for 4–14% of all strokes and is associated with high morbidity and mortality. The burden of stroke is higher in the developing countries and Asian countries report a much higher incidence of ICH compared to the west.

The morbidity associated with ICH is very high, with only 20% patients regaining independence

6 months post-stroke, which is why considerable interest has prevailed in finding outcome predictors after ICH. Various clinical, radiological, hematological, and biochemical parameters at time of onset of ICH have been investigated and found associated with outcome in these patients. The ICH score consisting of a 6-point calculation based on five clinical indicators: (1) Age >80 years, (2) GCS (Glasgow coma scale), (3) Volume of hematoma on baseline CT scan, (4) Location (infratentorial or supratentorial), and (5) The presence of intra-ventricular extension, is a validated tool which has been developed as a mortality predictor for patients with hemorrhagic stroke.

This prospective, observational 2-year study done at Government Medical College, Kota, Rajasthan was designed to study the clinical profile of acute ICH patients presenting to the hospital and to assess the predictors of mortality in them. In addition, they studied the utility of ICH score as an outcome predictor based on the mRS (modified Rankin Scale) score, at discharge, 30 days and 60 days follow-up.

Of the total 120 patients with acute ICH (108 supratentorial and 12 infratentorial), 48 (40%) patients died during hospitalization. Presence of vomiting, seizures, loss of consciousness, lower GCS (≤8), higher ICH score and requirement for mechanical ventilation were found to be statistically significant, independent predictors of increased mortality. Infratentorial location of ICH, higher midline shift, presence of hydrocephalus, intraventricular extension of ICH, and higher baseline hematoma volume were significant radiological predictors associated with increased mortality. Baseline ICH score showed a statistically significant correlation with mRS score at discharge, at 1 month and at 2 months of follow-up. Authors recommend that due to its high utility as an outcome predictor, ICH score assessment and documentation should become standard procedure in acute care and management of ICH.

Key Messages

- *Mortality and morbidity of ICH are substantially high.*
- *Knowledge about clinical and radiological predictors of mortality is essential for physicians so as to take timely and prompt action.*
- *Spontaneous intracerebral hemorrhage score assessment is a reliable and validated tool for outcome prediction in these patients.*

ARTICLE 4

Intensive blood pressure reduction with intravenous thrombolysis therapy for acute ischaemic stroke (ENCHANTED): an international, randomised, open-label, blinded-endpoint, phase 3 trial

Anderson CS, Huang Y, Lindley RI, Chen X, Arima H, Chen G, et al. Intensive blood pressure reduction with intravenous thrombolysis therapy for acute ischaemic stroke (ENCHANTED): an international, randomised, open-label, blinded-endpoint, phase 3 trial.
Lancet. 2019;393:877-88.

Abstract

Background: Systolic blood pressure (SBP) of >185 mm Hg is a contraindication to thrombolytic treatment with intravenous alteplase in patients with acute ischemic stroke, but the target SBP for optimal outcome is uncertain. We assessed intensive blood pressure (BP) lowering compared with guideline-recommended BP lowering in patients treated with alteplase for acute ischemic stroke.

Methods: We did an international, partial-factorial, open-label, blinded-endpoint trial of thrombolysis-eligible patients (aged ≥18 years) with acute ischemic stroke and SBP 150 mm Hg or more, who were screened at 110 sites in 15 countries. Eligible patients were randomly assigned (1:1, by means of a central, web-based program) within 6 hours of stroke onset to receive intensive (target SBP 130–140 mm Hg within 1 hour) or guideline (target SBP <180 mm Hg) BP lowering treatment over 72 hours. The primary outcome was functional status at 90 days measured by shift in mRS (modified Rankin Scale) scores, analyzed with unadjusted ordinal logistic regression. The key safety outcome was any intracranial hemorrhage. Primary and safety outcome assessments were done in a blinded manner. Analyses were done on intention-to-treat basis. This trial is registered with ClinicalTrials.gov, number NCT01422616.

Findings: Between March 3, 2012 and April 30, 2018, a total number of 2,227 patients were randomly allocated to treatment groups. After exclusion of 31 patients because of missing consent or mistaken or duplicate randomization, 2,196 alteplase-eligible patients with acute ischemic stroke were included: 1,081 in the intensive group and 1,115 in the guideline group, with 1,466 (67.4%) administered a standard dose among the 2,175 actually given intravenous alteplase. Median time from stroke onset to randomization was 3.3 hours [interquartile range (IQR) 2.6–4.1]. Mean SBP over 24 hours was 144.3 mm Hg [standard deviation (SD) 10.2] in the intensive group and 149.8 mm Hg (12.0) in the guideline group (p < 0.0001). Primary outcome data were available for 1,072 patients in the intensive group and 1,108 in the guideline group. Functional status (mRS score distribution) at 90 days did not differ between groups [unadjusted odds ratio (OR) 1.01; 95% confidence interval (CI) 0.87–1.17; p = 0.8702]. Fewer patients in the intensive group [160 (14.8%) of 1,081] than in the guideline group [209 (18.7%) of 1,115] had any intracranial hemorrhage (OR 0.75, 0.60–0.94; p = 0.0137). The number of patients with any serious adverse event did not differ significantly between the intensive group [210 (19.4%) of 1,081] and the guideline group [245 (22.0%) of 1,115; OR 0.86, 0.70–1.05; p = 0.1412]. There was no evidence of an interaction of intensive BP lowering with dose (low vs. standard) of alteplase with regard to the primary outcome.

Interpretation: Although intensive BP lowering is safe, the observed reduction in intracranial hemorrhage did not lead to improved clinical outcome compared with guideline treatment. These results might not support a major shift toward this treatment being applied in those receiving alteplase for mild-to-moderate acute ischemic stroke. Further research is required to define the underlying mechanisms of benefit and harm resulting from early intensive BP lowering in this patient group.

"To do or not to do, that is the question: Intensive blood pressure management after thrombolysis."

COMMENT

Intravenous thrombolysis remains the cornerstone of hyperacute reperfusion treatment for acute ischemic stroke patients with large vessel occlusion. Evidence suggests administration of IV alteplase within 4.5 hours of stroke onset for improved efficacy and safety; however, recommendations for blood pressure (BP) control during and after thrombolysis are conflicting and controversial.

Although guidelines advocate use of alteplase after reduction of systolic blood pressure (SBP) to >185 mm Hg, studies have observed poor outcomes with increased symptomatic intracerebral hemorrhage (ICH) post-thrombolysis in patients with BPs even below this threshold.

This study reports the results of the BP control assessment arm of the ENCHANTED (ENhanced Control of Hypertension and Thrombolysis Stroke Study) trial, which was an international, open-label, blinded-endpoint trial in adult patients with acute ischemic stroke eligible for thrombolysis, with a SBP >150 mm Hg or more. It aimed to compare intensive BP lowering regimen (target SBP 130–140 mm Hg) to standard guideline-recommended BP lowering regimen (target BP <180 mm Hg) in acute ischemic stroke patients treated with alteplase, within 60 minutes of randomization. The premise was based on the potential benefits related to a reduced risk of thrombolysis-related symptomatic

ICH versus a worsening of cerebral ischemia due to low BP and hypoperfusion.

Eligible patients were recruited and randomly assigned from 110 sites in 15 countries, within 6 hours of stroke onset, to receive either the intensive BP control or the guideline BP control treatment for 72 hours. Noninvasive BP monitoring was done, every 15 minutes for 1 hour, hourly from hours 1 to 6, and 6-hourly from hours 6 to 2, following thrombolysis. The functional status measured by shift in mRS (modified Rankin Scale) score at 90 days was assessed as the primary outcome, while any ICH was assessed as the key safety outcome. A total number of 2,196 eligible patients were allocated to the two treatment groups (1,081 in the intensive group and 1,115 in the guideline group) between March, 2012 and April, 2018. Median time from stroke onset to randomization was 3.3 hours [interquartile range (IQR) 2.6–4.1]. Mean SBP over 24 hours was 144.3 mm Hg in the intensive group and 149.8 mm Hg in the guideline group. No significant difference was noted in the functional status of patients at 90 days between the two groups; however, fewer patients in the intensive group than in the guideline group had any ICH.

The authors concluded that intensive BP lowering, although safe, did not lead to a translatable improvement in clinical outcomes when compared to guideline treatment. Further research is required to understand the underlying mechanisms of benefit and harm resulting from early intensive BP lowering in these patients.

Key Message

⊙ *Intensive BP lowering in acute ischemic stroke patients after IV thrombolysis, when compared to guideline recommended BP management, shows no measurable benefit.*

ARTICLE 5

Guillain–Barré syndrome in Indian population: a retrospective study

Jain RS, Kookna JC, Srivastva T, Jain R. Guillain–Barré Syndrome in Indian Population: A Retrospective Study. *J Assoc Physicians India. 2019;67:56-9.*

Abstract

Objectives: To study clinical characteristics of various forms of Guillain–Barré syndrome (GBS) in Indian adults.

Materials and methods: The epidemiological, clinical, cerebrospinal fluid (CSF), and electrophysiological data of 65 patients of GBS were reviewed in a retrospective study.

Results: Analysis of age distribution disclosed a high incidence (36.92%) in young adults between 18 and 29 years of age. Seasonal preponderance in winter and summer was found. Preceding events were identified in 22 (33.84%) cases. Motor weakness, areflexia, and facial weakness were the most common clinical features. CSF albuminocytological dissociation was present in 80% of patients. Utilizing clinical and electrophysiological data, these 65 patients with GBS were subclassified as acute demyelinating polyradiculoneuropathy 17 (26.15%), axonal form 17 (26.15%), Fisher's syndrome 2 (3.07%), and ataxic variant 1 (1.53). The remaining 28 (43.07%) patients were unclassified. Around 9 (13.8%) patients had recurrent GBS. Only 5 (7.7%) patients required mechanical ventilation. Follow-up available on 47 patients disclosed that all of them recovered satisfactorily. No patient was persistently disabled and no mortality occurred during hospitalization.

Conclusions: Guillain–Barré syndrome in Indian population from northwest India showed peculiar age, seasonal distribution, and high frequency of both AIDP and axonal subtypes. Both, axonal and demyelinating subtypes shared common clinical features and had good prognosis.

"Spectrum of Guillain–Barré syndrome and its variants: The Indian perspective."

COMMENT

This 2-year retrospective study from a tertiary care hospital in northwest India assesses the epidemiological, clinical, cerebrospinal, and electrophysiological profile of various forms of Guillain–Barré syndrome (GBS). Asbury and Cornblath's clinical diagnostic criteria was used to classify a total of 65 patients into acute demyelinating, axonal, ataxic, Fischer variant, and unclassified forms of GBS, of which the acute demyelinating and axonal forms were noted to have the highest frequency. Characteristic age distribution was present with high incidence in the young adults (18–29 years). Seasonal preponderance was also observed with increase in frequency in summer (April to June) and winter (October to January) months. Around 34% patients reported preceding events ranging between 11 and 45 days prior to the onset of weakness, all of which were infectious in nature. One patient notably had jaundice prior to weakness and tested positive for hepatitis A. Motor weakness, sensory symptoms, myalgias, and facial and bulbar weakness were the most frequently reported symptoms, respectively. Nine patients had history of a previous similar episode, with the interval between previous and present episode being >5 years in all patients. Cerebrospinal fluid (CSF) examination was done in 39 patients and albuminocytological dissociation was demonstrated in all patients beyond 2 weeks from disease onset.

The average duration of hospital stay was 12 (3–90) days. Patients were managed with immuno-globulin (25), steroids (16), and plasmapheresis (2) apart from general medical management. Eight patients developed respiratory distress out of which five patients required mechanical ventilation during course of hospital stay. By discharge, all patients showed improvement of at least one grade from the point of maximal weakness and no patient died during hospitalization. All patients showed good recovery on follow-up.

The typical presentation of progressive ascending and areflexic motor weakness with albuminocytological dissociation is the most frequently seen presentation of GBS. Electrophysiological tests help in confirming, characterizing into various subtypes, and prognosticating the disease. The available Indian data is sparse, of which the acute demyelinating form is attributed as the most common, compared to Central America, Japan, and China where the axonal forms are much more common. On the whole, GBS, even the axonal variants respond well to treatment and have a good prognosis.

Key Messages

⊙ *The typical presentation of GBS is that of an areflexic, ascending paralysis, although other presentations can be present.*

⊙ *Cerebrospinal fluid and electrophysiological tests are adjunctive in confirming, characterizing, and prognosticating the disease.*

⊙ *Guillain–Barré syndrome responds well to treatment and on the whole has a good prognosis.*

ARTICLE 6

An intracerebral hemorrhage care bundle is associated with lower case fatality

Parry-Jones AR, Sammut-Powell C, Paroutoglou K, Birleson E, Rowland J, Lee S, et al. An Intracerebral Hemorrhage Care Bundle Is Associated with Lower Case Fatality.
Ann Neurol. 2019;86:495-503.

Abstract

Objective: Anticoagulation reversal, intensive blood pressure lowering, neurosurgery, and access to critical care might all be beneficial in acute intracerebral hemorrhage (ICH). We combined and implemented these as the acute bundle of care (ABC) hyperacute care bundle and sought to determine whether, the implementation was associated with lower case fatality.

Methods: The ABC bundle was implemented from June 1, 2015 to May 31, 2016. Key process targets were set, and a registry captured consecutive patients. We compared 30-day case fatality before, during, and after bundle implementation with multivariate logistic regression and used mediation analysis to determine which care process measures mediated any association. Difference-in-difference analysis compared 30-day case fatality with 32,295 patients with ICH from 214 other hospitals in England and Wales using Sentinel Stroke National Audit Program data.

Results: A total of 973 ICH patients were admitted in the study period. Compared to before implementation, the adjusted odds of death by 30 days were lower in the implementation period [odds ratio (OR) 0.62, 95% confidence interval (CI) 0.38–0.97, p = 0.03), and this was sustained after implementation (OR 0.40; 95% CI 0.24–0.61; p < 0.0001). Implementation of the bundle was associated with a 10.8% point (95% CI –17.9 to –3.7; p = 0.003) reduction in 30-day case fatality in difference-in-difference analysis. The total effect of the care bundle was mediated by a reduction in do-not-resuscitate orders within 24 hours (52.8%) and increased admission to critical care (11.1%).

Interpretation: Implementation of the ABC care bundle was significantly associated with lower 30-day case fatality after ICH. *Ann Neurol. 2019;86:495-503.*

"The 'ABC' of improving outcomes after intracerebral hemorrhage."

COMMENT

Spontaneous intracerebral hemorrhage (ICH) is a significant cause of morbidity and mortality globally. Different studies have analyzed various causative factors and the effect of addressing the same toward mortality benefit in ICH. Patients on oral anticoagulants may present with spontaneous ICH with the added risk of early hematoma expansion. Prompt reversal of the anticoagulation effect has shown to improve outcomes. Similarly, rapid and intensive reduction of blood pressures within 6 hours of onset to a systolic pressure <140 mm Hg was shown to improve quality of life in the INTERACT2 (Intensive Blood Pressure Reduction in Acute Cerebral Hemorrhage Trial 2) study. Neurosurgical interventions to evacuate

hematoma or treat hydrocephalus have also shown benefit but uncertainty prevails regarding when and on whom to intervene.

This study combined all these strategies into the acute bundle of care ("ABC" care bundle) with the purpose to determine whether implementation of the same was associated with reduction in 30-day case fatality rates. Since individual randomization was considered unethical, a quasi-experimental design was used on data collected from local and national registries in the United Kingdom over a period of 1 year. Multivariate logistic regression was used to compare before, during, and after bundle implementation of 30-day case fatality rates.

Of the total 973 ICH patients admitted during the study period, 353 patients were in the before-implementation, 266 patients in the during-implementation, and 241 patients in the after-implementation groups, respectively. The adjusted odds of death were lower in the implementation period, a measure which continued to remain sustained in the postimplementation period as well. A significant reduction in 30-day case fatality rate was observed with the implementation of the "ABC bundle". Increase in rates of admission to critical care units and decrease in rates of do-not-resuscitate orders within 24 hours were noted.

This study proposes that the implementation of the "ABC bundle", if consistently delivered, may provide survival benefit in ICH; however, the clinical and cost effectiveness of the program needs to be established in a randomized trial design.

Key Messages

- ◉ *The "ABC bundle" combines prompt reversal of anticoagulation (if present), rapid and intensive reduction of systolic blood pressures, and urgent neurosurgical intervention (when required) into a single strategy to be implemented for patients with ICH.*
- ◉ *The "ABC bundle" may be beneficial for lowering case fatality and improving outcomes in ICH patients.*

ARTICLE 7

Lasmiditan for the acute treatment of migraine: subgroup analyses by prior response to triptans

Knievel K, Buchanan AS, Lombard L, Baygani S, Raskin J, Krege JH, et al. Lasmiditan for the acute treatment of migraine: subgroup analyses by prior response to triptans.
Cephalalgia. 2020;40:19-27.

Abstract*

Background: In two similarly designed Phase 3 trials (SAMURAI and SPARTAN), it was found that lasmiditan was superior to placebo for the acute treatment of migraine among adults patients who have moderate or severe migraine disability. In post-hoc integrated analyses, assessment of the efficacy of lasmiditan was done among patients in whom a good or insufficient response to triptans was reported and among patients who were triptan naive.

Materials and methods: This study included subgroups of patients who reported an overall good or poor/none response to the most recent use of a triptan at baseline (which was defined as good or insufficient responders, respectively) and a triptan naive subpopulation, which were taken from combined study participants. Randomization of the patients was done to receive lasmiditan 50 mg (SPARTAN only), 100 mg or 200 mg, or placebo, as the first dose. Comparison of outcomes (which included most bothersome symptom-freedom, headache pain-freedom, and headache-pain relief 2 hours post-first dose of lasmiditan) was done with placebo. Also, treatment-by-subgroup analyses evaluated whether there was a variation in therapeutic benefit as per the prior triptan response (good or insufficient).

Results: Irrespective of triptan response, higher efficacy was demonstrated by lasmiditan as compared to placebo; majority of the comparisons were statistically significant. On treatment by-subgroup analyses, it was observed that the benefit over placebo of lasmiditan was similar between those who have a good response and patients with an insufficient response to triptans. Lasmiditan had significantly higher efficacy as compared to placebo among triptan-naive patients.

Conclusion: Efficacy of lasmiditan was similar among patients in whom a good or insufficient response to prior triptan use was reported. Also, in patients who were triptan naïve, lasmiditan demonstrated efficacy. In patients who have migraine, lasmiditan can be a beneficial therapeutic option. *Redrafted abstract

"You shouldn't do things differently just because they're different: They need to be better."
—Elon Musk

COMMENT

Migraine has been ranked by the WHO as the second highest cause of disability worldwide as measured in years of life lost to disability. The unmet needs in many patients include headache-related disability and dissatisfaction with current acute medication regimen. Presently, triptans are the gold standard for acute treatment but they are not efficacious in all patients and are contraindicated in patients with coronary artery disease, peripheral vascular disease, uncontrolled hypertension and in patients with risk factors for undiagnosed coronary artery disease.

Our understanding of the pathophysiology of migraine has evolved from vasodilation to a brain disorder involving pain other sensory processing. The trigeminal nociceptors in the dura mater are sensitized by neuropeptide release such as calcitonin gene-related peptide (CGRP). 5-HT1F receptor agonists are a potential alternative to triptans. Lasmiditan is a drug that acts on these receptors as an agonist without vasoconstrictive activity. Lasmiditan has been shown to be effective in previous studies.

The authors have conducted a prospective, randomized, double-blind, placebo-controlled, multicenter phase 3 study of three doses of oral lasmiditan (200 mg, 100 mg, and 50 mg) for the acute treatment of a single migraine attack (with and without aura) in adults. A single dose was given with a second dose permitted between 2 and 24 hours after initial dosing, if needed, for rescue or recurrence of migraine. The primary objective was in achieving headache pain freedom and freedom from the most bothersome symptom (MBS), while secondary efficacy objectives included sustained pain freedom and freedom from individual symptoms associated with migraine and patient global impression of change. The safety objective was to assess safety and tolerability of lasmiditan through adverse events, physical examinations, vital signs, laboratory tests and ECGs.

The results were:
- The proportion of patients who were pain-free and MBS-free was significantly higher with 200 mg compared with placebo, which was also observed with the other two doses.
- A significant dose-related sustained pain freedom at 24 hours was observed with all three doses.
- There were significant dose-related improvements in global impression of "very much better" and "much better" across the groups.
- The majority of adverse effects were mild or moderate in severity, the most frequent being dizziness, somnolence and paresthesia.

Limitation of the study: The enrolled patients were primarily middle-aged white females and hence may not extrapolate to other patient populations, as ethnic differences are known in migraine.

Key Messages

- *Lasmiditan, a 5-HT1F receptor agonist, is an effective drug for acute treatment of migraine and is a welcome addition to the basket of acute migraine treatments. The response to the drug is dose-related.*
- *Lasmiditan because of its lack of vasoconstrictive properties may be useful in patients who cannot take triptans (e.g., coronary artery disease, uncontrolled hypertension).*
- *The least effective dose needs to be determined in our population by dedicated studies.*
- *In our country, the pricing of the drug when it is available will be a major determinant of its usage in practice.*

ARTICLE 8

Intensive vs standard treatment of hyperglycemia and functional outcome in patients with acute ischemic stroke: the SHINE randomized clinical trial

Johnston KC, Bruno A, Pauls Q, Hall CE, Barrett KM, Barsan W, et al. Intensive vs Standard Treatment of Hyperglycemia and Functional Outcome in Patients With Acute Ischemic Stroke: The SHINE Randomized Clinical Trial. *JAMA. 2019;322:326-35.*

Abstract*

Importance: Hyperglycemia during acute ischemic stroke is associated with poor functional outcomes. Intensive treatment of hyperglycemia could be a promising option in this setting, but the data are limited.

Objectives: To compare the efficacy of intensive treatment of hyperglycemia with the standard treatment during acute ischemic stroke, and to determine the functional outcome.

Design, setting, and participants: Adult patients with hyperglycemia (glucose concentration of >110 mg/dL if had diabetes, or ≥150 mg/dL if did not have diabetes) and acute ischemic stroke from 63 US sites between April, 2012 and August, 2018 and enrolled within 12 hours from stroke onset were included in the SHINE (Stroke Hyperglycemia Insulin Network Effort) randomized clinical trial. They were followed up till November, 2018. A total of 1,151 patients met eligibility criteria.

Interventions: Patients were randomly assigned one of the two groups. The intensive treatment group received (n = 581) continuous intravenous insulin using a computerized decision support tool [target blood glucose concentration of 80–130 mg/dL (4.4–7.2 mmol/L)]. The standard treatment group (n = 570) received insulin on a sliding scale that was administered subcutaneously [target blood glucose concentration of 80–179 mg/dL (4.4–9.9 mmol/L)]. Both the treatment continued for 72 hours.

Main outcomes and measures: The proportion of patients with a favorable outcome based on the 90-day mRS (modified Rankin Scale) score [a global stroke disability scale ranging from 0 (no symptoms or completely recovered) to 6 (death)], adjusted for baseline stroke severity was the primary efficacy outcome.

Results: Of the total 1,151 patients, 1,118 (97%) completed the trial. The mean age of the patients was 66 years [standard deviation (SD) 13.1 years]; 529 (46%) were women, and 920 (80%) were diagnosed to have diabetes. Enrollment was stopped for futility based on prespecified interim analysis criteria. During treatment, the mean blood glucose level was 118 mg/dL (6.6 mmol/L) and 179 mg/dL (9.9 mmol/L) in the intensive treatment and standard treatment group, respectively. About 119 out of 581 patients (20.5%) and 123 of 570 patients (21.6%) had a favorable outcome in the intensive treatment group and standard treatment group, respectively [adjusted relative risk 0.97 (95% CI 0.87–1.08), p = 0.55; unadjusted risk difference –0.83% (95% CI –5.72–4.06%)]. Hypoglycemia or other adverse events led to early stopping of treatment in 65 out of 581 patients (11.2%) in the intensive treatment group and in 18 out of 570 patients (3.2%) in the standard treatment group. Almost 15 patients in the intensive treatment group and none in the standard treatment group suffered from severe hypoglycemia [15/581 (2.6%); risk difference 2.58% (95% CI 1.29–3.87%)].

Conclusions and relevance: No significant difference in favorable functional outcome at 90 days was observed among patients with acute ischemic stroke and hyperglycemia, treated with intensive versus standard glucose control for up to 72 hours.

Trial registration: ClinicalTrials.gov identifier: NCT01369069. *Redrafted abstract

"Slow and steady wins the race—Intensive hyperglycemia control inadvisable in ischemic stroke."

COMMENT

Hyperglycemia in acute ischemic stroke is associated with poor clinical outcomes such as increase in infarct size as well as greater risk of hemorrhagic transformation. It has been postulated that increased blood sugar levels lead to increased oxidative stress, endothelial dysfunction, and altered fibrinolysis. Although present American Heart Association/American Stroke Association (AHA/ASA) guidelines recommend a blood glucose level in the range of 140–180 mg/dL; however, there is paucity of sufficient data for optimal blood sugar management in such patients from randomized controlled trials.

The SHINE (Stroke Hyperglycemia Insulin Network Effort) randomized clinical trial was conducted to compare the efficacy of intensive blood glucose management to standard blood glucose management in patients with acute ischemic stroke in improving clinical outcomes. Adult patients with acute ischemic stroke and hyperglycemia (blood glucose >110 mg/dL in patients known to have diabetes, or >150 mg/dL in patients not known to have diabetes) who were enrolled within 12 hours from stroke onset, from 63 US hospitals between April, 2012 and November, 2018 were included into the study.

Of the total 1,151 patients, 1,118 went on to complete the trial. Patients were randomized to the intensive treatment arm (n = 581; to receive continuous intravenous insulin) to a target blood glucose concentration of 80–130 mg/dL and to the standard treatment arm (n = 570; to receive insulin subcutaneously according to sliding scale) to a target blood glucose concentration of 80–179 mg/dL for up to 72 hours. The primary outcome assessed was the proportion of patients with a favorable outcome which was based on the 90-day mRS (modified Rankin Score) which was defined differently for different patients according to their baseline NIHSS (National Institutes of Health Stroke Scale) scores.

The mean blood glucose level in the intensive treatment arm was 118 mg/dL and 179 mg/dL in the standard treatment group. A favorable outcome occurred in 20.5% of patients in the intensive treatment arm compared to 21.6% patients in the standard treatment arm. Adverse events such as hypoglycemia occurred in 11.2% and 3.2% patients in the intensive and standard treatment arms respectively, requiring early discontinuation of treatment. This study concluded that the findings did not suggest a significant difference in favorable functional outcomes at 90 days between the two treatment arms and the authors thereby do not support using intensive glucose control among acute ischemic stroke patients.

Key Messages

- *Rapid intensive control of hyperglycemia when compared to standard treatment in patients with acute ischemic stroke showed no significant difference in functional outcomes between the two arms.*
- *Adverse events such as hypoglycemia occurred more in the intensive group.*
- *Intensive blood sugar control is not advisable at present in ischemic stroke.*

ARTICLE 9

Randomized trial of three anticonvulsant medications for status epilepticus

Kapur J, Elm J, Chamberlain JM, Barsan W, Cloyd J, Lowenstein D, et al. Randomized Trial of Three Anticonvulsant Medications for Status Epilepticus.
N Engl J Med. 2019;381:2103-13.

Abstract*

Background: Studies on the treatment choices for patients with status epilepticus that is refractory to benzodiazepines are scarce. Here, we compare the efficacy and safety of three drugs, namely levetiracetam, fosphenytoin, and valproate in children and adults with convulsive status epilepticus unresponsive to benzodiazepines.

Methods: A randomized, blinded, adaptive trial conducted for comparison of three intravenous anticonvulsive agents: Levetiracetam, fosphenytoin, and valproate. Absence of clinically evident seizures and improvement in the level of consciousness by 60 minutes after the start of drug infusion, without need of additional anticonvulsants, was taken as the primary outcome. The posterior probabilities that each drug was the most or least effective were calculated. Safety outcomes included life-threatening hypotension or cardiac arrhythmia, endotracheal intubation, seizure recurrence, and death.

Results: A total number of 384 patients were randomly assigned to receive levetiracetam (145 patients), fosphenytoin (118), or valproate (121). There were 16 additional instances of randomization due to re-enrollment of patients with a second episode of status epilepticus. The trial was stopped after a planned interim analysis in accordance with a prespecified stopping rule for futility of finding one drug to be superior or inferior. About 10% of the enrolled patients had psychogenic seizures. The primary outcome was achieved in 68 patients of levetiracetam group (47%; 95% credible interval 39–55), 53 patients of fosphenytoin group (45%; 95% credible interval 36–54), and 56 patients of valproate group (46%; 95% credible interval 38–55). The posterior probability that each drug was the most effective and that was 0.41, 0.24, and 0.35, respectively. Hypotension and intubation occurred were noted more in the fosphenytoin group and more deaths occurred in the levetiracetam group than in the other groups, but these differences were not statistically significant.

Conclusions: The three drugs led to cessation of seizures and improvement in alertness by 60 minutes in approximately 50% of the patients with status epilepticus refractory to benzodiazepines, and these were associated with similar incidences of adverse events [Funded by the National Institute of Neurological Disorders and Stroke; ESETT (Established Status Epilepticus Treatment Trial) ClinicalTrials.gov number, NCT01960075].
*Redrafted abstract

"Wider choices for the second-line treatment of generalized convulsive status epilepticus."

COMMENT

Status epilepticus is the most serious and dramatic expression of epilepsy and seizures. It is associated with high case fatality rates and many other life-threatening complications. In addition, the control of status epilepticus is critically dependent on the timely institution of parenterally administered anti-seizure medications. Time lost in instituting these treatments has devastating consequences. Indeed, status epilepticus is eminently responsive to treatment in the first 30 minutes or the so-called, "golden period", an expression derived from the emergency management of acute myocardial infraction or trauma but perhaps, more true for status epilepticus. Even within the first 30 minutes, the earlier the better. In recognition of this principle and also the expectation that emergency physicians would be influenced to institute treatments more swiftly, the time criteria in the definition of status epilepticus stands amended from 5 to 30 minutes.

Intravenous benzodiazepines are the first-line treatment for generalized convulsive status epilepticus based on sturdy evidence accumulated over several decades. Roughly 40% of status epilepticus episodes remain uncontrolled despite benzodiazepines. Moreover, a long-acting antiseizure medication needs to be administered after control of status with benzodiazepines in order to prevent further seizures and status epilepticus. Till about 10 years ago, loading doses of phenytoin (or fosphenytoin) or phenobarbital were the only options available. Across the world, availability of intravenous preparations of the two medications guided physician choice in the emergency management of status epilepticus. The availability of parenteral preparations of several antiseizure medications in the last two decades prompted the consideration of their use as a second-line agent in status epilepticus. Currently, intravenous formulations are available for valproate, levetiracetam, and lacosamide.

The ESETT (Established Status Epilepticus Treatment Trial)was a treatment trial of convulsive status epilepticus across 57 centers in the United States that compared intravenous fosphenytoin (20 mg phenytoin-equivalents), levetiracetam (60 mg/kg, maximum dose: 4,500 mg) and valproate (40 mg/kg, maximum dose: 3,000 mg) (**Fig. 1**). The primary outcome was cessation of the status episode and recovery of consciousness. All three medications achieved the primary outcome in roughly 50% cases, fulfilling criteria for noninferiority. Moreover, the adverse effect profiles were similar with respiratory depression being reported in approximately 10% cases.

What are the implications of the trial results for emergency physician practice? The findings of the trial mean that the three medications have equivalent efficacy and adverse effect profiles. Physicians, thus, have a wider choice available to them. In real-world situations, they now should feel empowered to manage their patients with status epilepticus with a variety of comorbidities with any of three options.

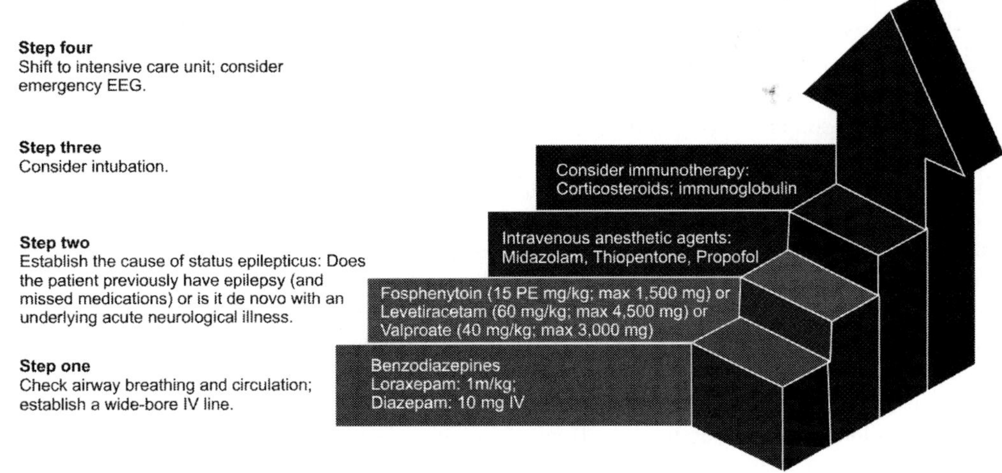

FIG. 1: Treatment algorithm for convulsive status epilepticus.

Key Messages

- *The ESETT was a multicentric trial of intravenous fosphenytoin (15 PE mg/kg), levetiracetam (60 mg/kg), and valproate (40 mg/kg) in generalized convulsive status epilepticus in adults and children.*
- *All three agents demonstrated similar efficacy and controlled status epilepticus in roughly 50% cases.*
- *Respiratory depression was the most common serious adverse event and similar in frequency of occurrence after all three agents.*

ARTICLE 10

Japanese encephalitis- and dengue-associated acute encephalitis syndrome cases in Myanmar

Kyaw AK, Ngwe Tun MM, Nabeshima T, Buerano CC, Ando T, Inoue S, et al. Japanese Encephalitis- and Dengue-associated Acute Encephalitis Syndrome Cases in Myanmar.
Am J Trop Med Hyg. 2019;100:643-6.

Abstract

This study was conducted to find the burden of dengue virus (DENV) and Japanese encephalitis virus (JEV) among children under the age of 13 years who presented with acute encephalitis syndrome at Mandalay Children Hospital in Myanmar in 2013. Molecular and serological investigations were performed on 123 cerebrospinal fluid (CSF) samples collected from these patients. By neutralization tests and/or virus isolation, four (3.3%) JEV- and one DENV-associated encephalitis cases (0.8%) were confirmed. Antibody titer against JEV genotype 3 was the highest among the laboratory-confirmed JEV cases. One strain of DENV-1 with genotype 1 was isolated from the CSF sample of the dengue encephalitis patient; this was similar to the virus circulating in the study area and neighboring countries. This study shows that flaviviruses are important pathogens causing encephalitis in Myanmar. Active disease surveillance, vector control, and vaccination programs should be enforced to reduce the morbidity and mortality caused by flavivirus encephalitis.

"Is Dengue Encephalitis a defined clinical entity?"

COMMENT

The National Vector Borne Disease Control Program of India estimated 136,000 cases of dengue across India. This is perhaps an underestimate and less than the number of reported cases in 2017. Nevertheless, dengue remains one of the most common infective disorders seen by physicians across most parts of India.

The manifestations of dengue are varied and form a spectrum—from asymptomatic cases to severe dengue shock and dengue hemorrhagic fever. Neurological manifestations can be placed somewhere midway between these extreme manifestations, albeit and fortunately, rare. These are rare perhaps because dengue virus (DENV) is not considered neurotropic akin to "Herpes" viruses and some other "Flaviviruses". Among the neurological manifestations, however, are myalgias, myositis, Guillain–Barré syndrome, acute disseminated encephalomyelitis, optic neuritis, and dengue-maculopathy. Two other conditions merit discussion: (1) Dengue encephalitis and (2) Dengue encephalopathy. The former is a condition characterized by fever (and/or other systemic features of dengue) and alteration in sensorium and seizures. When the altered mentation is on account of other conditions associated with dengue, e.g., hepatic encephalopathy or respiratory failure, the condition is known as "dengue encephalopathy". The distinction, however, between dengue encephalitis and dengue encephalopathy is somewhat imprecise. It is also imperative to rule out other CNS conditions such as Herpes encephalitis or Coxsackie encephalitis in all suspected cases of dengue encephalitis.

Japanese B encephalitis (JE) like dengue is caused by a flavivirus and transmitted by mosquito bites. In many parts of India, JE and dengue are co-endemic. In such circumstances, the distinction between dengue encephalitis and JE becomes critical.

Kyaw (2019) from Myanmar reported findings in cerebrospinal fluid (CSF) in cases of dengue encephalitis and JE. He first used an in-house immunoglobulin M (IgM)/immunoglobulin G (IgG)-capture enzyme-linked immunosorbent assay (ELISA) for JE and DENV in the CSF. The problem with the ELISA was the cross-reactivity with other *Flavivirus* species. Next, they employed a neutralization assay to detect the presence of the viruses in the CSF. The neutralization assays were more specific and included the focus-reduction neutralization test (FRNT), which distinguishes between all four strains of DENV and the plaque-reduction neutralization test for JE virus. The neutralization tests thus permitted the distinction between various flaviviruses. Lastly, they employed a reverse transcriptase polymerase chain reaction to isolate the viruses. Overall, the researchers met with success in less than in a handful of cases. Indeed, review of other published cases, likewise shows the low rates of detection of viral antibodies in the CSF in suspected cases of dengue encephalitis. We propose criteria for establishing a diagnosis of "dengue encephalitis" in **Box 1**.

Box 1: Proposed diagnostic criteria for "dengue encephalitis".

Feature

- Residence in/travel to a dengue endemic region
- Acute febrile illness
- Any of the following:
  - Aches and pains
  - Rash
  - Positive tourniquet test
  - Leukopenia
  - Thrombocytopenia
  - Hepatomegaly with elevated liver enzymes
- Altered sensorium or mentation including hyperactive or hypoactive delirium
- Convulsive seizures
- Absence of the any of the following features:
  - Severe hepatic failure
  - Severe renal failure
  - Severe respiratory failure as evidenced on blood gas studies
- Positive IgM ELISA in CSF sample

or

- Positive focus-reduction neutralization test to any one serotype of dengue virus in the CSF

or

- Demonstration of viral RNA using reverse transcriptase PCR in the CSF
- Absence of infective screen in the CSF using PCR for herpes virus, CMV, EBV, and other arboviruses (arthropod-borne virus)

(CMV: cytomegalovirus; CSF: cerebrospinal fluid; EBV: Epstein–Barr virus; IgM: immunoglobulin M; ELISA: enzyme-linked immunosorbent assay; PCR: polymerase chain reaction; RNA: ribonucleic acid)

Key Messages

- *Dengue encephalitis should be differentiated for other conditions including other causes for encephalopathy in dengue and other viral encepahlitides, e.g., JE.*

- *A positive antibody response in the CSF or the demonstration of viral RNA supports a diagnosis of "dengue encephalitis".*

- *Exclusion of other viral encepalitides, e.g., herpes simplex encephalitis and other arbovirus encephalitides is mandatory before diagnosing "dengue encephalitis".*

ARTICLE 11

Intermittent perilesional edema and contrast enhancement in epilepsy with calcified neurocysticercosis may help to identify the seizure focus

Jama-António JC, Yasuda CL, Cendes F. Intermittent perilesional edema and contrast enhancement in epilepsy with calcified neurocysticercosis may help to identify the seizure focus.
Epilepsia Open. 2019;4:351-4.

Abstract

Neurocysticercosis is a frequent cause of seizures in endemic countries. It is caused by the larvae of the tapeworm *Taenia solium*. The larvae once hosted in the cerebral parenchyma evolve into viable cysts, called the vesicular stage (with little or no inflammatory reaction), and may remain at this stage for years, or may enter in an inflammatory-degenerative process (colloidal phase) that ends with calcified nodules. Edema and magnetic resonance imaging (MRI) contrast enhancement associated with these calcifications have been described suggesting that it may be associated with seizures. However, most of these reports were either cross-sectional case-control series or case reports with a single time point MRI. Therefore, the clinical significance of recurring perilesional edema and contrast enhancement around calcified lesions is still uncertain. Here, we describe repeated MRIs of a patient with calcified neurocysticercosis over 4 years. The seizures were associated with edema and contrast enhancement that disappeared in the seizure-free periods, occurring only around one calcified nodule that coincided with the EEG findings and seizure semiology, although he had three additional calcifications. These findings support the association between pericalcification contrast enhancement and edema with recent seizures. This MRI finding may be a marker to define the epileptogenic focus in epilepsies with calcified neurocysticercosis.

"Neurocysticercosis: How long to treat with antiepileptic drugs?"

COMMENT

Neurocysticercosis remains one of most common attributable causes of seizures and epilepsy in India. The most common presentation of brain parasitic infestation is the solitary cysticercus granuloma (SCG) or the single, small (<10 mm), (ring or disk-shaped) enhancing lesion of computed tomography or magnetic resonance imaging (MRI). Despite, the well-known association between seizures and neurocysticercosis, several issues remain unsettled in consideration of the treatment of seizures and epilepsy in the setting of neurocysticercosis. One such crucial question is how long should the treatment with antiepileptic drugs be continued after presentation with the first seizure? Related to this question is the elucidation of factors that might predict the recurrence of seizures in patients presenting with a first seizure due to neurocysticercosis.

The SCG most often represents the granulomatous-nodular stage of cysticercosis (**Fig. 1A**).

This stage mostly resolves to a calcified-fibrous stage (**Fig. 1B**), which is traditionally considered the inactive stage of the parasite and hence need not be treated with antihelminthic drugs. However, follow-up studies have shown that roughly 35% of people with these calcified lesions will continue to have seizures over the next 5 years. Furthermore, what factors predict the occurrence of seizures in people with these calcified residues? A follow-up study from Peru, in which MRIs were performed in close temporal relationship to recurrent seizures found that roughly 50% of the calcified residues enhance upon administration of contrast and have surrounding brain parenchymal edema. Presumably, these calcified residues harbor some parasite remnants, which when released intermittently provoke seizures (**Figs. 2A** to **D**).

Jama-Antonio et al. in this elegant paper from Brazil, illustrate precisely that how the phenomenon of phasic contrast enhancement

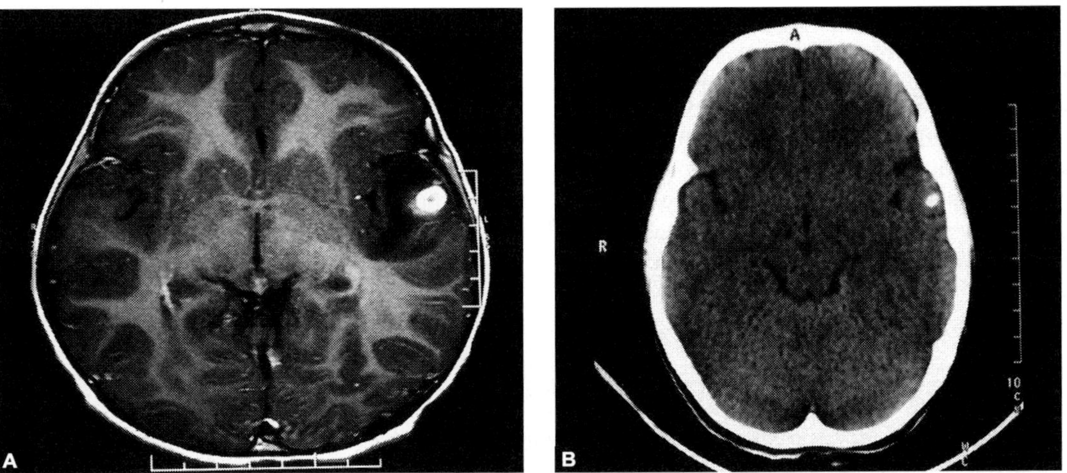

FIGS. 1A AND B: (A) Evolution of a cysticercus (B) to the calcified stage.

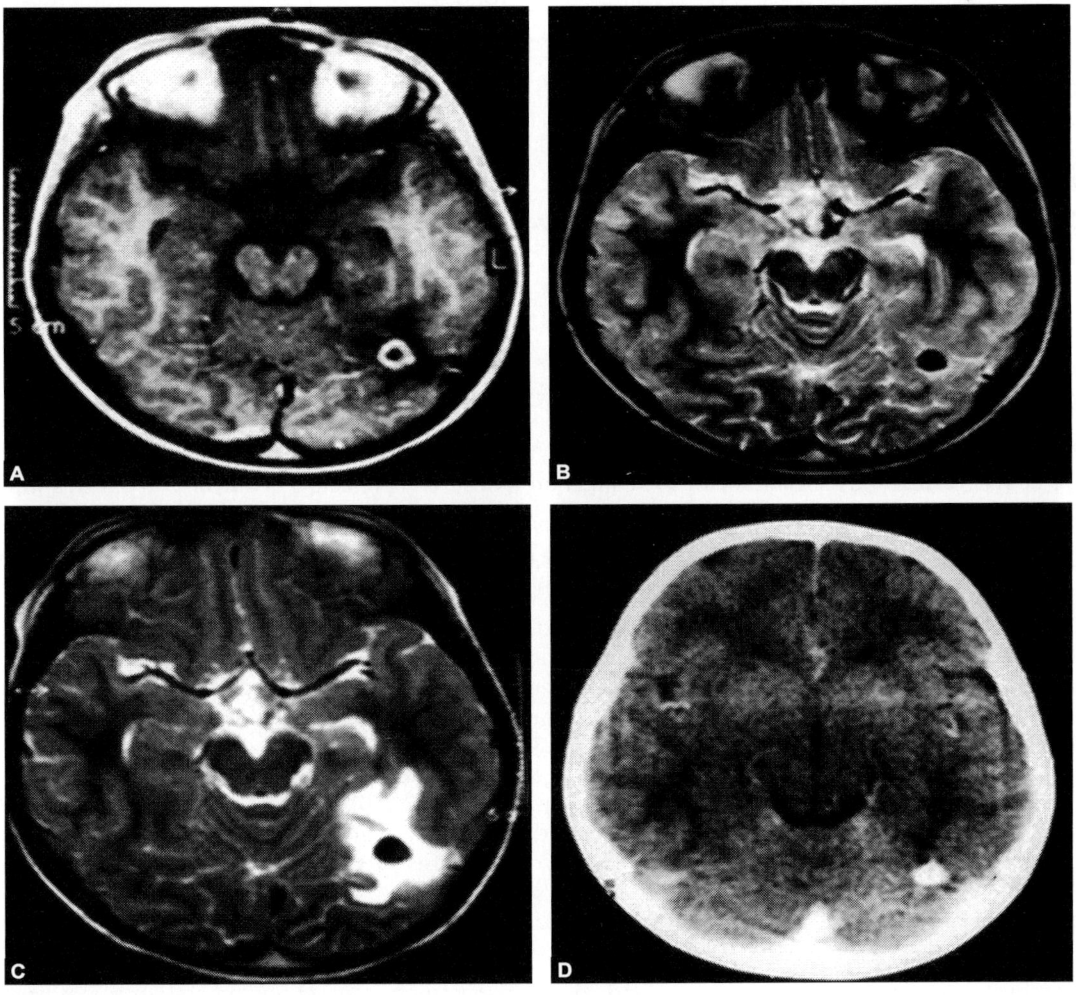

FIGS. 2A TO D: Serial images (A to D) showing the intermittent development of inflammatory edema around a calcified cysticercus.

in calcified neurocysticercosis is linked to the occurrence of seizures. They observed that when there are multiple cysticerci, the one that enhances can be considered to be responsible for seizures.

Coming back to the question of how long to treat with antiepileptic drugs and which are the patients, we should be treating with antiepileptic drugs in the long-term? It seems appropriate to continue treatment with antiepileptic drugs for long periods of time in those people who have residual calcified lesions. Roughly half of the recurrent seizure episodes in these people are on account of inflammatory reactions at the site of calcification. The next imminent question would be whether we can prevent the resolution of active cysticerci by calcifications? We do not have any pharmaceutical agent at present that can prevent calcification. However, given that much of the burden of seizures in neurocysticercosis is on account of the calcified lesions, the identification of measures to prevent calcification would be welcome.

Key Messages

⊙ *The calcified stage of neurocysticercosis traditionally represents the inactive stage of the parasite.*

⊙ *The calcified stage of neurocysticercosis is often associated with seizures.*

⊙ *In roughly 50% cases, seizures associated with the calcified stage of neurocysticercosis are related to the intermittent release of remnant antigenic material located within the calcified cysticercus.*

ARTICLE 12

Primary angiitis of the central nervous system: clinical profiles and outcomes of 45 patients

Sundaram S, Menon D, Khatri P, Sreedharan SE, Jayadevan ER, Sarma P, et al. Primary angiitis of the central nervous system: clinical profiles and outcomes of 45 patients.
Neurol India. 2019;67:105-12.

Abstract

Objective: To describe the clinical profile, treatment response, and predictors of outcome in patients with primary angiitis of the central nervous system (PACNS) from a single tertiary care center.

Methodology: Retrospective analysis of consecutive patients diagnosed with PACNS from January, 2000 to December, 2015. Outcome was defined as poor when the 6-month mRS (modified Rankin Scale) was ≥3.

Results: The median age of the 45 patients included in this study was 36 (range 19–70) years at disease onset and 31 (68.9%) were males. The initial presentation was ischemic stroke in 15 (33.3%), hemorrhagic stroke in 4 (8.9%), headache in 11 (24.4%), seizures in 8 (17.8%), and cognitive dysfunction in 5 (11.1%) patients. Diagnosis was confirmed by a four-vessel cerebral digital subtraction angiography (DSA), biopsy and by both biopsy and DSA in 26 (57.8%), 15 (33.3%), and 4 (8.9%) patients, respectively. All patients received glucocorticoids and 14 patients received in addition either cyclophosphamide or azathioprine as their first treatment. The median duration of follow-up was 33.1 (0.7-356) months. A poor 6-month outcome was observed in 12 (26.7%) patients. Relapse occurred in 25 (55.6%) patients and 7 (15.6%) died. Predictors of a poor outcome consisted of cognitive dysfunction at diagnosis (80% vs. 20%; p = 0.014) and the NIHSS (National Institutes of Health Stroke Scale) ≥5 (62.5% vs. 37.5%; p < 0.0005). None of the patients with a normal EEG had a poor outcome (p = 0.046). Predictors of relapse were a higher NIHSS at admission (p = 0.032) and a normal DSA (p = 0.002).

Conclusion: In this cohort, severe deficits and cognitive symptoms at onset and an abnormal EEG were associated with a poor 6-month outcome.

"Primary CNS Vasculitis: An Update."

COMMENT

Primary central nervous system (CNS) vasculitis is an inflammatory vasculitis restricted to the CNS. A diagnosis of primary CNS vasculitis excludes involvement of the cerebral blood vessels in systemic large, medium, and small vessel vasculitides, of which the list is long and not covered herein.

A series of patients reported by Sundaram et al. (2002) draws attention to an esoteric but underdiagnosed condition. A diagnosis of primary CNS vasculitis is often overlooked or not considered on account of its nonspecific features and also because the tools to conform the diagnosis are not easily accessible. The authors report a series of 45 patients diagnosed with primary CNS vasculitis at a single center. The presentations were with stroke (predominantly occlusive but also hemorrhagic), headache, and seizures. Of course, these presentations are nonspecific and hence, a high index of diagnostic suspicion is required to consider the diagnosis. The strokes are often multiple and occur in different vascular territories. Headaches are often of the thunderclap type, i.e., begin and peak within seconds. Some patients present with stepwise progression of cognitive deficits. This presentation was noted in 11% in the current series. There are many atypical manifestations and these are captured by this relatively large series: Presentation with a mass lesion and myelopathy. The condition usually affects people above 50 years of age and in this regard the series differs as the median age at diagnosis was in the 30s.

Magnetic resonance angiography is often performed in patients presenting with ischemic and hemorrhagic stroke and thunderclap headaches but it may or may not raise suspicion of the diagnosis. Focal constrictions at multiple sites might raise consideration of the diagnosis. The utility of novel magnetic resonance imaging technique and known and cerebral blood vessel wall imaging in raising suspicion of the diagnosis is patently brought about by this report. The imaging might reveal focal vessel wall thickening and enhancement.

The gold standards for establishing a diagnosis of primary CNS vasculitis are either a digital subtraction angiography (DSA) or meningeal biopsy. In the reported series, both DSA and meningeal biopsy confirmed the diagnoses in nearly two-third of the cases and in many cases independent of each. Hence, there were some cases in which the DSA was abnormal and others in which the DSA was normal but the meningeal biopsy clinched the diagnosis.

A number of conditions need to be considered in the differential diagnosis; reversible cerebral vasoconstriction, a condition presenting with thunderclap headaches and is related often to the use of several medications, is foremost among the differential diagnosis. The treatment comprises corticosteroid and cyclophosphamide administration and the good response to this treatment emphasizes the need to suspect the condition more often in clinical practice.

Key Messages

- *Primary CNS vasculitis is an underdiagnosed condition on account of its nonspecific manifestations and difficulties in establishing the diagnosis.*
- *The diagnosis is established either by DSA or meningeal biopsy.*
- *It is crucial to suspect the diagnosis because the treatment strategy comprises corticosteroids and cyclophosphamide, quite distinct from the usual treatment of stroke.*

ARTICLE 13

Scrub typhus-associated opsoclonus: clinical course and longitudinal outcomes in an Indian cohort

Ralph R, Prabhakar AT, Sathyendra S, Carey R, Jude J, Varghese GM. Scrub typhus-associated opsoclonus: clinical course and longitudinal outcomes in an Indian Cohort.
Ann Indian Acad Neurol. 2019;22:153-8.

Abstract

Context: Opsoclonus, a rare neurological manifestation in scrub typhus, causes significant distress and disability. There is a paucity of clinical data and outcomes in these patients.

Aim: This study aims to describe the clinical and laboratory profile and longitudinal outcomes in a scrub typhus patient cohort with opsoclonus.

Settings and designs: This retrospective study was conducted in a 2,700-bed teaching hospital in South India, in scrub typhus patients with opsoclonus over a 5-year period.

Patients and methods: Clinical, laboratory, and radiological data and outcomes at discharge and 6- and 12-weeks postdischarge were documented.

Results: Of 1,650 scrub typhus patients, 18 had opsoclonus. About 17 had opsoclonus at presentation, while one patient developed opsoclonus on the 5th admission day, 1-day post-defervescence. Opsoclonus was first noted after a median interval of 11 (7–18) days from fever onset. It was associated with myoclonus in 94% (17/18), cerebellar dysfunction in 67% (12/18), extrapyramidal symptoms (EPS) in 33% (6/18), and aseptic meningitis in 17% (3/18) patients. Mean cerebrospinal fluid (CSF) white blood cell (WBC) count was 9 ± 2.7 cells/mm^3, with mean CSF protein 118.5 ± 53.9 mg% and mean CSF glucose 97 ± 13 mg% in 1l/15 patients. Brain magnetic resonance imaging was unremarkable in 75% (9/12). Case-fatality rate was 5.5% (1/18). Complete resolution of the index neurological syndrome occurred at 12-week postdischarge.

Conclusion: Opsoclonus is a rare neurological manifestation in scrub typhus, usually occurring in association with myoclonus, cerebellar dysfunction, or EPS. It appears to occur during the resolving febrile phase, with neurological deficits completely resolving at 12 weeks.

"The neurology of scrub typhus: Must know for all physicians."

COMMENT

Scrub typhus is a tick-borne infectious disorder characterized mostly by a nonspecific febrile illness but also by multisystemic involvement including renal, hepatic, hematological, and pulmonary systems. The multisystem involvement is on account of an immune-mediated endotheliitis. The organism responsible for the infection is *Orientia tsutsugamushi*.

Neurological manifestations occur but are not well described so far (**Table 1**). Meningitis and encephalitis are the most common neurological manifestations. Prabhakar et al. (2020), report a rare but characteristic neurological manifestation of scrub typhus. Opsoclonus myoclonus is a rare but characteristic manifestation of scrub typhus. It is a distinctive condition with rapid (shock-like), chaotic, multidirectional conjugate eye movements with asymmetric myoclonus of the limbs. These patients are often sick and many require assisted ventilation.

In the series of cases of opsoclonus myoclonus numbering 18 out of 1,650 patients with scrub typhus admitted to Christian Medical College, Vellore, Prabhakar et al. draw our attention to this rare but distinctive manifestation of the infectious disorder. In most patients, the neurological illness began on or after day 10 of fever. These patients were treated with doxycycline and corticosteroids

TABLE 1: Neurological manifestations of scrub typhus.

Systems	Manifestations
Central nervous system manifestations	• Encephalitis • Meningitis • Opsoclonus myoclonus
Peripheral nervous system manifestations	• Guillain–Barré syndrome • Brachial neuritis • Mononeuritis • Myositis

and the neurological condition remitted in all patients by week 12.

Opsoclonus myoclonus is associated with a variety of etiological conditions, most often infectious and paraneoplastic disorders. It is important that these disorders be ruled out before attributing the condition to scrub typhus. Nonetheless, this report adds to the list of neurological manifestations of scrub typhus. All physicians in susceptible geographical areas should be aware of these common and uncommon manifestations.

Key Messages

◉ *Opsoclonus myoclonus is a rare but characteristic condition characterized by chaotic conjugate shock-like movements of the eyes and limb myoclonus.*

◉ *Among the varied etiologies, paraneoplastic disorders and viral infections are common.*

◉ *Scrub typhus should be added to the list of infective etiologies of opsoclonus myoclonus.*

ARTICLE 14

Acute migraine therapy with external trigeminal neurostimulation (ACME): a randomized controlled trial

Chou DE, Shnayderman Yugrakh M, Winegarner D, Rowe V, Kuruvilla D, Schoenen J. Acute migraine therapy with external trigeminal neurostimulation (ACME): a randomized controlled trial.
Cephalalgia. 2019;39:3-14.

Abstract*

Objective: This study aimed at evaluating the safety and efficacy of external trigeminal nerve stimulation for acute pain relief during migraine attacks with or without aura through a sham-controlled trial.

Methods: This double-blind, randomized, sham-controlled study was carried out at three headache centers in the US. Study population included adult patients with an acute migraine attack with or without aura; the recruitment of participants was done on site and they were randomized 1:1 to receive either verum or sham external trigeminal nerve stimulation treatment (CEFALY Technology) for 1 hour. Visual analog scale (VAS) (0 = no pain to 10 = maximum pain) was used for measuring pain intensity. The primary outcome measure in the study was the mean change in pain intensity at 1 hour as compared with the baseline.

Results: In the duration of February 1, 2016 to March 31, 2017, screening of 109 participants was done. Among these, 106 patients were randomized and enrolled in the intention-to-treat analysis (verum, n = 52; sham, n = 54). As compared to the sham group, there was a significant reduction in primary outcome measure in the verum group [3.46 ± 2.32 vs. −1.78 ± 1.89 (p < 0.0001), or −59% vs. −30% (p < 0.0001)]. In terms of migraine subgroups, a significant difference was noted between verum and sham for "migraine without aura" attacks (mean VAS reduction at 1 hour: Verum group vs. sham group, −3.3 ± 2.4 vs. −1.7 ± 1.9, p = 0.0006). In case of "migraine with aura" attacks, there was higher pain reduction in verum than sham;

however, not statistically significant (mean VAS reduction at 1 hour: Verum group vs. sham group, -4.3 ± 1.8 vs. -2.6 ± 1.9, p = 0.060).

There were no serious adverse events in the participants; in the verum group, five minor adverse events were noted.

Conclusion: For the treatment of migraine attacks, 1 hour treatment with external trigeminal nerve stimulation caused significant relief in headache pain relief in comparison to sham stimulation, it was well-tolerated also. This indicates that 1 hour treatment with external trigeminal nerve stimulation can be a safe as well as effective acute treatment for migraine attacks. *Redrafted abstract

"The life so short, the craft so long to learn."

—Hippocrates

COMMENT

Currently available acute migraine treatments are mainly pharmacologic therapies comprising analgesics and "migraine-specific' drugs such as ergots and triptans. But these medications are not totally efficacious and have several side effects and contraindications. Moreover, many patients go on to consuming them excessively sometimes resulting in medication overuse headache.

External trigeminal nerve stimulation has been shown in the past to be effective for sedation and in the prevention of episodic migraine. It has also been shown in the past to have good tolerability and patient satisfaction.

The acute migraine therapy with external trigeminal neurostimulation (eTNS) (ACME) study is a randomized controlled trial based on the above findings in previous studies. It was prospective, double-blind, randomized, sham-controlled clinical trial done on adults aged between 18 and 65 years. The eTNS session was for 1 hour. The device used was the Cefaly device (CEFALY Technology, Belgium). The pulse frequency used was 100 Hz and pulse width 250 µs.

The intensity of the stimulation increases linearly to reach a maximum of 16 mA after 14 minutes and then remains constant for 46 minutes. The transcutaneous stimulation was via a supraorbital bipolar self-adhesive electrode placed on the forehead designed to excite the supratrochlear and supraorbital nerves.

The mean change in pain score at 1 hour was significantly decreased in the treated group (p < 0.0001). The pain reduction was also significant at 2 hour and 24 hour time periods. The efficacy results were more robust than prior studies which used shorter eTNS sessions (20 and 30 minutes).

Limitations of the study: Small sample size (52 and 54 in the two arms) and the execution of the study in a clinic setting. These need to be verified with a better plan and executed in the "real-world" context. It also remains to be seen if it would be effective in a domestic setting. A good aspect was that there were no severe SAEs. Moreover, a direct comparison would also be necessary between pharmacotherapy and eTNS.

Key Message

⊙ *Pharmacotherapy continues to be the primary choice for treatment of patients with an acute migraine attack. Although we now have a wider range of drugs including the newer drugs targeting the calcitonin gene-related peptide (CGRP) pathway, it is at times frustrating to manage patients who do not respond to these drugs or become intolerant to them.*

The availability of eTNS devices will be a welcome addition to the arsenal we already have but which prove inadequate. In particular, such devices might be easily used by patients at home or office (if they have it handy) and can help reduce disability significantly.

ARTICLE 15

Parkinson's disease in intensive care unit: an observational study of frequencies, causes, and outcomes

Paul G, Paul BS, Gautam PL, Singh G, Kaushal S. Parkinson's Disease in Intensive Care Unit: An Observational Study of Frequencies, Causes, and Outcomes.
Ann Indian Acad Neurol. 2019;22:79-83.

Abstract

Objective: To analyze the frequency, causes, and outcomes of admission to the intensive care unit (ICU) among Parkinson's disease (PD) population so that preventive measures can be developed.

Methods: We prospectively observed patients with diagnosis of PD admitted to ICU from January, 2014 to December, 2016. Based on etiology for hospital admission, they were divided into two groups—related to PD (further divided into direct or indirect) or not associated with PD at all. Etiology for hospitalization was determined from history and investigational data. The primary outcome was death or discharge from the hospital. Factors contributing to ICU admission were analyzed by comparing these patients with a cohort of 50 PD patients admitted to the neurology ward during the same study period. All values were expressed as mean (standard deviation) and percentages using SPSS version 16.0.

Results: Fifty-three (36%) out of a total of 146 patients required ICU admission. Most common causes leading to admission in decreasing order of frequency were fever (34%), delirium (16%), falls (12%), encephalopathy (8%), gastrointestinal emergencies (6%); while direct disease-related severe dyskinesias were seen only in two patients (4%). About 13.7% needed mechanical ventilation and mean duration of ventilation was 5.94 days with mortality rate of 20%. Significant factors predicting ICU admission, and thus, poor outcomes were age >65 years, history of previous admission within the last 12 months, delirium, and hypoalbuminemia. There was no significant association between the incidence of ICU admission and duration of disease or severity of the disease.

Conclusion: Poor outcome in PD patients is due to systemic causes, hence multidisciplinary teamwork may improve outcome in these patients.

> *"Hope sees the invisible, feels the intangible, and achieves the impossible."*
>
> —Helen Keller

COMMENT

Parkinson's disease (PD) affects approximately 51.3–176.9/100,000 persons of all age groups in the Asian population with a predilection for the elderly. With increasing life expectancy worldwide, the incidence is increasing as well. As the disease advances, motor and nonmotor fluctuations, levodopa-induced dyskinesias, falls, psychiatric issues, infections and complications of immobility set in and are causes of considerable morbidity and at times mortality.

Hospitalization and the need for institutional care are reported to be 1.5 times higher than the general population. Since it is a disease primarily of the elderly, comorbidities play a role too in the need for intensive care.

The authors have conducted a prospective observational study in a tertiary care teaching hospital in Northern India over a 3-year period. They have classified patients who needed intensive care unit (ICU) admission into two broad categories: (i) Those due to PD per se and (ii) Those due to comorbidities.

Category (i) included those directly related to PD such as motor complications, severe motor fluctuations, and dyskinesias as well as indirect causes (but contributed largely by PD) such as falls, delirium, infections, aspiration pneumonia, severe gastrointestinal tract (GIT) disturbance, and electrolyte disturbances.

The salient features of the results of the study are:

- Most patients requiring ICU care were in H&Y stage 2 or 3 (82%).
- The mean duration of PD was 4.9 + or – 2.89 years, meaning that it did not occur only after prolonged disease.
- Parkinson's disease was diagnosed de novo in 4%.
- Eight percent had history of previous hospitalization.
- Eighty percent had PD-related causes—of these, 95% had indirect causes, the most common being fever and delirium.
- About 42% had comorbid conditions—diabetes mellitus, hypertension, coronary artery disease being the common ones.
- Mortality rate among the PD patients in ICU was 20%.
- The statistically significant factors that predicted ICU admission were age, history of previous hospitalization, delirium, and hypoalbuminemia.
- The most common cause of ICU admission was infections—lung infections followed by urinary tract infections.
- Twelve percent of patients were admitted with trauma causing head injury or limb fractures.

Key Messages

It is very important to remember and also inform patients and caregivers that:

⊙ *Patients with PD are more likely to have serious complications related to the disease itself.*

⊙ *The immobility and poor swallowing reflex can predispose to aspiration pneumonitis*

⊙ *The impairment of sphincter relaxation can lead to urinary tract infections, which are often mistaken to be due to an enlarged prostate in the elderly.*

⊙ *Trauma is very likely due to postural instability, dyskinesias and motor fluctuations including freezing of gait.*

⊙ *These complications can occur as early as 4 years after onset and can occur in H&Y stage 2 itself.*

It is important to diagnose PD early so the patients can be started on symptomatic treatment early to avoid serious complications such as falls and infections.

Proper attention to nutrition and exercises are important aspects of management of PD patients.

ARTICLE 16

Association of serum levels of calcitonin gene-related peptide and cytokines during migraine attacks

Han D. Association of serum levels of calcitonin gene-related peptide and cytokines during migraine attacks. *Ann Indian Acad Neurol. 2019;22:277-81.*

Abstract

Background: During a migraine attack, trigeminal activation results in the release of calcitonin gene-related peptide (CGRP), which stimulates the release of inflammatory cytokines playing an important role in migraine.

Objective: We analyze the relation between CGRP and cytokines during attacks to explore the possible mechanism of migraine.

Materials and methods: Migraine patients and healthy control were recruited at the Department of Neurology, the Sixth People's Hospital of Fuyang City, between March, 2018 and July, 2018. The protein levels of interleukin (IL)-1β, IL-2, IL-6, IL-10, tumor necrosis factor-alpha (TNF-α), and CGRP were determined from the sera of patients with migraine and control subjects by enzyme-linked immunosorbent assay kits. Spearman's rank correlation coefficient was also determined to calculate the correlation between CGRP and inflammatory factors levels.

Results: The level of IL-1β, IL-6, TNF-α, and CGRP in migraine group were significantly higher than normal group ($p < 0.05$). The level of CGRP was significantly correlated with IL-1 β ($r = 0.30$, $p < 0.05$) and IL-6 ($r = 0.94$, $p < 0.05$), but not significantly correlated with IL-2 ($r = -0.047$, $p = 0.75$), IL-10 ($r = 0.12$, $p = 0.43$), and TNF-α ($r = 0.05$, $p = 0.72$).

Conclusion: In our study, we found migraine patients had a higher IL-6, IL-1β, and TNF level than healthy controls and the level of CGRP was related significantly with the level of IL-1β and IL-6. In conclusion, our results suggest that IL-1β and IL-6 may be involved in the pathogenesis of migraine attacks and CGRP related with the secretion of cytokines.

"Symptoms are the body's mother tongue; signs are in a foreign language."

—**John Brown**

COMMENT

Migraine is considered a neuromuscular disorder whose mechanism remains unclear despite numerous studies and hypothesis. It is a major cause of disability and loss of manpower in the world. Many studies have favored the trigeminal neurovascular reflex theory which believed that the migraine is due to neurogenic inflammation induced by vasoactive peptides released by the peripheral nerves. During an attack of migraine, trigeminal activation occurs which in turn results in the release of calcitonin gene-related peptide (CGRP). The CGRP induces neurogenic inflammation and leptomeningeal vasodilation giving rise to the typical pain of migraine.

■ CALCITONIN GENE-RELATED PEPTIDE AND CYTOKINES IN ACUTE MIGRAINE

More than 50% of trigeminal neutrons produce CGRP. CGRP release has been shown to occur after stimulation of the gasserian ganglion. During an acute attack of migraine, CGRP levels are elevated in the cranial circulation and triptans have been shown to reverse this elevation in CGRP levels. Calcitonin gene-related peptide induces the release of inflammatory cytokines such as tumor necrosis factor-alpha (TNF-α), interleukin (IL)-1β, and IL-6 from human lymphocytes in vitro studies. Hence, it is possible that pain is related to these molecules.

The authors have done a case–control study analyzing jugular venous blood samples obtained within 2 hours from the onset of the migraine and compared with healthy controls. The levels of IL-1β, IL-6, TNF-α, and CGRP were found to be significantly elevated in the group with migraine (irrespective of whether it was with or without aura). They have postulated that the pain is related to the release of CGRP and its ability to induce cytokine secretion from white cells, platelets, and endothelium. They further suggest that IL-1β and IL-6 may be involved in the pathogenesis of migraine attacks and CGRP in the secretion of the cytokines.

Key Message

⊙ *Calcitonin gene-related peptide antagonists are now available for treatment of acute attacks. The findings and hypothesis proposed in this study, if proven by a larger study, may lead to the development of treatment aimed at reducing the impact of the cytokines as they could be the final pathway mediating the pain in acute attacks of migraine.*

ARTICLE 17

Randomized delayed-start trial of levodopa in Parkinson's disease

Verschuur CVM, Suwijn SR, Boel JA, Post B, Bloem BR, van Hilten JJ, et al. Randomized Delayed-Start Trial of Levodopa in Parkinson's Disease.
N Engl J Med. 2019;380:315-24.

Abstract*

Background: Levodopa, the primary drug for treatment·of symptoms of Parkinson's disease, may also has a disease-modifying effect. This effect of levodopa, if proven, will allow us to modify its time of introduction in the treatment plan during the course of disease.

Methods: A multicenter, double-blind, placebo-controlled, delayed-start trial, was conducted on 445 patients of early Parkinson's disease. They were randomly assigned one of the two groups: One group received levodopa (100 mg three times per day) and carbidopa (25 mg three times per day) for 80 weeks (early-start group), and the other group received placebo for 40 weeks followed by levodopa and carbidopa for 40 weeks (delayed-start group). The difference between the mean change in the total score on the UPDRS (Unified Parkinson's disease rating scale), taken from baseline to week 80 of both the groups, was taken as the primary outcome. Progression of symptoms, as measured by the UPDRS score, between weeks 4 and 40 and the noninferiority of early initiation of treatment to delayed initiation between weeks 44 and 80, with a noninferiority margin of 0.055 points per week, were also analyzed.

Results: A total of 222 and 223 patients were assigned early-start group and delayed-start group, respectively. In the early-start group, the mean ($\pm$SD) UPDRS score at baseline was 28.1 ± 11.4 points and, the change in score from baseline to week 80 was -1.0 ± 13.1 points. In the delayed-start group, the scores were 29.3 ± 12.1 points, and -2.0 ± 13.0 points, respectively. No significant between-group difference at week 80 was observed [difference 1.0 point; 95% confidence interval (CI) -1.5–3.5; p = 0.44] implying that levodopa had no disease-modifying effect. The rate of progression of symptoms, as measured in UPDRS points per week, between weeks 4 and 40, was 0.04 ± 0.23 in the early-start group and 0.06 ± 0.34 in the delayed-start group (difference -0.02; 95% CI -0.07–0.03). Between 44 and 80 weeks, the corresponding rates were 0.10 ± 0.25 and 0.03 ± 0.28 (difference 0.07; two-sided 90% CI 0.03–0.10). The difference in the rate of progression between weeks 44 and 80 did not meet the criterion for noninferiority of early receipt of levodopa to delayed receipt. Also, no significant difference between the rates of dyskinesia and levodopa-related fluctuations in motor response was observed between the two groups.

Conclusion: Treatment with levodopa and carbidopa did not show any disease-modifying effect in early Parkinson's disease evaluated over 80 weeks. (Funded by the Netherlands Organization for Health Research and Development and others; LEAP Current Controlled Trials number, ISRCTN30518857.) *Redrafted abstract

"Does levodopa have disease-modifying effect if given early in Parkinson's disease?"

COMMENT

Parkinson's disease is a degenerative disease caused by a deficiency of dopamine in the basal ganglia. It is now becoming known that there are other neurotransmitters implicated in the pathogenesis of some of the manifestations of the disease. The mainstay of treatment of Parkinson's disease is levodopa. The other options include dopamine agonists, anticholinergics, monoamine oxidase-B (MAO-B) inhibitors, catechol-o-methyl transferase (COMT) inhibitors, and amantadine.

The motor complications due to levodopa are often held against the early usage of the drug in the disease. Of late, studies have shown that this levodopa phobia among prescribers needs to be given up as the motor complications especially dyskinesias appear to be better correlated with the duration of the disease than the duration of levodopa therapy. It should be remembered that levodopa is the gold standard of treatment of Parkinson's disease and all patients with Parkinson's disease would require it at some stage, preferably early. The time lost and hence the impairment in quality of life due to avoidance of levodopa far outweighs the erstwhile supposed benefit obtained by means of delaying dyskinesias and motor complications due to it. Today, the nonmotor symptoms of Parkinson's disease is a hot topic and much work is going on to identify and manage them as they contribute to significant disability by themselves.

For long there has been a debate about whether levodopa given early in the disease is toxic or protective. There have been suggestions that it could be toxic too but not proven.

The *LEAP* study was a multicentric, randomized delayed-start trial of levodopa in patients who had not been started on any therapy for the Parkinson's disease. There were two arms of the study: One had an early start and was followed up for 80 weeks while the other received a placebo for 40 weeks and then levodopa (with carbidopa) for 40 weeks. The patients were evaluated with the UPDRS (Unified Parkinson's disease rating scale) score at baseline and at 80 weeks. At the end of 80 weeks, the UPDRS score did not a statistically significant difference in score implying that levodopa had no disease-modifying effect. However, the rate of progression of the symptoms between weeks 4 and 40 was higher in the delayed-start group with a p-value of 0.02, whereas, the corresponding rates between weeks 44 and 80 did not show much difference. There was also no significant difference in rates of dyskinesia and levodopa-related fluctuations between the two groups.

Key Messages

So what do we learn from this study and how is it likely impact our prescription pattern while managing patients with Parkinson's disease? The key messages from the study are:

- *Starting levodopa early does not have any disease-modifying effect on Parkinson's disease.*
- *Starting levodopa (whenever it is started) helps in decreasing the symptoms of the disease.*
- *There was no advantage with respect to delaying of dyskinesias or fluctuations by delaying the start of levodopa.*

Hence, the key message is that levodopa can be started early in the course of Parkinson's disease for good symptomatic benefit (and thereby improvement in quality of life) but do not expect a disease-modifying effect.

A quick guide to treatment initiation can hence be:

- *At any age—start with levodopa with carbidopa or benserazide—start low and go slow.*
- *Tremor-predominant subtype—may be started on anticholinergics, except in the more elderly.*
- *If levodopa-intolerant—other drugs like dopamine agonists.*

ARTICLE 18

Association of statin use with Parkinson's disease: dose-response relationship

Jeong SM, Jang W, Shin DW. Association of statin use with Parkinson's disease: dose-response relationship. *Mov Disord. 2019;34:1014-21.*

Abstract

Background: There have been conflicting results on the association between statin use and Parkinson's disease (PD) incidence.

Objectives: This study investigated the association between time-varying status of statin use and incidence of PD while considering the dose-response relationship and total cholesterol level.

Methods: Using the database of the Korean National Health Insurance Service from 2002 to 2015, we examined 76,043 subjects (≥60 years old) free of PD, dementia, and stroke at baseline. The dose of statin use was classified into the following four 6-month categories (<180, 180–365, 365–540, and ≥540 days) for each 2-year interval. The incidence of PD was identified by the prescription records for any anti-PD medication with a diagnosis of PD.

Results: During 10 years of follow-up, 1,427 PD cases occurred. Statin "ever use" was significantly associated with a high risk of PD incidence (adjusted hazard ratio 1.28; 95% confidence interval 1.12–1.46) when compared with statin nonuse. In terms of a dose-response relationship, although a duration of statin use <365 days was associated with a higher risk of PD, the duration of statin use ≥365 days was not significantly associated with an increased risk of PD.

Conclusion: Statin use was associated with an elevated risk of PD, but long-term and adherent statin use was not significantly associated with elevated PD risk. However, there was no evidence of benefit with any statin treatment related to PD risk. Our study suggests that there is a complex relationship among cholesterol level, statin use, and PD risk that warrants further studies. © 2019 International Parkinson and Movement Disorder Society.

"Statins and Parkinson's disease—dose-response relationship."

COMMENT

The relationship between statin use and the incidence of Parkinson's disease (PD) has always been tenuous with studies reporting all types of associations—increase, decrease or neutral effect of statins on PD.

This often befuddles the physician since statins are very commonly used in practice to decrease cardiovascular morbidity.

Parkinson's disease has many underlying mechanisms of neurodegeneration such as free radicals, mitochondrial dysfunction, excitotoxicity, neuroinflammation, and the autophagy-lysosomal pathway. All these lead to the final common pathway of accumulation of toxic and misfolded proteins. Based on this, many neuroprotective candidates such as coenzyme Q10, calcitriol, erythropoietin, and statins have been reported to have neuroprotective effects in PD.

Statins competitively inhibit 3-hydroxy-3-methylglutaryl coenzyme A (HMG-CoA) and reduce plasma cholesterol levels. In addition, they have been demonstrated to have anti-inflammatory effect, apoptosis regulation, reduction of oxidative damage, and autophagy modulation. This has led to the hypothesis that statins are neuroprotective against neurodegenerative diseases. Statins also decrease the α-synuclein burden and dopaminergic cell death in animal and cell models of PD. A clinical trial of simvastatin in PD is ongoing. A meta-analysis showed that statin use decreases PD risk but individual studies have shown varied results. There are different biases such as unadjusted cholesterol level, statin indication and immortal time bias which when adjusted for, nullified the protective effect.

The authors have done a retrospective analysis using the elderly cohort database in South Korea. They have assessed statin use in three ways: (1) Any use, (2) Cumulative duration of use, and (3) Cumulative dose of use. The incidence of PD was assessed from the usage of any anti-PD medication. The important results that they found were:

- Low cholesterol (<160 mg/dL) levels were associated with high PD incidence risk.
- Statin use at any time was significantly associated with a high risk.
- The cumulative duration of use showed an inverse J-shaped association with PD risk.
  - Cumulative duration <365 days was associated with a higher risk.
  - Durations of 365–540 days was associated with a decreased risk.
  - Durations >540 days similar to statin non-users.

In effect, the results were:

- A low cholesterol level was associated with an increased PD risk and when adjusted for initial cholesterol level and confounding factors, statin use significantly increased PD risk.
- With increasing duration and adherence, this risk disappeared.
- Statins and low cholesterol could increase PD risk.
- High cholesterol levels might attenuate the processes of neurodegeneration in PD. Cholesterol stabilizes lysosomal membranes and prevents lysosomal permeability which leads to cell death.
- Statin therapy which lowers low-density lipoprotein (LDL) to 70–130 mg/dL can increase PD risk.
- Statins could reduce coenzyme Q10, a neuroprotective agent.
- The risk of PD is increased in the short-term (probably also due to unmasking of early PD symptoms).
- Long-term usage was associated with a lower risk of PD incidence.

Key Messages

So, what should we do as physicians—use statins or not? The key messages for practice would be:

- ◉ *Statins should continue to be used.*
- ◉ *Caution may be exercised if the total cholesterol levels fall below 160 mg/dL.*
- ◉ *Signs of PD may appear in the short-term—this may be unmasking of early underlying PD.*
- ◉ *Continued adherence and long-term usage reduces the incidence of PD.*

Lastly, we must remember that this is a retrospective study and these findings need to be substantiated by a well-designed randomized controlled trial. Till then, let us use statins, but be aware of the association with PD.

ARTICLE 19

Refractory epilepsy and nonadherence to drug treatment

Henning O, Lossius MI, Lima M, Mevåg M, Villagran A, Nakken KO, et al. Refractory epilepsy and nonadherence to drug treatment.
Epilepsia Open. 2019;4:618-23.

Abstract*

Nonadherence to antiepileptic drug (AED) treatment can have serious implications in patients with refractory epilepsy, sometimes resulting in sudden death. This study was conducted to analyze the extent of intentional and unintentional nonadherence in Norwegian patients with refractory epilepsy and to identify the associated risk factors. An anonymous survey was done on 333 consecutive adult in- and out-patients of the National Centre for Epilepsy in Norway, having refractory epilepsy. While, 22% of them admitted that they sometimes or often forget taking drugs as prescribed, 19% reported that they, rarely, sometimes or often intentionally did not follow the agreed AED treatment plan. Young age and depression were observed to be the two most common reasons for unintentional nonadherence. Intentional nonadherence was most commonly associated with young age (36 years or younger). In conclusion, about 20% of the patients with refractory epilepsy showed nonadherence to the agreed drug treatment plan, either intentionally or unintentionally. To improve seizure control, measures should be taken to reduce the nonadherence among the patients. *Redrafted abstract

"Medication nonadherence in epilepsy: A costly affair!"

COMMENT

In no known chronic disorder in humans is medication adherence more rigorously required than in epilepsy, a disorder defined by an enduring predisposition to recurrent seizures. Most chronic disorders such as hypertension and diabetes are beleaguered by poor medication adherence. In epilepsy, however, missing just a single dose of the prescribed antiepileptic medication can lead to seizures and even sudden unexpected death in epilepsy (SUDEP).

Henning et al. (2019) report the results of a cross-sectional anonymous survey on medication adherence among people with drug-resistant epilepsy. The latter is a special group among all people with epilepsy because they have very frequent seizures and are often on complex regimens comprising several different antiepileptic drugs (AEDs) to be taken multiple times in a day. Medication adherence is to be all the more strictly followed in people with drug-resistant epilepsy to ensure good seizure control but on the contrary, adherence is rather poor in this group of people. Henning et al. report that nearly 20% of their patient population admitted to medication nonadherence. To our mind this just represents the tip of the iceberg. Medication nonadherence is perhaps much more common, only not recognized by people using these medications. Indeed, people with epilepsy are often unaware that they have missed their medications. They simply loose count of the medications they are taking.

Medication nonadherence is classified as intentional and nonintentional. The later, i.e., nonintentional nonadherence was far more common among the respondents. The other, i.e., intentional nonadherence is, however, more serious. It requires considerable efforts on the part of healthcare providers to counsel intentional nonadherers and bring about a change in their attitudes. Two questions from the care provider might help in identifying intentional nonadherence:

1. When you feel fine (i.e., your seizures are controlled), do you often stop or miss your medications?
2. Do you miss or stop your medications when you have side-effects?

It is imperative that medication adherence should be discussed in ample detail during follow-up visits. The clinician should try to obtain an insight regarding the underpinnings of nonadherence and should emphasize the importance of methods to improve adherence. This applies to a number of chronic medical conditions but most of all to epilepsy.

Key Messages

⊙ *Medication adherence is the key to successful treatment of a number of chronic disorders including epilepsy.*

⊙ *Medication nonadherence is common in epilepsy and occurs in nearly 20% cases of drug-resistant epilepsy.*

⊙ *Medication nonadherence can be either intentional or nonintentional.*

ARTICLE 20

Placebo-controlled trial of an oral BTK inhibitor in multiple sclerosis

Montalban X, Arnold DL, Weber MS, Staikov I, Piasecka-Stryczynska K, Willmer J, et al. Placebo-Controlled Trial of an Oral BTK Inhibitor in Multiple Sclerosis.
N Engl J Med. 2019;380:2406-17.

Abstract*

Background: The recognition of the role of B cell in pathogenesis of multiple sclerosis has led to the development of Bruton's tyrosine kinase (BTK) inhibitors for therapeutic purpose. Evobrutinib, a selective oral BTK inhibitor inhibits B-cell activation by acting on B-cell receptor signaling pathway.

Methods: In a double-blind phase 2 trial, patients with relapsing multiple sclerosis were randomly assigned to five groups: Placebo, evobrutinib 25 mg, 75 mg once-daily, 75 mg twice-daily, and open-label of dimethyl fumarate (DMF). T1-weighted magnetic resonance imaging done at 12, 16, 20, and 24 weeks identified gadolinium-enhancing lesions and their total (cumulative) number was taken as primary endpoint. The annualized relapse rate and change in EDSS (Expanded Disability Status Scale) scores were the key secondary endpoints.

Results: A total of 267 patients were randomly assigned to one of the trial groups. The mean ($\pm$SD) total number of gadolinium-enhancing lesions during weeks 12 through 24 was 3.85 $\pm$ 5.44 in the placebo group, 4.06 $\pm$ 8.02 in the evobrutinib 25-mg group, 1.69 $\pm$ 4.69 in the evobrutinib 75-mg once-daily group, 1.15 $\pm$ 3.70 in the evobrutinib 75-mg twice-daily group, and 4.78 $\pm$ 22.05 in the DMF group. The total number of lesions over time were 1.45 in the evobrutinib 25-mg group (p = 0.32), 0.30 in the evobrutinib 75-mg once-daily group (p = 0.005), and 0.44 in the evobrutinib 75-mg twice-daily group (p = 0.06), after baseline adjustment of rate ratios. The unadjusted annualized relapse rate at week 24 was 0.37 in the placebo group, 0.57 in the evobrutinib 25-mg group, 0.13 in the evobrutinib 75-mg once-daily group, 0.08 in the evobrutinib 75-mg twice-daily group, and 0.20 in the DMF group. There was no significant effect of trial group on the no change from baseline in the EDSS score was observed across the trial groups. Use of evobrutinib was associated with elevations in liver aminotransferase levels.

Conclusion: There were fewer enhancing lesions in 75 mg of evobrutinib once daily group during 12–24 weeks as compared to placebo. No significant difference was noted with placebo for either the 25-mg once-daily or 75-mg twice-daily dose of evobrutinib. Similarly, the annualized relapse rate and disability progression at any dose were not significantly associated with trial groups. To establish the efficacy and safety profile, larger trials and of longer duration are needed. (Funded by EMD Serono; ClinicalTrials.gov number, NCT02975349.) *Redrafted abstract

"New, newer and more newer medications for multiple sclerosis."

COMMENT

Multiple sclerosis is the prototype demyelinating disorder of the central nervous system with neurological relapses and remissions, eventually evolving to a secondary progressive stage. The goals of treatment are to improve the chances of complete remission following a relapse and prevention of further relapses. The former is mostly well-achieved with the use of corticosteroids. The prevention of relapses and eventually evolution to a secondary progressive stage with considerable irreversible neurological disability is an area of considerable research. Several agents have now been evaluated and approved for the prevention of relapses, i.e., as disease-modifying treatments. The question for newer agents, however, continues—and for several reasons. One reason is that none of agents approved thus far are completely efficacious in preventing relapses. The efficacy varies from 33% for some of the interferons to nearly 70% for Tysabri. Several other immunological agents are available between the efficacy spectrum of interferons and Tysabri. To name a few—teriflunomide, DMF, and fingolimod. None is perfect, though and many are associated with serious adverse effects, often life-threatening. Hence, there is an unmet need for developing and evaluating newer agents.

Most agents rely on either B-cell or T-cell mechanisms to prevent relapses and maintain remission in multiple sclerosis. Bruton's tyrosine kinase (BTK) is a chemical agent involved in B-cell signaling through specified receptors. It is involved in the pathogenesis of several immunological disorders including rheumatoid arthritis, systemic lupus erythematosus, and multiple sclerosis. BTK inhibitors are being evaluated in a number of immunological disorders.

Montalban et al. reported the results of a placebo-controlled trial of evobrutinib, an oral BTK inhibitor in relapsing-remitting multiple sclerosis. The results of the trial were only modestly encouraging. While the number of demyelinating lesions on magnetic resonance imaging decreased with treatment with certain dosing schedules of evobrutinib, the agent did not seem to significantly alter the annualized relapse rate in comparison to placebo or another active comparator drug. Moreover, they were serious adverse effects, notably an increase in liver aminotransferases.

While the results of the evobrutinib trial are not really very encouraging, the need for developing more agents is underscored. There is an immense need to evaluate agents with greater efficacy and lesser side-effects than the currently available disease-modifying agents. The quest continues...........

Key Messages

⊙ *Disease-modifying agents are the mainstay to prevent relapses and disease progression in relapsing-remitting multiple sclerosis.*

⊙ *An oral BTK inhibitor was found to be modestly efficacious in the treatment if relapsing-remitting multiple sclerosis.*

⊙ *The pursuit of newer disease-modifying agents for multiple sclerosis is justified because none available is totally efficacious and most have serious adverse effects.*

Section Editor: Rohini Handa

Associate Editors: Aman Sharma, Durga Prasanna Misra

ARTICLE 1

How the weather affects the pain of citizen scientists using a smartphone app

Dixon WG, Beukenhorst AL, Yimer BB, Cook L, Gasparrini A, El-Hay T, et al. How the weather affects the pain of citizen scientists using a smartphone app.
NPJ Digit Med. 2019;2:105.

Abstract

Patients with chronic pain commonly believe their pain is related to the weather. Scientific evidence to support their beliefs is inconclusive, in part due to difficulties in getting a large dataset of patients frequently recording their pain symptoms during a variety of weather conditions. Smartphones allow the opportunity to collect data to overcome these difficulties. Our study *"Cloudy with a Chance of Pain"* analyzed daily data from 2,658 patients collected over a 15-month period. The analysis demonstrated significant yet modest relationships between pain and relative humidity, pressure and wind speed, with correlations remaining even when accounting for mood and physical activity. This research highlights how citizen–science experiments can collect large datasets on real-world populations to address long-standing health questions. These results will act as a starting point for a future system for patients to better manage their health through pain forecasts.

"Emerging evidence links changes in weather pattern to pain."

COMMENT

Patients with rheumatic diseases commonly report that several environmental factors influence their pain. Dietary factors and climatic conditions top the list. Patients do subscribe to the belief that cold, damp conditions or changes in barometric pressure can exacerbate pain, stiffness, and swelling of their joints. Physicians who deal with chronic painful conditions, including rheumatologists, will attest to observations from patients that their pain varies with changes in weather patterns. However, objective validation of these subjective observations was lacking. A recent observational cohort evaluated more than 2,500 individuals with chronic painful conditions from the United Kingdom, whose pain and functionality were assessed daily using a dedicated smartphone application and linked with meteorological data regarding temperature, barometric pressure, humidity and wind speed at their geographic location. The study observed increased pain with increase in wind speed or humidity and decrease in barometric pressure. This study provides the first large-scale validation of the influences of weather patterns on chronic painful conditions. Another notable feature is the demonstration of the feasibility of using real-life data from smartphone applications to answer scientific questions regarding dynamic daily occurences.[1] Another cross-sectional study with >2,300 participants from different European nations also revealed a significant association of environmental temperature and relative humidity with physical activity in patients with osteoarthritis.[2] Smaller scale studies have identified worsening of fibromyalgia pain with decrease in barometric pressure and increase in humidity.[3] Other rheumatic diseases such as Raynaud's phenomenon, seen in association with diseases such as systemic sclerosis or mixed connective tissue disease, are known to worsen with colder weather.[4] Physicians require to be aware of environmental influences on severity of the symptomatology of rheumatic diseases to enable them to adequately counsel patients regarding the same. This study also brings to the forefront the concept of "citizen science", which alludes to the public participation and collaboration in scientific research to augment scientific knowledge. Through citizen science, patients can proactively contribute to data monitoring and collection programs, which in turn are likely to improve patient satisfaction by addressing issues that patients perceive as important.

Key Messages

- *Increases in relative humidity and decreases in atmospheric pressure may exacerbate chronic painful conditions.*
- *Patients should be counselled regarding potential worsening of pain during colder, windier days.*
- *Patients should be encouraged to partner in citizen science experiments.*

ARTICLE 2

Nintedanib for systemic sclerosis-associated interstitial lung disease

Distler O, Highland KB, Gahlemann M, Azuma A, Fischer A, Mayes MD, et al.; SENSCIS Trial Investigators. Nintedanib for systemic sclerosis-associated interstitial lung disease.
N Engl J Med. 2019;380:2518-28.

Abstract

Background: Interstitial lung disease (ILD) is a common manifestation of systemic sclerosis and a leading cause of systemic sclerosis-related death. Nintedanib, a tyrosine kinase inhibitor, has been shown to have antifibrotic and anti-inflammatory effects in preclinical models of systemic sclerosis and ILD.

Methods: We conducted a randomized, double-blind, placebo-controlled trial to investigate the efficacy and safety of nintedanib in patients with ILD associated with systemic sclerosis. Patients who had systemic sclerosis with an onset of the first non-Raynaud's symptom within the past 7 years and a high-resolution computed tomographic scan that showed fibrosis affecting at least 10% of the lungs were randomly assigned, in a 1:1 ratio, to receive 150 mg of nintedanib, administered orally twice daily, or placebo. The primary endpoint was the annual rate of decline in forced vital capacity (FVC), assessed over a 52-week period. Key secondary endpoints were absolute changes from baseline in the modified Rodnan skin score and in the total score on the St. George's Respiratory Questionnaire (SGRQ) at week 52.

Results: A total of 576 patients received at least one dose of nintedanib or placebo; 51.9% had diffuse cutaneous systemic sclerosis, and 48.4% were receiving mycophenolate at baseline. In the primary endpoint analysis, the adjusted annual rate of change in FVC was −52.4 mL per year in the nintedanib group and −93.3 mL per year in the placebo group [difference, 41.0 mL per year; 95% confidence interval

(CI), 2.9–79.0; p = 0.04]. Sensitivity analyses based on multiple imputation for missing data yielded p values for the primary endpoint ranging from 0.06 to 0.10. The change from baseline in the modified Rodnan skin score and the total score on the SGRQ at week 52 did not differ significantly between the trial groups, with differences of −0.21 (95% CI, −0.94 to 0.53; p = 0.58) and 1.69 [95% CI, −0.73 to 4.12 (not adjusted for multiple comparisons)], respectively. Diarrhea, the most common adverse event, was reported in 75.7% of the patients in the nintedanib group and in 31.6% of those in the placebo group.

Conclusion: Among patients with ILD associated with systemic sclerosis, the annual rate of decline in FVC was lower with nintedanib than with placebo; no clinical benefit of nintedanib was observed for other manifestations of systemic sclerosis. The adverse-event profile of nintedanib observed in this trial was similar to that observed in patients with idiopathic pulmonary fibrosis; gastrointestinal adverse events, including diarrhea, were more common with nintedanib than with placebo. (Funded by Boehringer Ingelheim; SENSCIS ClinicalTrials.gov number, NCT02597933.)

"Nintedanib may be useful for ILD associated with scleroderma."

COMMENT

Therapeutic options that modify the disease course of systemic sclerosis (SSc) are few. Even biologic disease-modifying antirheumatic drugs (DMARDs) have not consistently demonstrated a benefit in reducing interstitial lung disease (ILD) associated with SSc.[5] In a prior randomized controlled trial of 663 patients with idiopathic pulmonary fibrosis (IPF), a disease that has generally been proven to have very little effective medical therapy, patients receiving nintedanib showed reduction in decline in forced vital capacity (FVC) over 52 weeks compared to placebo-treated patients.[6] However, no add-on benefit to nintedanib could be demonstrated with sildenafil (a phosphodiesterase 5 inhibitor) in another controlled trial of patients with IPF.[7] The present study randomized 288 individuals each with SSc-related ILD (with area of lung involvement at least 10% on high-resolution computerized tomography) to receive nintedanib or placebo for 52 weeks, as add-on therapy. Patients receiving nintedanib had lesser decline in FVC over 1 year compared to placebo (41 mL more). Other SSc-related manifestations such as skin involvement were not significantly different between groups. Diarrhea with nintedanib was the significant dose-limiting side effect.[8] While this might appear a small improvement, in the context of disease-modifying therapies in SSc, this is a notable achievement and holds promise for further evaluation. Although a prespecified subgroup analysis showed lower FVC decline in the nintedanib arm irrespective of mycophenolate mofetil (MMF) use, the trial was not designed or powered to calculate the efficacy of nintedanib over and above background MMF. While assessing the effect of addition of antifibrotic therapy in SSc-ILD, the trial design adopted by Scleroderma Lung Study (SLS)-III seems more pragmatic. (https://clinicaltrials.gov/ct2/show/NCT03221257).

Key Messages

- *Definitively proven therapeutic modalities for SSc ILD are few.*
- *Nintedanib, an orally administered tyrosine kinase inhibitor, might prevent progression of interstitial lung disease associated with SSc.*

ARTICLE 3

Trial of anifrolumab in active systemic lupus erythematosus

Morand EF, Furie R, Tanaka Y, Bruce IN, Askanase AD, Richez C, et al.; TULIP-2 Trial Investigators. Trial of anifrolumab in active systemic lupus erythematosus.
N Engl J Med. 2020;382:211-21.

Abstract

Background: Anifrolumab, a human monoclonal antibody to type I interferon receptor subunit 1 investigated for the treatment of systemic lupus erythematosus (SLE), did not have a significant effect on the primary endpoint in a previous phase III trial. The current phase III trial used a secondary endpoint from that trial as the primary endpoint.

Methods: We randomly assigned patients in a 1:1 ratio to receive intravenous anifrolumab (300 mg) or placebo every 4 weeks for 48 weeks. The primary endpoint of this trial was a response at week 52 defined with the use of the British Isles Lupus Assessment Group (BILAG)-based Composite Lupus Assessment (BICLA). A BICLA response requires reduction in any moderate-to-severe baseline disease activity and no worsening in any of nine organ systems in the BILAG index, no worsening on the Systemic Lupus Erythematosus Disease Activity Index, no increase of 0.3 points or more in the score on the Physician Global Assessment of disease activity [on a scale from 0 (no disease activity) to 3 (severe disease)], no discontinuation of the trial intervention, and no use of medications restricted by the protocol. Secondary endpoints included a BICLA response in patients with a high interferon gene signature at baseline; reductions in the glucocorticoid dose, in the severity of skin disease, and in counts of swollen and tender joints; and the annualized flare rate.

Results: A total of 362 patients received the randomized intervention: 180 received anifrolumab and 182 received placebo. The percentage of patients who had a BICLA response was 47.8% in the anifrolumab group and 31.5% in the placebo group (difference, 16.3 percentage points; 95% confidence interval, 6.3–26.3; p = 0.001). Among patients with a high-interferon gene signature, the percentage with a response was 48.0% in the anifrolumab group and 30.7% in the placebo group; among patients with a low interferon gene signature, the percentage was 46.7% and 35.5%, respectively. Secondary endpoints with respect to the glucocorticoid dose and the severity of skin disease, but not counts of swollen and tender joints and the annualized flare rate, also showed a significant benefit with anifrolumab. Herpes zoster and bronchitis occurred in 7.2% and 12.2% of the patients, respectively, who received anifrolumab. There was one death from pneumonia in the anifrolumab group.

Conclusions: Monthly administration of anifrolumab resulted in a higher percentage of patients with a response (as defined by a composite endpoint) at week 52 than did placebo, in contrast to the findings of a similar phase III trial involving patients with SLE that had a different primary endpoint. The frequency of herpes zoster was higher with anifrolumab than with placebo. (Funded by AstraZeneca; ClinicalTrials.gov number, NCT02446899.)

"Anifrolumab in lupus—promising, but needs validation."

COMMENT

The role of type I interferons in the pathogenesis of systemic lupus erythematosus (SLE) has been known for a while. However, until now, clinical trials targeting type I interferons for treatment of lupus have had mixed results.[9] The latest agent being investigated in this regard is anifrolumab, a monoclonal antibody against the type I interferon receptor. A phase III clinical trial of anifrolumab in >450 patients with lupus demonstrated no significant benefit versus placebo when outcomes were assessed using the composite SLE responder index 4 (SRI 4), and also in secondary outcome measures such as improvement in cutaneous lupus, reduction of corticosteroid dose, or relapses of disease.[10] Another recently published trial evaluated the role of anifrolumab in SLE by randomizing 181 patients to receive anifrolumab and 184 patients to receive placebo four weekly for the study duration of 48 weeks. Although the endpoint proposed at the beginning of the trial was superiority with respect to the SRI-4, this was changed midway by the investigators to the British Isles Lupus Assessment Group-based Composite Lupus Assessment (BICLA). Based on this new endpoint of BICLA, 48% patients achieved the primary endpoint with anifrolumab versus 31.5% in placebo at 52 weeks of observation, a difference that was statistically significant, as well as better outcomes in various other secondary endpoints such as reduction in corticosteroid dose, cutaneous activity, and relapses.[11] While these findings appear promising for the use of anifrolumab in lupus, the change of primary endpoint is a concerning feature, which still leaves open the question regarding the efficacy of anifrolumab in lupus. Internists should be aware that changing endpoints of trials mid-way through the trial, even if adequately justified (as in this case), is not good practice and brings into question the reputation of the trial results.[12]

Key Messages

- *Anifrolumab is a monoclonal antibody targeting the type I interferon receptor.*
- *Two recent clinical trials of anifrolumab in lupus have shown mixed results. There may be potential beneficial effects on disease activity. However, further studies are required.*

ARTICLE 4

Evaluation of remission definitions for systemic lupus erythematosus: a prospective cohort study

Golder V, Kandane-Rathnayake R, Huq M, Louthrenoo W, Luo SF, Wu YJJ, et al.; Asia Pacific Lupus Collaboration. Evaluation of remission definitions for systemic lupus erythematosus: a prospective cohort study.
Lancet Rheumatol. 2019;1: e103-10.

Abstract*

Introduction: For systemic lupus erythematosus (SLE), validated outcome measures are required from which treatment strategies are derived. But, there is no widely adopted definition of remission for SLE. A framework is proposed by the Definitions of Remission in Systemic Lupus Erythematosus (DORIS) group, which has various potential definitions of remission. This study aimed to evaluate the attainability as well as effect on disease outcomes of the DORIS definitions of remission, in comparison to the lupus low disease activity state (LLDAS), among patients who have SLE.

Materials and methods: This prospective cohort study included patients with SLE from 13 international centers, which are part of the Asia Pacific Lupus Collaboration. Patients who were >18 years of age and fulfilled one of two classification criteria for SLE (1997 American College of Rheumatology Criteria or the 2012 Systemic Lupus International Collaborating Clinics Criteria) were enrolled. Visits were as per clinical need; frequency was at least one visit per 6 months. Achievement of remission was assessed based on the eight DORIS definitions of remission, which varied with respect to glucocorticoid use, immunosuppressive agents use, and serological activity; achievement of LLDAS; and disease flares at every visit. Annually, irreversible organ damage accrual was recorded. Primary aim of the study was to evaluate patients' exposure to each of the remission definitions or LLDAS. The primary outcome measure was to assess the respective association of these states with accrual of irreversible organ damage. Key secondary outcome was occurrence of disease flares. Time-dependent Cox proportional hazards models and generalized linear models were used for evaluating DORIS definitions of remission as well as LLDAS with respect to their association with damage accrual and disease flares.

Results: From May 1, 2013 to December 31, 2016, total 1,707 patients with SLE were enrolled; patients were followed for a mean (±SD) of 2.2 (±0.9) years, totaling 12,689 visits. Remission, based on DORIS definition, was attained in 4.6% (n = 581) to 35.8% (n = 4,546) of 12,689 visits. Spending ≥50% of observed time in any remission state was found to be associated with a significant decrease in damage accrual, with the exception for the two most stringent remission definitions, for which the frequency of achievement was lowest. Remission definitions disallowing serological activity were observed to be associated with the highest decreases in disease flares. LLDAS was more achievable as compared to any remission definition; it was found to be associated with a comparable magnitude of protection from disease flares as well as damage accrual. LLDAS and sustained remission were associated with a wider spread of effect sizes for decrease in risk of damage. On evaluating patients who met the definition for LLDAS but not remission, it was observed that there was a significant association between LLDAS and damage accrual reduction, independent of all definitions of remission, with the exception of the least stringent.

Conclusion: An association was seen between achievement of remission with significant decreases in disease flares and damage accrual. LLDAS was more attainable as compared to remission on the basis of DORIS criteria; however, it was similarly protective. Remission definitions with less stringency might be inadequately different from LLDAS for substantially affecting outcome measures. Further studies should be conducted for differentiating the protective effects of the several remission definitions.

Funding: UCB, GlaxoSmithKline, Janssen, Bristol-Myers Squibb, and AstraZeneca. *Redrafted abstract

"Remission in lupus—the holy grail!"

COMMENT

Remission refers to disappearance of disease symptoms or a halt of disease activity. Unlike rheumatoid arthritis, the concept of remission in lupus is more difficult to define. This stems from the heterogeneity inherent in systemic lupus erythematosus (SLE). Patients may experience remission in one organ like the skin while continuing to be active in other organs like the kidney. Definitions of remission in SLE have yet to be standardized. In 2016, an international panel (the Definition of Remission in Systemic Lupus Erythematosus, DORIS project) proposed three definitions of remission in SLE: (1) Complete remission (with negative serology), (2) clinical remission on therapy (clinical ROT), and (3) complete ROT. A commonly used composite measure of disease activity in SLE is the SLE Disease Activity Index, 2000 (SLEDAI-2K), which considers features of activity in various organ systems as well as some serological parameters

such aslike complement levels and titeres of antibodies to double-stranded deoxy ribonucleic acid (dsDNA). Various definitions of remission in lupus have used SLEDAI-2K ≤4, with or without low dose prednisolone or hydroxychloroquine.[13,14] However, the relevance of a low disease activity is not yet clear. In this context, a recent cohort study of >1,700 lupus patients from different Asian centers evaluated remission based on different criteria, including the low lupus disease activity state (LLDAS) and SLEDAI-2K. Overall, patients attained remission ranging from 4.6 to 35.8% of their clinical visits. Those who attained remission sustained lesser features of end-organ damage over the follow-up period.[15] This paper suggests that remission in lupus is a feasible target. Disease activity measurement in lupus, although cumbersome, should be done routinely in the clinic. The target should be to attain remission to improve long-term outcomes.

Key Messages

⊙ *Remission in SLE is achievable.*

⊙ *Various definitions are used for remission in lupus.*

⊙ *Attaining remission leads to better long-term outcomes in lupus by minimizing damage accrual.*

ARTICLE 5

Use of combined hormonal contraceptives among women with systemic lupus erythematosus with and without medical contraindications to oestrogen

Mendel A, Bernatsky S, Pineau CA, St-Pierre Y, Hanly JG, Urowitz MB, et al. Use of combined hormonal contraceptives among women with systemic lupus erythematosus with and without medical contraindications to oestrogen. *Rheumatology (Oxford). 2019;58:1259-67.*

Abstract*

Objectives: This study aimed at assessing the prevalence of combined hormonal contraceptives (CHCs) among women of reproductive-age having systemic lupus erythematosus (SLE) with and without possible contraindications. Factors associated with the use of CHCs were also determined in the presence of possible contraindications.

Methods: This was a observational cohort study, which included premenopausal women belonging to 18–45 years of age enrolled in the Systemic Lupus International Collaborating Clinics (SLICC) registry ≤15 months after onset of SLE, with annual assessments during 2000–2017. At each study visit, WHO category 3 or 4 contraindications to CHCs [e.g., antiphospholipid (aPL) and hypertension] were evaluated. High disease activity [i.e., Systemic Lupus Erythematosus Disease Activity Index (SLEDAI) score >12 or use of >0.5 mg/kg/day of prednisone] was taken as a relative contraindication.

Results: Total 927 SLE women were included. Overall 6,315 visits were contributed by subjects; out of these, 60% (n = 3,811) took place the setting of ≥1 possible contraindication to CHCs. During 8% (n = 512) visits, women used CHCs; out of these, 55% (n = 281) occurred in the presence of ≥1 possible contraindication. The most common contraindications included aPL in 52% patients, followed by hypertension and migraine with aura in 34% and 22%, respectively. As compared to women with no contraindications [9% (95% CI 8, 10)], women with ≥1 contraindication were slightly less taking CHCs [7% of visits (95% CI 7, 8)].

Conclusion: Compared to general population estimates (>35%), CHC use was low; minimum one possible contraindication was present in more than half of CHC users. Several factors were not measured in present study, such as patient preferences, which may have led to these findings. Further studies should be conducted for assessing outcomes associated with such exposure. *Redrafted abstract

"Contraception methods should always be discussed with females in lupus."

COMMENT

Connective tissue diseases (CTDs) like systemic lupus erythematosus (SLE) disproportionately affect females, more so young females in the reproductive age group in the case of lupus. Adequate control of disease activity for at least the 6 months preceding pregnancy is highly recommended in SLE. Otherwise, the risk of fetal complications such as intrauterine death and fetal growth retardation, as well as maternal outcomes such as pre-eclampsia, flare of disease, and thrombotic events is much higher. Hence, planning a pregnancy in a young female with SLE is of paramount importance. Contraceptive measures that are to be used in such patients also require caution, since some forms of oral contraceptive pills (OCPs) such as those containing estrogen increase the risk of thrombotic events in general, more so in patients with antiphospholipid (aPL) antibodies. Other contraindications to OCP use include presence of systemic hypertension and migraine.[16,17] A large international cohort of >900 patients with SLE recently reported prevalence and appropriateness of combined OCP (estrogen and progesterone) use in pregnant females with SLE. Over >6,300 visits, nearly 8% used combined OCPs. However, combined OCP use was prevalent despite the use of the aforementioned contraindications in more than one-half of the study population.[18] Clinicians should be aware of pregnancy risks as well as appropriate contraceptive use in females with lupus to avoid both unplanned pregnancies as well as the unwanted adverse effects of OCP use in those with contraindications.

Key Messages

- *Contraception use in lupus needs to address disease features such as hypercoagulable state, before using hormonal contraceptives.*

- *Always discuss the issue of contraception with females with lupus in reproductive age group, as unplanned pregnancies during periods of high disease activity can be catastrophic for both mother and child.*

ARTICLE 6A

Dose tapering and discontinuation of biological therapy in rheumatoid arthritis patients in routine care—2-year outcomes and predictors

Brahe CH, Krabbe S, Østergaard M, Ørnbjerg L, Glinatsi D, Røgind H, et al. Dose tapering and discontinuation of biological therapy in rheumatoid arthritis patients in routine care—2-year outcomes and predictors.
Rheumatology (Oxford). 2019;58:110-9.

Abstract*

Objectives: A cohort of routine care patients with rheumatoid arthritis (RA) in sustained remission had biological disease-modifying antirheumatic drugs (bDMARDs) tapered as per a treatment guideline. This study aimed at studying—the number of patients in whom tapering or discontinuation of bDMARD could be done successfully; unwanted outcomes of tapering/discontinuation; and potential baseline predictors of successful tapering as well as discontinuation.

Methods: Total 143 patients with sustained disease activity score 28-C-reactive protein (DAS28-CRP) 2.6 or less and no radiographic progression the previous year were enrolled. Total 91% patients received tumor necrosis factor (TNF) inhibitor and 9% a non-TNF inhibitor. At baseline, bDMARD was decreased to two-thirds of standard dose, half after 16 weeks, and discontinued after 32 weeks. Tapering was stopped in patients who flared (that was defined as either DAS28-CRP 2.6 or more and ΔDAS28-CRP 1.2 or more from baseline, or erosive progression on X-ray and/or MRI); these patients were escalated to the previous dose level.

Results: Two-year follow-up was completed in 141 patients. At 2 years, 62% patients (n = 87) successfully tapered bDMARDs; 18% (n = 26) received two-thirds of standard dose, 28% (n = 39) half dose, and 16% (n = 22) discontinued. Total 38% (n = 54) received full dose. ΔDAS28-CRP0-2years was 0.1[(−0.2) −0.4] [median (interquartile range)] and mean ΔTotal-Sharp-Score0-2years was 0.01 (1.15) [mean (SD)]. In 7% (n = 9) patients, radiographic progression was noted. Successful tapering was independently predicted by—male gender, <1 previous bDMARD, low baseline MRI combined inflammation score, or combined damage score. Successful discontinuation was predicted by negative immunoglobulin M-rheumatoid factor (IgM-RF).

Conclusion: On implementation of a clinical guideline, successful tapering was achieved in 62% of patients with RA in sustained remission in routine care, including successful discontinuation in 16% patients at 2 years. Radiographic progression was rarely found. The independent predictors for successful tapering included male gender, maximum one bDMARDs, and low baseline MRI combined inflammation and combined damage scores. *Redrafted abstract

ARTICLE 6B

Gradual tapering TNF inhibitors versus conventional synthetic DMARDs after achieving controlled disease in patients with rheumatoid arthritis: first-year results of the randomised controlled TARA study

van Mulligen E, de Jong PHP, Kuijper TM, van der Ven M, Appels C, Bijkerk C, et al. Gradual tapering TNF inhibitors versus conventional synthetic DMARDs after achieving controlled disease in patients with rheumatoid arthritis: first-year results of the randomised controlled TARA study.
Ann Rheum Dis. 2019;78:746-53.

Abstract

Objectives: The aim of this study is to evaluate the effectiveness of two tapering strategies after achieving controlled disease in patients with rheumatoid arthritis (RA), during 1 year of follow-up.

Methods: In this multicentre single-blinded (research nurses) randomized controlled trial, patients with RA were included who achieved controlled disease, defined as a disease activity score (DAS) $\leq$2.4 and a swollen joint count (SJC) $\leq$1, treated with both a conventional synthetic disease-modifying antirheumatic drugs (csDMARD) and a tumor necrosis factor (TNF) inhibitor. Eligible patients were randomized into gradual tapering csDMARDs or TNF inhibitors. Medication was tapered, if the RA was still under control, by cutting the dosage into half, a quarter, and thereafter it was stopped. Primary outcome was proportion of patients with a disease flare, defined as DAS >2.4 and/or SJC >1. Secondary outcomes were DAS, European Quality of Life-5 Dimensions (EQ5D) and functional ability [Health Assessment Questionnaire Disability Index (HAQ-DI)] after 1 year and over time.

Results: A total of 189 patients were randomly assigned to tapering csDMARDs (n = 94) or tapering anti-TNF (n = 95). The cumulative flare rates in the csDMARD and anti-TNF tapering group were, respectively, 33% (95% CI, 24% to 43%) and 43% [95% CI, 33% to 53% (p = 0.17)]. Mean DAS, HAQ-DI, and EQ-5D did not differ between tapering groups after 1 year and over time.

Conclusion: Up to 9 months, flare rates of tapering csDMARDs or TNF inhibitors were similar. After 1 year, a nonsignificant difference was found of 10% favoring csDMARD tapering. Tapering TNF inhibitors was, therefore, not superior to tapering csDMARDs. From a societal perspective, it would be sensible to taper the TNF inhibitor first, because of possible cost reductions and less long-term side effects.

Trial registration number: NTR2754.

"Tapering DMARDs in RA is feasible."

COMMENT

Patients with rheumatoid arthritis (RA) often require long-term medical therapy. While clinical outcomes have significantly improved in the past two decades with the advent of biological disease-modifying antirheumatic drugs (DMARDs), it is still a matter of debate when and how fast to taper DMARDs, whether conventional or biological, and what are the long-term outcomes of this in terms of radiological damage to the joints.[19] Two recent studies have addressed this issue. In a cohort of 141 individuals with RA who were on biological DMARDs with disease activity in remission for at least 1 year, protocolized tapering regimen of the biologic DMARD was followed. Dose was initially reduced to two-thirds, thereafter to one-half after for 16 weeks, and stopped at 32 weeks, if feasible. At the end of the observation period of 2 years, nearly two-thirds patients had managed to tolerate taper of biological DMARD, and one-sixth had discontinued the drug successfully. Such a regimen of tapering did not result in radiographic damage progression in >90%

patients. Patients, who were males, had used up to a single biological DMARD previously, and had evidence of low radiological disease activity at baseline, were more successful in tapering their biological DMARD successfully.[20] The other open-label clinical trial being discussed randomized patients with RA in remission who were on both conventional and biological DMARD, to initiate taper of either conventional DMARD (in 94) or the biologic DMARD, i.e., anti-tumor necrosis factor-alpha agent (in 95). Irrespective of which agent was tapered, similar proportions of patients (33% conventional DMARD, 43% biological DMARD) relapsed by the time point of 1 year, with similar disease activity scores and quality of life indices in both groups at the end of the observation period.[21] These two studies indicate that tapering of DMARDs with discontinuation in a small proportion of patients is feasible, with careful monitoring for relapse of disease activity. It may be suitable to taper either of conventional or biological DMARD with similar effectiveness.

Key Messages

⊙ *It is feasible to reduce dose of DMARDs (whether biological or conventional) in patients with RA who are in remission, with careful monitoring during tapering to detect relapses of disease at the earliest.*

⊙ *Tapering DMARDs in RA does not necessarily lead to worse clinical or radiographic outcomes or quality of life.*

ARTICLE 7

Effectiveness of different combinations of DMARDs and glucocorticoid bridging in early rheumatoid arthritis: two-year results of CareRA

Stouten V, Westhovens R, Pazmino S, De Cock D, Van der Elst K, Joly J, et al.; CareRA Study Group. Effectiveness of different combinations of DMARDs and glucocorticoid bridging in early rheumatoid arthritis: two-year results of CareRA. *Rheumatology (Oxford). 2019;58:2284-94.*

Abstract*

Objectives: This study aimed at evaluating whether combination of methotrexate (MTX) with an additional disease-modifying antirheumatic drug (DMARD) as well as bridging glucocorticoids as initial treatment in patients, who have early rheumatoid arthritis (RA), induces an effective long-term response.

Methods: The care in early RA study, an investigator-initiated pragmatic multicenter randomized trial, was conducted for duration of 2 years. Stratification of the early RA patients, who were naïve to DMARDs and glucocorticoids, was done on the basis of prognostic factors. The high-risk patients were randomized to either COBRA-Classic (n = 98): MTX, sulfasalazine, prednisone step-down from 60 mg; or COBRA-Slim (n = 98): MTX, prednisone step-down from 30 mg; or COBRA-Avant-Garde (n = 93): MTX, leflunomide, prednisone step-down from 30 mg. The low-risk patients were randomized to either tight step-up (TSU) (n = 47): MTX without prednisone; or COBRA-Slim (n = 43). Assessment of clinical and radiological outcomes at 2 years, sustainability of response, safety, and treatment adaptations was done.

Results: In the 98 patients of high-risk group, 72% (n = 71) achieved a DAS28-CRP <2.6 with COBRA-Slim as compared to 64/98 (65%) with COBRA-Classic and 74% (n = 69) with COBRA-Avant-Garde (p = 1.00). There was no significant difference between other clinical/radiological outcomes and sustainability of response. Less therapy-related adverse events were caused by COBRA-Slim treatment in comparison to COBRA-Classic (p = 0.02) or COBRA-Avant-Garde (p = 0.005). In the 43 patients of low-risk group, 67% (n = 29) patients on COBRA-Slim and 72% (n = 34) on TSU achieved a DAS28-CRP <2.6 (p = 1.00). On COBRA-Slim, low-risk patients were observed to have lower longitudinal DAS28-CRP scores over 2 years; a lower requirement for glucocorticoid injections; and a similar safety profile in comparison to TSU.

Conclusion: In patients with early RA, all the regimens combining DMARDs with glucocorticoids were found to be effective up to 2 years. The best balance between efficacy and safety was provided by the COBRA-Slim regimen, MTX monotherapy with glucocorticoid bridging, regardless of the prognosis of patients.

Trial registration: ClinicalTrials.gov, http://www.clinicaltrials.gov, NCT01172639. *Redrafted abstract

> *"Low disease activity or remission should be the goal of RA treatment, no matter how it is achieved."*

COMMENT

Understanding regarding the use of conventional disease-modifying antirheumatic drugs (DMARDs) has gradually evolved over the years.[22] A recent study from Belgium evaluated different regimens of conventional DMARDS, with or without glucocorticoids, in patients with rheumatoid arthritis (RA) in the 1st year of their disease. First, the patients were stratified into high- and low-risk groups. High-risk group (289 RA patients) were those who had erosive disease with presence of rheumatoid factor (RF) or anti-citrullinated peptide antibody (ACPA) with or without moderate-to-high disease activity at baseline, or non-erosive disease with both RF/ACPA positivity and moderate-to-high disease activity at baseline; the rest 90 patients were categorized as low-risk patients. High-risk patients were randomized to one of three treatment arms—COBRA-Classic (weekly methotrexate 15 mg/kg, daily sulfasalazine 2 g/day, and prednisolone 60 mg daily tapered to 7.5 mg daily by 7 weeks), COBRA-Slim (weekly methotrexate 15 mg/kg and prednisolone 30 mg daily tapered to 5 mg daily by 6 weeks), or COBRA-Avant Garde (weekly methotrexate 15 mg/kg, daily leflunomide 10 mg and prednisolone 30 mg daily tapered to 7.5 mg daily by 6 weeks). Low-risk RAs were randomized to receive either COBRA-Slim or methotrexate 15 mg/week without glucocorticoid. At the end of this 2-year open label study, all the three high-risk treatment strategies and two low-risk treatment strategies had similar attainment of remission (defined as disease activity score in 28 joints using C-reactive protein: DAS28-CRP ≤2.6—ranging from 65 to 74% in different groups) and similar functional status assessed using health assessment questionnaire scores. With respect to safety, COBRA-Slim had lesser adverse events than the other two groups for the high-risk RA patients; whereas for low-risk individuals, both groups were similar with regards to safety.[23] This study reinforces the message that good control of disease activity is achievable in patients with RA using conventional DMARDs. Irrespective of the treatment regimen used, the attainment of remission or low disease activity should be the lodestar.[22]

Key Messages

◉ *Varying combinations of conventional DMARDs, with or without prednisolone, were able to attain remission in more than two-thirds of early RA patients.*

◉ *Risk stratification into high- and low-risk based on disease activity at baseline, seropositivity for RF/ACPA or presence of erosions might help to identify suitable treatment strategies in RA.*

ARTICLE 8

Safety and effectiveness of upadacitinib or adalimumab plus methotrexate in patients with rheumatoid arthritis over 48 weeks with switch to alternate therapy in patients with insufficient response

fleischmann RM, Genovese MC, Enejosa JV, Mysler E, Bessette L, Peterfy C, et al. Safety and effectiveness of upadacitinib or adalimumab plus methotrexate in patients with rheumatoid arthritis over 48 weeks with switch to alternate therapy in patients with insufficient response.
Ann Rheum Dis. 2019;78:1454-62.

Abstract*

Background: In SELECT-COMPARE, which was a randomized double-blind study, upadacitinib 15 mg once daily was found to be superior to placebo or adalimumab on background methotrexate (MTX) in treatment of signs and symptoms of rheumatoid arthritis (RA) and inhibited radiographical progression compared to placebo at 26 weeks. In this study, 48-week safety and efficacy was reported among patients who remained on the original medication or were given the alternative medication due to unsatisfactory response.

Methods: For 48 weeks, patients on MTX were either given upadacitinib 15 mg, placebo, or adalimumab. In the case of patients who had <20% improvement in tender joint count (TJC) or swollen joint count (SJC) (in weeks 14/18/22) or Clinical Disease Activity Index (CDAI) >10 (in week 26), rescue without washout occurred from placebo/adalimumab to upadacitinib or upadacitinib to adalimumab. At week 26, the remaining placebo patients were switched to upadacitinib. Analysis of efficacy was done in randomized group (nonresponder imputation), and separately in rescued patients (as noted). Treatment-emergent adverse events per 100 patient-years were summed up.

Results: Consistent with responses through week 26, from 26th to 48th week, responses by randomized group comprising clinical remission, low disease activity, and improvements in pain as well as function persisted superior for upadacitinib in comparison with adalimumab. Radiographical progression was decreased for upadacitinib compared to placebo (linear extrapolation). Both switch groups responded; however, a greater number of patients rescued to upadacitinib from adalimumab attained CDAI 10 or less at 6 months post-switch compared to patients who were rescued from upadacitinib to adalimumab. There was no significant difference in safety at week 48th compared to week 26th.

Conclusion: As compared to adalimumab + MTX, upadacitinib + MTX showed superior clinical and functional responses as well as maintained inhibition of structural damage compared to placebo + MTX through week 48th. In patients who did not have a sufficient response to adalimumab or upadacitinib, clinically meaningful responses were achieved safely following switching to the alternative medication without washout.

Trial registration: ClinicalTrials.gov NCT02629159. *Redrafted abstract

"David challenges Goliath—Small molecules (end of observation period of 48) versus the big boys—the Biologics (mAbs and Cepts)."

COMMENT

Tyrosine kinase inhibitors are orally administered targeted synthetic disease-modifying anti-rheumatic drugs (DMARDs) (also called small molecules), which have revolutionized the management of rheumatoid arthritis (RA).[24] One such selective Janus kinase 1 (JAK1) inhibitor, upadacitinib (15 mg daily), was recently evaluated in a large multicentric trial of RA patients against standard of care anti-tumor necrosis factor (TNF) agent adalimumab (40 mg subcutaneous 2 weekly injections) or placebo, with background stable dose of methotrexate (MTX) in all groups. All patients had active disease at baseline, and had seropositivity or radiographically demonstrable erosive disease. About 651 patients each received upadacitinib or placebo, and 327 received adalimumab. At 26 weeks, those on upadacitinib with inadequate disease activity control were switched to adalimumab and vice-versa. By the end of observation period of 48 weeks, patients on upadacitinib had significantly better improvements in disease activity as demonstrated by the American College of Rheumatology (ACR) 20% (ACR 20), 50% (ACR 50), and 70% (ACR 70) criteria. Similar results were also obtained by using other measures of disease activity in RA. Radiographic joint damage progression was similar in upadacitinib and adalimumab groups, both better than placebo.[25] While other JAK inhibitors like tofacitinib have shown similar improvements compared to gold standard of biologic drugs like adalimumab,[26] demonstration of superior control of disease activity compared to biologic drugs, as in this case with upadacitinib is unheard of.[25] Hence, the promise of upadacitinib in treating RA needs further exploration, particularly in refractory disease states such as long-standing RA.

Key Messages

- Upadacitinib is a selective JAK1 inhibitor.
- In this trial, upadacitinib attained better control of disease activity in RA patients than adalimumab or placebo, and with similar degree of radiographic damage retardation as adalimumab.
- Targeted synthetic DMARDs such as upadacitinib pose stiff challenge to the biologics.

ARTICLE 9

Methotrexate achieves major cDAPSA response, and improvement in dactylitis and functional status in psoriatic arthritis

Appani SK, Devarasetti PK, Irlapati RVP, Rajasekhar L. Methotrexate achieves major cDAPSA response, and improvement in dactylitis and functional status in psoriatic arthritis.
Rheumatology (Oxford). 2019;58:869-73.

Abstract*

Objective: Although methotrexate (MTX) is widely used in the psoriatic arthritis (PsA), limited efficacy is indicated by the data from published randomized controlled studies. This study aimed at assessing the efficacy of MTX.

Methods: This open-label, prospective study included patients meeting the ClASsification criteria for Psoriatic ARthritis (CASPAR) study criteria for PsA who received MTX in doses of ≥15 mg/week during the 9 months follow-up period. Disease activity was measured, at baseline and at 3, 6, and 9 months follow-up periods, across several domains by physician and patient global evaluation; tender and swollen joint count; Disease activity score (DAS28) erythrocyte sedimentation rate (ESR); minimal disease activity; leeds dactylitis instrument basic; Leeds Enthesitis Index (LEI); Clinical Disease Activity Index for PsA (cDAPSA); Psoriasis Area and Severity Index (PASI); and Health Assessment Questionnaire (HAQ) (CRD Pune version). Disease Activity Index for PsA (cDAPSA) response, European League Against Rheumatism (EULAR) DAS28 ESR, HAQ response, and PASI75 were used to assess response to therapy. MTX dose escalation as well as the usage of combination disease-modifying anti-rheumatic drugs (DMARDs) was dictated by the disease activity.

Results: Study population included 73 patients; the mean (±SD) age was 44 (±9.7) years. The mean (±SD) dose of MTX was 17.5 (±3.8) mg/week. Additional DMARDs [leflunomide (LEF)/sulphasalazine (SSZ)] were given to 7 patients. There was a significant improvement in the global activity, tender and swollen joint count, DAS-28ESR, cDAPSA, PASI, Leeds Dactylitis Index basic, LEI, and HAQ at the end of 9 months (p < 0.05). In 58.9% patients, major cDAPSA response was achieved. EULAR DAS28 moderate response was achieved in 74% patients and good response in 6.8% patients. In 63% patients, minimal Disease Activity was noted. A PASI75 response was observed in 67.9% patients and HAQ response in 65.8% patients.

Conclusion: A significant improvement was observed in the skin, joint, dactylitis, enthesitis, and functional domains of PsA after initiation of MTX ≥15 mg/week with targeted escalation. *Redrafted abstract

"OLD IS GOLD—Methotrexate improves joint disease, enthesitis, and skin disease in psoriatic arthritis."

COMMENT

While conventional disease-modifying anti-rheumatic drugs (DMARDs) have been proven effective beyond reasonable doubt in rheumatoid arthritis (RA),[22] the same is not the case with psoriatic arthritis (PsA), another commonly encountered inflammatory arthritis in the clinic. PsA is seen in up to one-fourth of patients with psoriasis. The joint diseases follow skin psoriasis in nearly 70% of the patients. In 15% of the patients, the arthritis and skin manifestations come up simultaneously, while the arthritis precedes skin disease in 15% of patients. PsA is also more heterogeneous than RA. Apart from skin, nails, and joints, the other domains include dactylitis, enthesitis, and axial disease. The oral drugs used to treat PsA are divided into two categories—conventional synthetic DMARDs such as methotrexate (MTX), leflunomide (LEF), cyclosporine, etc. and targeted synthetic DMARDs such as tofacitinib and apremilast. Biologics, which are administered parenterally, include the bio-originators and biosimilars. MTX is effective against both the skin and articular manifestations. Biologics, despite being effective, are infrequently used in developing countries because of cost issues. MTX is the most commonly used DMARD in PsA. A major clinical trial published a few years back compared MTX at a dose of 15 mg/week (111 patients) with placebo (112 patients) in PsA, and could not demonstrate significant differences in joint disease activity, despite better improvements in active skin disease with MTX.[27] A limitation of this study was that the dose of MTX was probably not escalated to the currently accepted optimum dose of 25 mg/week.[27] In this context, a recent open label clinical trial from India reported the effectiveness of MTX in 73 patients with PsA. Nearly 60% patients, treated with a mean dose of 17.5 mg/week MTX (few received additional LEF or sulfasalazine), attained significant improvements in joint disease activity at 9 months. At this same time point, about two-thirds patients attained significant improvements in enthesitis, skin disease activity, as well as quality of life.[28] In a resource-constrained setting like ours where access to biologic drugs is often limited, this study reinforces the utility of MTX in the therapeutic armamentarium for psoriatic arthritis.

Key Messages

- *Methotrexate is a useful conventional DMARD for PsA management.*
- *Nearly two-thirds PsA patients attain improvement in joint and skin disease and quality of life with MTX.*

ARTICLE 10

A multicenter, randomized, placebo-controlled trial of atorvastatin for the primary prevention of cardiovascular events in patients with rheumatoid arthritis

Kitas GD, Nightingale P, Armitage J, Sattar N, Belch JJF, Symmons DPM, et al. A multicenter, randomized, placebo-controlled trial of atorvastatin for the primary prevention of cardiovascular events in patients with rheumatoid arthritis. *Arthritis Rheumatol. 2019;71:1437-49.*

Abstract

Objective: Rheumatoid arthritis (RA) is associated with increased cardiovascular event (CVE) risk. The impact of statins in RA is not established. We assessed whether atorvastatin is superior to placebo for the primary prevention of CVEs in RA patients.

Methods: A randomized, double-blind, placebo-controlled trial was designed to detect a 32% CVE risk reduction based on an estimated 1.6% per annum event rate with 80% power at p < 0.05. RA patients age >50 years or with a disease duration of >10 years who did not have clinical atherosclerosis, diabetes, or myopathy received atorvastatin 40 mg daily or matching placebo. The primary endpoint was a composite of cardiovascular death, myocardial infarction, stroke, transient ischemic attack, or any arterial revascularization. Secondary and tertiary endpoints included plasma lipids and safety.

Results: A total of 3,002 patients (mean age 61 years; 74% female) were followed up for a median of 2.51 years [interquartile range (IQR) 1.90, 3.49 years] (7,827 patient-years). The study was terminated early due to a lower than expected event rate (0.70% per annum). Of the 1,504 patients receiving atorvastatin, 24 (1.6%) experienced a primary endpoint, compared with 36 (2.4%) of the 1,498 receiving placebo [hazard ratio (HR) 0.66; {95% confidence interval (CI) 0.39, 1.11}; p = 0.115 and adjusted HR 0.60 (95% CI 0.32, 1.15);

p = 0.127]. At trial end, patients receiving atorvastatin had a mean ± SD low-density lipoprotein cholesterol (LDL-C) level 0.77 ± 0.04 mmol/L lower than those receiving placebo (p < 0.0001). C-reactive protein level was also significantly lower in the atorvastatin group than the placebo group [median 2.59 mg/L (IQR 0.94, 6.08) vs. 3.60 mg/L (IQR 1.47, 7.49); p < 0.0001]. CVE risk reduction per mmol/L reduction in LDL-C was 42% (95% CI −14%, 70%). The rates of adverse events in the atorvastatin group [n = 298 (19.8%)] and placebo group [n = 292 (19.5%)] were similar.

Conclusion: Atorvastatin 40 mg daily is safe and results in a significantly greater reduction of LDL-c level than placebo in patients with RA. The 34% CVE risk reduction is consistent with the Cholesterol Treatment Trialists' Collaboration meta-analysis of statin effects in other populations.

"Atorvastatin—safe for CVD prevention in RA, but its efficacy requires to be established."

COMMENT

It is a well-known fact that rheumatoid arthritis (RA) is the most common inflammatory polyarthritis encountered in clinical practice. Much less appreciated is the fact that what hurts in RA is the "joint" but what kills is the "heart". Accumulating evidence over the past few years has demonstrated unequivocally that cardiovascular disease is the major killer in RA. Pari passu, there is the growing realization that inflammation is the prime driver for atherosclerosis. Atherosclerosis is now viewed as an active immunoinflammatory disease rather than an inert metabolic disease. Inflammatory rheumatic diseases like RA and lupus offer a fertile ground, where, novel and traditional risk factors congregate resulting in an increased risk of premature atherosclerosis. It has been established beyond doubt that RA is associated with an increased risk of cardiovascular disease (CVD). The increase in CVD risk with RA is equivalent, if not more, than that with diabetes.[29] A recent clinical trial has attempted to explore primary preventative strategies for CVD in patients with RA. In the present study, patients without prior CVD were randomized to either receive atorvastatin (40 mg/day, in 1,504) or placebo (in 1,498), and followed up for a median 2.5 years. Numerically lesser number of patients (24 CVD events) on atorvastatin developed CVD as opposed to placebo (36 CVD events). Adjusted for potential confounders, the hazard ratio for CVD events with atorvastatin compared with placebo was 0.6 (95% 0.32–1.15). While a statistically significant difference was not attained between groups, the study was underpowered due to a markedly lesser number of CVD events than expected (434 CVD events). Hence, potential reduction in the risk of developing a CVD event might have occurred with a larger number of events. Atorvastatin was not associated with any major adverse events in patients with RA when compared with placebo.[30] While the trial could not prove the hypothesis that atorvastatin reduces the risk of incident CVD events in a high-risk population of RA patients, this issue requires further exploration. Meanwhile, standard measures to reduce CVD risk such as healthy diet, appropriate body weight, and exercise should be recommended for patients with RA.[31]

Key Messages

- *Rheumatoid arthritis is associated with increased CVD risk (at least to the same extent as diabetes).*
- *Primary preventative strategies for CVD such as atorvastatin are being explored in RA.*

ARTICLE 11A

Myocardial inflammation, measured using 18-fluorodeoxyglucose positron emission tomography with computed tomography, is associated with disease activity in rheumatoid arthritis

Amigues I, Tugcu A, Russo C, Giles JT, Morgenstein R, Zartoshti A, et al. Myocardial inflammation, measured using 18-fluorodeoxyglucose positron emission tomography with computed tomography, is associated with disease activity in rheumatoid arthritis.
Arthritis Rheumatol. 2019;71:496-506.

Abstract

Objective: To determine the prevalence and correlates of subclinical myocardial inflammation in patients with rheumatoid arthritis (RA)

Methods: RA patients (n = 119) without known cardiovascular disease underwent cardiac 18-fluoro-deoxyglucose (FDG) positron emission tomography with computed tomography (PET-CT). Myocardial FDG uptake was assessed visually and measured quantitatively as the standardized uptake value (SUV). Multivariable linear regression was used to assess the associations of patient characteristics with myocardial SUVs. A subset of RA patients who had to escalate their disease-modifying antirheumatic drug (DMARD) therapy (n = 8) underwent a second FDG PET-CT scan after 6 months, to assess treatment-associated changes in myocardial FDG uptake.

Results: Visually assessed FDG uptake was observed in 46 (39%) of the 119 RA patients, and 21 patients (18%) had abnormal quantitatively assessed myocardial FDG uptake [i.e., mean of the mean SUV (SUV_{mean}) ≥ 3.10 units; defined as 2 SD above the value in a reference group of 27 non-RA subjects]. The SUV_{mean} was 31% higher in patients with a Clinical Disease Activity Index (CDAI) score of ≥ 10 (moderate-to-high disease activity) as compared with those with lower CDAI scores (low disease activity or remission) (p = 0.005), after adjustment for potential confounders. The adjusted SUV_{mean} was 26% lower among those treated with a non-tumor necrosis factor-targeted biologic agent compared with those treated with conventional (nonbiologic) DMARDs (p = 0.029). In the longitudinal substudy, the myocardial SUV_{mean} decreased from 4.50 units to 2.30 units over 6 months, which paralleled the decrease in the mean CDAI from a score of 23 to a score of 12.

Conclusion: Subclinical myocardial inflammation is frequent in patients with RA, is associated with RA disease activity, and may decrease with RA therapy. Future longitudinal studies will be required to assess whether reduction in myocardial inflammation will reduce heart failure risk in RA.

ARTICLE 11B

Correlation of inflammatory markers and disease severity with cardiovascular autonomic dysfunction in indian patients with rheumatoid arthritis

Saminathan MB, Sharma R, Gogna A, Rani A, Kapoor R. Correlation of inflammatory markers and disease severity with cardiovascular autonomic dysfunction in Indian patients with rheumatoid arthritis.
Indian J Rheumatol. 2019;14:123-6.

Abstract*

Introduction: Cardiovascular disease is accountable for >40% of mortality in rheumatoid arthritis (RA); the cardiovascular autonomic nervous system dysfunction (CAD) is generally noted. There is a scarcity of studies related to the status of cardiac autonomic function in RA; therefore, this study is aimed to assess the same among patients with RA and to find the correlation of cardiac autonomic function with the level of inflammatory markers as well as disease severity. This study is also determined to assess the heart rate variability (HRV) and inflammatory markers in patients with RA and controls, and to evaluate the correlation of inflammatory markers and disease severity with HRV.

Materials and methods: This study included 35 patients who were diagnosed cases of RA and 35 controls. Short-term HRV was considered as an index of autonomic function. Assessment of tumor necrosis factor (TNF)-α and interleukin (IL)-10 was done in 3 mL overnight fasting serum. DAS28 score was used for assessing RA severity.

Result: Disease severity of RA was found to be low. Among patients with RA, LF, NN50, and RANGE were significantly reduced, and TNF-α was significantly increased. There was significant positive correlation of TNF-α with LF/HF ratio. Correlation of DAS28 with RMSSD, NN50, and HF was also significantly positive.

Conclusion: Among patients with RA, there is a significant correlation of CAD with inflammatory activity as well as disease severity. HRV can act as an effective method for monitoring patients with RA for early signs of autonomic dysfunction, and may aid immensely in minimizing future morbidity and mortality.
*Redrafted abstract

ARTICLE 11C

Non-ischemic cardiomyopathy: role of immunologic work-up and cardiac MRI in etiologic diagnosis and outcomes

Malgutte D, Waghmare I, Bhute V, Joshi A, Gokhale Y. Non-ischemic cardiomyopathy: role of immunologic work-up and cardiac MRI in etiologic diagnosis and outcomes.
J Assoc Physicians India. 2019;67:30-4.

Abstract

Objective: To study etiology of non-ischemic cardiomyopathy (NICMP) and role of cardiac MRI in diagnosis and outcomes

Methods: Prospective observational study.

Inclusion criteria: (1) Clinical feature of cardiac failure; (2) 2D echo systolic dysfunction, ejection fraction (EF) <45% or diastolic dysfunction without regional wall motion abnormality; (3) absent ischemic changes on electrocardiogram (ECG) and/or coronary angiography. Exclusion—valvular and congenital heart disease, cor pulmonale, and renal failure. Patient were subjected to complete blood count (CBC) with absolute eosinophil count (AEC), erythrocyte sedimentation rate (ESR), Urine-r/m, N-terminal pro-b-type natriuretic peptide (NT-ProBNP), antinuclear antibody (ANA), anti-neutrophil cytoplasmic antibodies (ANCA), angiotensin-converting enzyme (ACE), bone marrow, amyloid fat pad biopsy, etc., chest X-ray, and 2DE. High-resolution CT (HRCT) chest and coronary angiography, and cardiac MRI by 3-Tesla MRI machine. Patients were treated with antic-failure drugs and as per etiology, and followed at 6-week clinically [New York Heart Association (NYHA)] and 2DE.

Result: Forty four patients, mean age 36 years F:M (22:22), many patients had feature other than cardiac failure like Raynaud's phenomenon (3), joint pain (10), oral ulcer (4), leg ulcer (1), recent delivery (4), and neurological weakness (4). ESR elevated in 30, urine r/m abnormal—12, eosinophilia—4, hypothyroidism—9, ANA positive—5, ANCA positive—4, and serum ACE elevated in 2 patients. Diagnosis established in 36 patients. Raised ESR with p value (0.0001) and abnormal urine r/m predicted systemic cardiomyopathy. Cardiac MRI detected two HOCMP missed on 2DE, 1 sarcoid (abnormal delayed enhancement, non-necrotic mediastinal lymph node), and scarring (predictor of poor prognosis). Out of 44 patient, 30 received additional specific treatment with which clinical NYHA class of symptom (p value = 0.001) and EF improvement (p value = 0.0023) by 20% in 14 and >10% in 9, as compared to idiopathic dilated cardiomyopathy (DCMP) patients on antifailure treatment only.

Conclusion:

- For etiology of cardiac failure features like fever, joint pain, Raynaud's phenomenon, oral/leg ulcer, high ESR, abnormal urine microscopy points toward systemic immune disease.
- In cardiomyopathy patient with treatable cause, specific treatment in addition to antifailure drugs gives significant clinical and EF improvement.

"Unexplained cardiac failure—always look for underlying rheumatic diseases."

COMMENT

There is an increasing understanding of the heightened risk of cardiovascular events in patients with rheumatic diseases, in part driven by the effects of the inflammatory milieu. Such cardiac and cardiovascular involvement might be asymptomatic for years until it presents with features of overt heart failure, coronary artery disease (CAD), or cardiac arrhythmias.[31] A recent study of 44 patients with cardiomyopathy in the absence of CAD from India emphasizes this point. Nearly one half of patients had a rheumatic disease, including systemic lupus erythematosus (SLE), granulomatosis with polyangiitis (GPA), microscopic polyangiitis (MPA), eosinophilic granulomatosis with polyangiitis (EGPA), medium-vessel vasculitis, large-vessel vasculitis (Takayasu arteritis), and sarcoidosis. Cardiac magnetic resonance imaging (cMRI) with gadolinium contrast was undertaken in 28 patients, and a significant proportion of these patients had detectable abnormalities on cMRI. For those 30 patients where specific etiologies for cardiac abnormalities were amenable to treatment, specific therapies resulted in improvement in ejection fraction by >10% in 23 patients.[32] This study drives home the point that underlying rheumatic diseases should be sought for in the differential diagnosis of a patient with cardiac failure in the absence of demonstrable vascular disease.

Cardiac MRI is increasingly being recognized as a tool to aid the diagnosis of subclinical cardiovascular disease in patients with inflammatory rheumatic diseases. This generally requires the administration of intravenous gadolinium-based contrast agents. Abnormalities might be visible in myocardial involvement (in the form of early or late gadolinium enhancement, myocardial fibrosis, or edema), coronary vascular involvement (main vessels or smaller penetrating vessels), pericardial involvement, as well as the noninvasive assessment of ejection fraction and other cardiac functions. Stress-induced myocardial perfusion abnormalities might also be demonstrable.[33] A recent study of 50 patients with systemic sclerosis (19 of whom were asymptomatic for cardiac disease) identified abnormalities in a large proportion of the cohort on cMRI. Those patients with demonstrable cMRI abnormalities had a higher propensity to develop future clinical cardiac disease over the next couple of years.[34] A study of 35 patients with rheumatoid arthritis (RA) from India demonstrated higher cardiac autonomic dysfunction (abnormal heart rate variability) in patients compared to a similar number of healthy controls, more so in those with active joint disease. Such autonomic dysfunction also correlated with level of the inflammatory cytokine tumor necrosis factor-alpha.[35] Similar abnormalities might also be demonstrated by positron emission tomography computerized tomography (PET-CT). As noted in a recent study of 119 patients with RA, about 40% had demonstrable 18-fluorodeoxyglucose (18-FDG) uptake in the myocardium. Those with higher clinical joint disease activity had greater 18-FDG enhancement in the myocardium compared to those without, and such increased uptake also reduced with concomitant decrease in clinical disease activity on follow-up.[36]

To summarize, subclinical cardiac and cardiovascular disease is prevalent in rheumatic diseases, including common inflammatory arthritides such as RA. Such abnormalities might manifest or be detectable in the form of cardiac dysautonomia, abnormalities on cMRI or 18-FDG PET-CT. Underlying systemic rheumatic disease should be sought for in patients with unexplained cardiac failure.

Key Messages

- ⊙ *Subclinical cardiac and cardiovascular disease might occur with rheumatic diseases.*
- ⊙ *Such subclinical involvement might be detectable by autonomic function testing, cMRI, or PET-CT.*
- ⊙ *These abnormalities might associate with high disease activity states.*

ARTICLE 12

Comparative cardiovascular risk of allopurinol versus febuxostat in patients with gout: a nation-wide cohort study

Kang EH, Choi HK, Shin A, Lee YJ, Lee EB, Song YW, et al. Comparative cardiovascular risk of allopurinol versus febuxostat in patients with gout: a nation-wide cohort study.
Rheumatology (Oxford). 2019;58:2122-9.

Abstract

Objective: To compare cardiovascular (CV) risk among gout patients initiating allopurinol versus febuxostat.

Methods: Using 2002–2015 Korean National Health Insurance Service data for the entire Korean population, we conducted a cohort study on gout patients initiating allopurinol or febuxostat. The primary outcome was a composite CV endpoint of myocardial infarction, stroke/transient ischemic attack, or coronary revascularization. Secondary outcomes were individual components of the primary outcome and all-cause mortality. We used propensity score matching with a 4:1 ratio for allopurinol and febuxostat initiators to control for confounding. Competing risk analyses were done for nonfatal outcomes accounting for deaths.

Results: We included 39,640 allopurinol initiators propensity score matched on 9,910 febuxostat initiators. The mean age was 59.1 years and 78.4% were male. The incidence rate per 100 person-years for the primary outcome was 1.89 for allopurinol and 1.84 for febuxostat initiators. The corresponding hazard ratio comparing allopurinol versus febuxostat initiators was 1.09 [95% confidence interval (CI) 0.90, 1.32]. No significant difference was found for the secondary outcomes, including all-cause mortality [hazard ratio (HR) 0.96; 95% CI 0.79, 1.16]. Subgroup analyses limited to those at high CV risk and to equipotent-dose initiators (i.e., allopurinol ≥300 mg/day vs. febuxostat ≥40 mg/day) showed similar results.

Conclusion: Overall, this large Korean population-based study suggests no difference in the risk of non-fatal CV events and all-cause mortality between allopurinol and febuxostat initiators. These findings are consistent with the recent US Medicare population study, although the current study population consisted of younger Asians.

"Febuxostat and allopurinol—possibly both have similar cardiovascular safety?"

COMMENT

Gout is one of the most common forms of inflammatory arthritis seen in the clinic. Urate lowering drugs, allopurinol, and febuxostat are commonly used for the management of patients with gout. Febuxostat has the advantage of being able to be used in those with more advanced renal failure, which forms a significant proportion of patients with gout. The cardiovascular safety of febuxostat was brought into question when a large randomized controlled trial (RCT) involving >6,000 patients compared cardiovascular outcomes in patients with gout and concomitant cardiovascular disease treated with febuxostat or allopurinol. The investigators reported greater all-cause mortality and cardiovascular mortality in patients treated with febuxostat when compared with allopurinol. While these findings received widespread attention and were followed by the United States Food and Drug Administration issuing a black box warning against febuxostat for cardiovascular events, the trial had its limitations due to a large proportion of patients being lost to follow-up.[37] Thereafter, the cardiovascular safety of febuxostat has been an area of active investigation.

In this context, the present article utilized a national healthcare database from South Korea and identified a retrospective cohort of nearly 40,000 gout patients treated with allopurinol and nearly 10,000 gout patients treated with febuxostat. Comparability between groups was ensured by propensity-matched scoring. Followed up over a mean period of 10 months, both groups had similar rates of cardiovascular events as well as cardiovascular mortality.[38] Another recent retrospective cohort of patients with gout from Hong Kong compared 276 patients treated with febuxostat with 828 patients with allopurinol. Both groups had similar rates of major cardiovascular events.[39] Some studies have also shown contrary results. A national health insurance database from Taiwan compared rates of cardiovascular events in nearly 44,000 patients treated each with febuxostat and allopurinol, and found greater rates of heart failure and cardiovascular death in those treated with febuxostat.[40] A recent systematic review compiled 10 studies of patients treated with allopurinol or febuxostat. Patients on allopurinol between doses of 100 and 300 mg compared with those on 40 mg daily febuxostat had similar blood pressure, cardiovascular events (myocardial infarction and stroke), and cardiovascular mortality.[41] Thus, at this stage there is little definitive evidence that febuxostat has worse cardiovascular outcomes than febuxostat. However, it is imperative to understand that patients with gout are at a greater risk of cardiovascular events, and need careful monitoring for both cardiovascular risk as well as management of such cardiovascular risk factors.

Key Messages

- Risk of cardiovascular events is increased in gout. However, there is little definitive evidence to conclusively support increase in cardiovascular risk with febuxostat compared with allopurinol.
- Physicians should actively seek and manage cardiovascular risk in patients with gout.

ARTICLE 13

Diagnosis of osteoporosis in statin-treated patients is dose-dependent

Leutner M, Matzhold C, Bellach L, Deischinger C, Harreiter J, Thurner S, et al. Diagnosis of osteoporosis in statin-treated patients is dose-dependent.
Ann Rheum Dis. 2019;78:1706-11.

Abstract*

Objective: It is still not completely understood whether inhibition of 3-hydroxy-3-methyl-glutaryl-coenzyme A (HMG-CoA)-reductase, which is the primary mechanism of statins, has a role in the pathogenesis of osteoporosis. This study was conducted for assessing the association of different types and dosages of statins with osteoporosis. It was hypothesized that the inhibition of the cholesterol synthesis could have an impact on the sex hormones and thus the diagnosis of osteoporosis.

Methods: This study included medical claims data of all Austrians from 2006 to 2007 for recognizing the patients who were treated with statins to calculate their daily defined dose averages of six different kinds of statins. Multiple logistic regression was applied for evaluating the dose-dependent risks of being diagnosed with osteoporosis for each statin individually.

Results: In the general study population, when compared to controls, statin treatment was found to be associated with an over-representation of diagnosed osteoporosis [odds ratio (OR) 3.62; 95% confidence interval (CI) 3.55–3.69; p < 0.01]. A highly nontrivial dependence of statin dosage was observed with the ORs of osteoporosis. Osteoporosis was under-represented in low-dose statin treatment (0–10 mg/day), consisting of lovastatin (OR 0.39; CI 0.18–0.84; p < 0.05); pravastatin (OR 0.68; 95% CI 0.52–0.89; p < 0.01); simvastatin (OR 0.70; 95% CI 0.56–0.86; p < 0.01); and rosuvastatin (OR 0.69; 95% CI 0.55–0.87; p < 0.01). The exceeding of the 40 mg threshold for simvastatin (OR 1.64; 95% CI 1.31–2.07; p < 0.01), and the exceeding of a 20 mg threshold for atorvastatin (OR 1.78; 95% CI 1.41–2.23; p < 0.01) and for rosuvastatin (OR 2.04; 95% CI 1.31–3.18; p < 0.01) was associated with an over-representation of osteoporosis.

Conclusion: It can be concluded that in statin-treated patients, the diagnosis of osteoporosis is dose-dependent. Therefore, in low-dose treatment, osteoporosis is under-represented; in high-dose statin treatment, osteoporosis is over-represented. This indicates the significance of future studies considering dose-dependency while examining the association between statins and osteoporosis. *Redrafted abstract

"Statin therapy and osteoporosis—may coexist, but not necessarily causal!"

COMMENT

Osteoporosis is the most common metabolic bone disease seen in the community, while statins are one of the most commonly used drugs for both primary and secondary prevention of cardiovascular disease. The effect of statin therapy on bone health may be dose-related. Data is available to show that low doses of statins are associated with a reduced risk for osteoporosis. However, high doses have been linked to an increased risk of the bone disease. A recent study from health claims data from Austria assessed whether statin use and osteoporosis were related.

The study revealed that overall, the use of statins was associated with a significantly higher odd of more than three and a half times of also being co-diagnosed with osteoporosis. The association between statin use and osteoporosis was dose-dependent. While the lowest dose ranges of statins did not associate the osteoporosis (rather was associated with lesser odds of osteoporosis), those individuals treated with at least 20 mg of atorvastatin or rosuvastatin or at least 40 mg of pravastatin had greater odds of having also received a concomitant diagnosis of osteoporosis.[42]

Information regarding statin use and osteoporosis/bone health is controversial. Another recent cohort study actually identified a lesser risk of vertebral fractures in those individuals with rheumatoid arthritis treated with statins.[43] Mechanistic links also exist to explain the positive association of lower levels of low-density lipoprotein cholesterol (LDL-C) with higher bone mass.[44,45] With lower dosages of statins, the osteoprotective effect of bone morphogenetic protein 2 (BMP-2) could be one of the reasons for the lower rates of osteoporosis. At higher dosages, statins lower cholesterol, from which estrogen is derived. This could be a possible explanation for the deleterious effect on bone health. However, there could well be other factors at play. When comorbidities requiring statin therapy coexist with osteoporosis, it is difficult to link causally statin use with osteoporosis. Physicians should be aware about the need to manage adequately all existing comorbid conditions in their patients.

Key Messages

- *Comorbid conditions such as cardiovascular disease and osteoporosis might coexist.*
- *It is essential to detect and treat all comorbid conditions in the individual patient.*

ARTICLE 14

Fibrotic cytokine interplay in evaluation of disease activity in treatment naïve systemic sclerosis patients from Western india

Khadilkar PV, Khopkar US, Nadkar MY, Rajadhyaksha AG, Chougule DA, Deshpande SD, et al. Fibrotic cytokine interplay in evaluation of disease activity in treatment naïve systemic sclerosis patients from Western India. *J Assoc Physicians India. 2019;67:26-30.*

Abstract

Background: Systemic sclerosis (SSc) is a demyelinating disease of skin, subcutaneous tissue, muscles, and internal organs, with fibrosis as an important pathological event.

Aim: To understand cytokine interplay of interleukin (IL)-1β, IL-4, and IL-6 and their association with disease activity in treatment naïve active cases of SSc from Western India.

Methods: Twenty-five SSc patients as per ACR-EULAR 2013 criteria (classified based on pulmonary fibrosis and generalized fibrosis) and 25 age–sex-matched controls were enrolled. Serum cytokine levels of IL-1β, IL-4, and IL-6 were assessed by multiplex bead based immunoassay.

Results: Ten patients had interstitial lung disease (ILD); whereas, 16 patients had generalized fibrosis. Antinuclear antibodies were seen in 22 patients (88%), antiScl70 in 15 patients (60%), and anticentromere antibodies in 5 patients (20%). Serum levels of IL-1β in patients were significantly higher than healthy controls (p = 0.0006). IL-4 levels in all SSc patients were marginally raised (p = 0.0102), while IL-6 levels were significantly raised (p < 0.0001). IL-4 was found to be significantly raised in SSc patients with ILD (p = 0.021) as compared to patients without ILD. IL-1β (p = 0.0293) and IL-4 (p < 0.0001) were significantly higher in SSc patients with fibrosis. On the contrary, IL-6 levels in patients with fibrosis were found to be lower than in patients without fibrosis.

Conclusion: Significantly raised cytokine levels among treatment naïve SSc patients were found to be associated with higher disease severity in our study. Higher levels of IL-1β and IL-6 indicated an active inflammatory status, whereas significantly raised IL-4 levels indicated at higher fibrotic activity.

"IL-6—a cytokine for targeting in systemic sclerosis?"

| COMMENT |

Systemic sclerosis (SSc) is an uncommon systemic fibrosing disease. Apart from skin, internal organ involvement like the lungs, heart, kidneys, or the gastrointestinal tract is common and influences outcome. A major cause of morbidity is interstitial lung disease (ILD). The exact pathobiology of this disease continues to be enigmatic. Cytokines are known to play a role in driving fibrosis, and reflect differing polarization of T lymphocytes and other immune cells. A study from India reported levels of cytokines interleukin (IL)-1β, IL-4, and IL-6 in 25 patients with SSc compared to 25 healthy controls. Patients with SSc-associated ILD had higher levels of IL-4 and IL-1β, with lower levels of IL-6. Overall, the study was limited and had a small sample size; however, SSc is a rare disease.[46]

A previous report comparing 93 patients with SSc with 33 healthy controls indicated higher levels of the cytokines IL-6, IL-17, and transforming growth factor-beta (TGF-β) in patients with SSc ILD compared to those without.[47] Cytokines play an important role in disease pathogenesis of SSc. This has become more evident by the successful targeting of cytokines to ameliorate disease processes associated with SSc, such as IL-6 targeting by tocilizumab.[5] However, given the multiplicity of cytokines involved, targeting of any one cytokine is unlikely to provide sustained relief.

Key Messages

◉ *Cytokine abnormalities underlie pathogenesis of SSc.*

◉ *Drugs targeting cytokines such as IL-6 pathway blockade with tocilizumab might help in treatment of SSc.*

ARTICLE 15A

Standardizing initial dilution titers of antinuclear antibodies for the screening of systemic lupus erythematosus

Rao JS, Shobha V, Thomas T, Kini U. Standardizing initial dilution titers of antinuclear antibodies for the screening of systemic lupus erythematosus.
Indian J Rheumatol. 2019;14:211-7.

Abstract*

Background: Systemic lupus erythematosus (SLE) is a systemic autoimmune disease; diagnosis of SLE is done by correlation of clinical features with a positive antinuclear antibody (ANA) test. For screening of SLE, ANA detection is done by indirect immunofluorescence (IIF), which depends on initial dilution titers that need population-specific standardization. For the population of South India, there is a lack of exclusive commercial kits; therefore, standardization of initial screening dilution titers for ANA is essential for differentiating SLE and other rheumatic diseases from the healthy.

Methods: This was a prospective study that included newly diagnosed SLE patients of 18–60 years of age and healthy controls from South India; the study was conducted for duration of 8 months (from September, 2015 to April, 2016). According to kit recommendations, serum samples were subjected to ANA-IIF in dilution titers of 1:40, 1:80, and 1:100. Clinical correlation of IIF intensity and staining patterns was performed; statistically analysis was done.

Results: In 2.1% of healthy controls, ANA positivity in dilutions of 1:40 and 1:80 was noted and was negative at 1:100. Nearly 97.9% patients with SLE were found to be positive at 1:100 dilution. The most common patterns were speckled pattern (in 52.1% patients) and homogeneous (37.4%). The patterns were best appreciated in 1:100 dilution; a high significant measure of agreement of kappa was noted between the two pathologists for patterns as well as intensity at all three dilutions.

Conclusion: For differentiating SLE patterns from normal healthy individuals, the best screening dilution is 1:100. Its major benefit is the delineation of different patterns of ANA when positive, particularly when mixed at this lower dilution. *Redrafted abstract

ARTICLE 15B

Clinical use of anti-DFS70 autoantibodies

Kang SY, Lee WI, Kim MH, Jeon YL. Clinical use of anti-DFS70 autoantibodies.
Rheumatol Int. 2019;39:1423-9.

Abstract

The dense fine speckled (DFS) nuclear pattern is one of the most common indirect immunofluorescence (IIF) patterns detected during routine antinuclear antibody (ANA) screening. There is a negative association between anti-DFS70 status and systemic autoimmune rheumatic disease (SARD), especially in the absence of concomitant SARD-specific autoantibodies. The purpose of this study was to determine the need for confirming anti-DFS70 status when a DFS pattern is observed in IIF-ANA. The frequency of anti-DFS70 detection on Western blot and the positive rate of connective tissue disease (CTD)-related autoantibody screening with a fluorescence-based enzyme immunoassay was evaluated in DFS (n = 182) and non-DFS (n = 359) groups. Specific autoantibodies against 15 autoantigens were identified by line immunoassay. We evaluated the frequency of cases of DFS mistaken for non-DFS and non-DFS cases mistaken for DFS, as well as the clinical impacts of these misinterpretations. Among cases of IIF-ANA with an observable DFS pattern, 68.1% had only anti-DFS70 without CTD-related autoantibodies, 20.3% were false positive for IIF-ANA, and the remaining 11.5% had CTD-related autoantibodies independent of anti-DFS70 status. These results indicated that CTD-related autoantibodies may be present with or without anti-DFS70 even if a DFS pattern is observed in IIF-ANA. Among patients who are ANA negative or have a low probability of SARD, an anti-DFS70 confirmation test has no clinical benefit and cannot replace specific tests for detecting CTD-related autoantibodies. Specific tests to detect CTD-related autoantibodies should be performed instead of anti-DFS70 confirmation tests when a DFS pattern is observed in IIF-ANA.

"Significance of newer ANA patterns like dense fine speckled needs to be elucidated."

COMMENT

Antinuclear antibodies (ANAs) are a key investigation to diagnose connective tissue diseases (CTDs). Patients with systemic lupus erythematosus (SLE) almost always have presence of ANA. ANA can be detected by various means. However, the gold standard remains the use of indirect immunofluorescence (IIF). IIF helps to detect the pattern of fluorescence based on pattern of binding of ANA in serum to targets in the nucleus, on cells with large nuclei such as Hep2 cells.[48] ANA is sometimes also reported using enzyme-linked immunosorbent assay (ELISA). While this technique is easy to do, it has associated fallacies, due to the loss of native structure of nuclear antigens while coating them on a microtiter plate, instead of retaining their native structure on the nucleus of the cell as in the case of detection by IIF.[49] Detection of ANA by IIF requires considerable skill on the behalf of the examiner, as well as the need to establish population-specific cut-offs for dilution of sera.[49] A previous study from North India had proposed a cut-off of 1:80 dilution;[50] however, the study was conducted nearly a decade back, during which period detection kits for ANA by IIF have undergone significant improvements to increase sensitivity and specificity.

In this context, a recent study from South India evaluated ANA by IIF in 238 patients with SLE compared with 300 healthy controls. Speckled pattern of ANA and homogenous pattern were the most common patterns seen in lupus. An optimal dilution was 1:100 (area under the curve was 97%). At a 1:100 dilution, speckled ANA pattern at 2+ intensity of fluorescence had 98% sensitivity and 100% specific for the diagnosis of lupus in this cohort.[51] This study emphasizes the need to validate the optimal dilution of ANA in a population before adopting for clinical use as well as repeat this exercise from time-to-time, since such figures might vary from population to population.

A recently described ANA pattern has been the anti-dense fine speckled (anti-DFS) antibody pattern. This pattern was initially thought to be present only, in those without a definitive connective tissue disease (CTD).[52] However, information in this area is still evolving. A recent study from South Korea compared 182 patients with an anti-DFS antinuclear antibody pattern on immunofluorescence on Hep-2 cells with 359 individuals without an anti-DFS ANA pattern. Furthermore, line immunoassay, a more specific technique, was used to confirm the presence of anti-DFS70 antibodies. The study identified that anti-DFS ANA pattern on immunofluorescence could be identified in a small proportion of patients with connective tissue diseases (CTDs) like lupus and Sjögren's syndrome also, although a majority did not have CTD. The presence of anti-DFS ANA pattern did not perfectly correlate with presence of anti-DFS 70 antibodies by line immunoassay.[53] Thus, some patients with presence of anti-DFS ANA pattern on immunofluorescence might still have CTDs. It is important to reiterate that the clinical judgment of the treating physician should always take precedence rather than relying on investigation parameters to detect and treat CTDs.

Key Messages

- ⊙ *Optimum titer for dilution of sera for testing antinuclear antibodies needs to be established in different populations and revised over time. In a South Indian population, an optimum dilution might be 1:100.*
- ⊙ *Dense fine speckled pattern is a newly described ANA pattern. Although in some Western populations, it has been noted to have little significance for connective tissue diseases; its significance in an Indian population remains to be determined.*

ARTICLE 16A

Prescribing patterns and safety of biologics in immune-mediated rheumatic diseases: Karnataka biologics cohort study group experience

Shobha V, Rao V, Desai AM, Jois R, Srikantiah C, Dharmanand BG, et al. Prescribing patterns and safety of biologics in immune-mediated rheumatic diseases: Karnataka biologics cohort study group experience.
Indian J Rheumatol. 2019;14:17-20.

Abstract*

Introduction: For treatment of autoimmune rheumatologic diseases (AIRDs), biologics are extensively used. But, overemphasis cannot be laid on the requirement to collect real-life data, which measures indications and adverse reactions.

Methods: This was a cross-sectional ambidirectional multicenter study, which was conducted by members of the Karnataka Rheumatology Association in 12 Tertiary Care Rheumatology Centers in Karnataka, India. The study was carried out for a period of 8 months (from January, 2016 to August, 2016).

Results: Tumor necrosis factor antagonist etanercept was the biologic that was most commonly prescribed. The most common indication for biologics was spondyloarthropathy group of disorders. Clinical improvement was stated as the most common cause for stopping biologics by patients. Discontinuation of biologics was present in only 4.8% of patients because of adverse drug reactions (ADRs).

Conclusion: In all the centers, the patterns of prescription, method of use, prebiologics screening methods, and adverse event profile were comparable. Across all the centers, consistency in prescreening for latent tuberculosis (TB) was observed. TB prophylaxis is effective in prevention of its reactivation.
*Redrafted abstract

ARTICLE 16B

Incidence of infection other than tuberculosis in patients with autoimmune rheumatic diseases treated with bDMARDs: a real-time clinical experience from India

Chandrashekara S, Shobha V, Rao V, Desai A, Jois R, Dharmanand BG, et al. Incidence of infection other than tuberculosis in patients with autoimmune rheumatic diseases treated with bDMARDs: A real-time clinical experience from India. *Rheumatol Int. 2019;39:497-507.*

Abstract

Biologic disease-modifying antirheumatic drugs (bDMARD) have transformed the treatment paradigm of chronic autoimmune rheumatic diseases (ARDs), but they are often associated with adverse drug reactions. The present study evaluated the frequency, characteristics, and type of infections, other than tuberculosis (TB), in ARD patients receiving bDMARDs. The multicentre, cross-sectional, retrospective, observational study was conducted across 12 centers in Karnataka, India, between January and August, 2016. The study included patients receiving bDMARD therapy for various ARDs. Outcome variables considered were any infection, minor infections, and major infections, other than TB. Clinical variables were compared between infection and no infection group, and the increase in the likelihood of infection with respect to various clinical variables was assessed. The study involved 209 subjects with a median (range) age of 41 (16–84) years and male to female ratio of 0.97:1. A total of 29 (13.88%) subjects developed infection following bDMARD therapy, out of whom a majority had minor infection (n = 26). The likelihood of developing any infection was noted to be more in subjects receiving anti-tumor necrosis factor (TNF) (golimumab, p = 0.03) and those on three or more conventional synthetic (cs) DMARDs (p < 0.01). Infection risk was higher in patients with systemic lupus erythematosus (p = 0.04), other connective tissue disease (p < 0.01), and in patients with comorbidities (p = 0.13). The risk of infection was associated with the use of anti-TNF therapy and more than three csDMARDs, comorbidities and Adds such as systemic lupus erythematosus and connective tissue disease.

"Remember, infections—tuberculosis and others—may occur with biological DMARDs!"

COMMENT

Biological disease-modifying antirheumatic drugs (DMARDs) directly target pathological biological processes, and form an important component of the armamentarium for the treatment of various rheumatic diseases. Increasing availability of biosimilar DMARDs in India as well as the reducing costs of biologic DMARDs have resulted in overall greater accessibility to biologic DMARDs across India.[54] Two recent multicentric studies from a collaborative effort from Southern India assessed the real-life patterns of biological drugs use as well as safety signals associated with the use of these drugs. The first study reported 411 patients treated with biological DMARDs. Most common biological agents used were antitumor necrosis factor-alpha agents, the most often used was etanercept, possibly related to its administration by the subcutaneous route. The diseases for which biological DMARDs were used most commonly were spondyloarthropathies, followed by rheumatoid arthritis, psoriatic arthritis, systemic lupus erythematosus (SLE), and vasculitis. Despite SLE and vasculitis being relatively uncommon diseases, still they feature prominently in the list of diseases for which biological DMARD was used in this cross-sectional data. All patients had been screened for latent tuberculosis infection (LTBI) with either a Mantoux test or interferon gamma release assay (IGRA), along with a chest radiograph. The 8% detected to have LTBI were treated with anti-tubercular therapy in prophylactic doses. Despite this, 4% developed tuberculosis infection after biological therapy. However, it was reassuring that none of those who received prophylactic antitubercular therapy developed tuberculosis reactivation.[55]

The other study from the same collaborative effort described patterns of infections other than tuberculosis in 209 patients on biological DMARD therapy. Of these, 14% developed infective episodes during follow-up, and most of these were minor infections. The authors identified a greater risk of infection in those treated with anti-TNF agents, those with SLE and other connective tissue diseases as the indication for biological DMARD, presence of comorbid conditions such as diabetes and chronic renal impairment, and those concomitantly receiving three or more conventional DMARDs in addition.[56] These findings emphasize the relative safety of biological DMARDs in Indian population, while enhancing the need to be aware of the propensity of these patients to develop infections and monitor for this.

Key Messages

- Infections (tuberculosis and others) might occur in patients on biological DMARDs, although these occur only in a minority.
- Always screen for latent tuberculosis before starting any biological DMARD in a patient in India.
- Clinicians should surveil patients for infections while on any DMARD therapy and appropriately treat the same.

ARTICLE 17

Physicians perception of rheumatology practice and training in India

Misra DP, Ravindran V, Sharma A, Wakhlu A, Negi VS, Chaturvedi V, et al. Physicians perception of rheumatology practice and training in India.

J Assoc Physicians India. 2019;67:38-43.

Abstract

Objective: To assess physicians' perception and their felt competence in dealing with patients with rheumatic complaints.

Methods: We assessed the quantum of rheumatological disorders seen by physicians in India, their felt competency in dealing with such patients, and their perceived adequacy of undergraduate and postgraduate medical training in rheumatology by means of an anonymized questionnaire conducted at the annual national conference of internal medicine specialists.

Results: Our analysis of 333 respondents revealed that while they saw an average of 10 patients with rheumatic complaints every month, the felt competence in dealing with such cases was only a median of 6/10 (interquartile range 5–7). About 75% professed little or no exposure to rheumatology as undergraduates, whereas, only 20% perceived adequacy of training during internal medicine residency to treat such diseases confidently. About 78.37% and 67.7% perceived an inadequacy of rheumatology training at undergraduate and postgraduate level respectively, and 83% felt the need for further training or sensitization in rheumatology.

Conclusion: There remains an unmet need to enhance existing undergraduate and postgraduate internal medicine curricula in India to impart greater skills in the diagnosis and management of rheumatic diseases. Initiatives and government funding to establish short-term training courses in rheumatology for established internal medicine faculty, to enable them to provide basic rheumatology services at their respective hospitals, are urgently needed.

"Rheumatology curriculum at the undergraduate and postgraduate training level in India needs improvement."

COMMENT

Rheumatic diseases are one of the most common causes of morbidity in the community. Up to 10–15% of the Indian population suffer from musculoskeletal complaints. Hence, training in diagnosis and management of rheumatic diseases is important for the general physician and for an internal medicine specialist.[57,58] However, there exists a substantial unmet need in this area. Patient numbers are huge and trained rheumatologists are a tiny number. Against this backdrop, Misra et al. have scientifically and systematically captured real-world information on the conditions prevalent in India. Refreshing feature of the survey is that the authors have not only outlined the problems but also listed possible solutions.

The present survey conducted at the national medical conference in 2018 assessed the perspectives of internists regarding the burden of musculoskeletal complaints seen by them as well as the perceived adequacy of rheumatology training at the undergraduate and postgraduate medical training levels. The authors surveyed >300 physicians, a majority of whom had been in practice for <5 years. Nearly 80% of the physicians felt that undergraduate rheumatology training was inadequate, whereas two-thirds felt that postgraduate rheumatology training was inadequate. Most of the surveyed physicians felt a need to enhance undergraduate and postgraduate curricula in rheumatology. This could be achieved by including mandatory questions related to rheumatology and including basic joint examination in the final MBBS examination, as well as having long cases related to rheumatology in the final MD/DNB medicine examinations. Such measures might help to enhance the outreach of rheumatology services in the community, since formal subspecialty training courses in this specialty remain few and far between.[59,60]

Key Messages

- *Patients with rheumatic diseases are often seen by the internist in daily practice.*

- *A majority of the sampled internists professed a lack of exposure to rheumatology at the undergraduate curriculum and during postgraduate internal medicine curricula.*

- *Stakeholders should consider improving the representation of rheumatology during undergraduate and postgraduate medical training.*

ARTICLE 18

Mycophenolate mofetil versus cyclophosphamide for remission induction in ANCA-associated vasculitis: a randomised, non-inferiority trial

Jones RB, Hiemstra TF, Ballarin J, Blockmans DE, Brogan P, Bruchfeld A, et al.; European Vasculitis Study Group (EUVAS).
Mycophenolate mofetil versus cyclophosphamide for remission induction in ANCA-associated vasculitis: a randomised, non-inferiority trial.
Ann Rheum Dis. 2019;78:399-405.

Abstract*

Objective: For the treatment of antineutrophil cytoplasmic antibody (ANCA)-associated vasculitis (AAV), cyclophosphamide induction regimens are reported to be effective. However, these are associated with infertility, infections, and malignancies. In small studies of AAV, mycophenolate mofetil (MMF) has demonstrated high-remission rates.

Methods: This randomized controlled trial evaluated whether for remission induction in AAV, MMF was noninferior than cyclophosphamide. Total 140 diagnosed patients were included, which were randomized to receive either MMF or pulsed cyclophosphamide. Same oral glucocorticoid regimen was given to all patients, who were switched to azathioprine after remission. The primary endpoint in the study was remission by 6 months needing compliance with the tapering of the glucocorticoid regimen. Exclusion criteria included patients who had estimated glomerular filtration rate (eGFR) <15 mL/min.

Results: Among groups, at baseline, there were no significant differences in terms of ANCA subtype, disease activity, and organ involvement. For the primary remission endpoint, noninferiority was showed, which was present in 67% (n = 47) patients in the MMF group and 61% (n = 43) patients in the cyclophosphamide group [risk difference 5.7%; 90% confidence interval (CI) −7.5% to 19%]. After remission, there were more relapses in the MMF group (33%, n = 23) than the cyclophosphamide group (19%, n = 13) (incidence rate ratio 1.97; 95% CI 0.96 to 4.23; p = 0.049). In patients of myeloperoxidase (MPO)-ANCA group, relapses were present in 12% and 15% patients of the cyclophosphamide group and MMF group, respectively. In patients of PR3-ANCA group, relapses were present in 24% and 48% patients of the cyclophosphamide group and MMF group, respectively. There was no significant difference in serious infections between groups (MMF vs. cyclophosphamide group, 26% vs. 17%) [odds ratio (OR) 1.67; 95% CI 0.68–4.19; p = 0.3].

Conclusion: It can be concluded that although MMF was noninferior to cyclophosphamide for remission induction in AAV, it led to higher relapse rate.

Trial registration number: NCT00414128. *Redrafted abstract

"MMF might not be good for induction of remission in ANCA-associated vasculitis!"

COMMENT

Vasculitis refers to systemic diseases associated with inflammation of the vessels. Antineutrophil cytoplasmic antibody (ANCA)-associated vasculitis (AAV) is a form of small vessel vasculitis associated with lung nodules, pulmonary hemorrhage, glomerulonephritis, palpable purpura, and mononeuritis multiplex as its predominant manifestations. Patients with AAV require high degree of immunosuppressive therapy in the form of cyclophosphamide or rituximab for systemic manifestations, along with high-dose corticosteroids.[61]

Cyclophosphamide can be used orally or as intravenous infusion. Despite being effective, oral cyclophosphamide is infrequently used because of the higher cumulative dose delivered by oral administration. There is an increasing tendency among rheumatologists to limit exposure to cyclophosphamide given its long-term toxicity. Many rheumatologists use monthly cyclophosphamide pulses to induce remission and switch over to maintenance therapies after 6 months. Rituximab is employed as an alternative to cyclophosphamide in organ-threatening or life-threatening AAV. The agents used for maintenance therapy in AAV include rituximab, azathioprine, methotrexate, or mycophenolate mofetil (MMF).

A recent study evaluated MMF as an alternative induction agent in patients with AAV. In a population with predominantly milder disease, the proportion of patients attaining remission in cyclophosphamide and MMF groups was similar. However, patients on MMF were more likely to relapse, particularly if they positive for antiproteinase 3 (anti-PR3) antibodies (which produce a cytoplasmic pattern on neutrophils on immunofluorescence).[62] In the authors' opinion, MMF should only be considered as an agent for induction of remission in milder presentations of AAV, with cyclophosphamide or rituximab reserved for more severe manifestations. However, MMF might be used as a reserve agent for maintenance of remission in AAV, with preferable agents being rituximab or azathioprine for which the evidence is more robust.[63]

Key Messages

◉ *Cyclophosphamide or rituximab remains the agents of choice for remission induction in AAV.*

◉ *Mycophenolate mofetil might be suitable for induction of remission in those with milder AAV.*

REFERENCES (Rheumatology and Immunology)

1. Dixon WG, Beukenhorst AL, Yimer BB, Cook L, Gasparrini A, El-Hay T, et al. How the weather affects the pain of citizen scientists using a smartphone app. NPJ Digit Med. 2019;2:105.

2. Timmermans EJ, van der Pas S, Dennison EM, Maggi S, Peter R, Castell MV, et al. The Influence of Weather Conditions on Outdoor Physical Activity Among Older People With and Without Osteoarthritis in 6 European Countries. J Phys Act Health. 2016;13:1385-95.

3. Fagerlund AJ, Iversen M, Ekeland A, Moen CM, Aslaksen PM. Blame it on the weather? The association between pain in fibromyalgia, relative humidity, temperature and barometric pressure. PLoS One. 2019;14:e0216902.

4. Cutolo M, Smith V, Furst DE, Khanna D, Herrick AL. Points to consider-Raynaud's phenomenon in systemic sclerosis. Rheumatology (Oxford). 2017;56:v45-8.

5. Misra DP, Ahmed S, Agarwal V. Is biological therapy in systemic sclerosis the answer? Rheumatol Int. 2020;40:679-94.

6. Flaherty KR, Wells AU, Cottin V, Devaraj A, Walsh SLF, Inoue Y, et al. Nintedanib in Progressive Fibrosing Interstitial Lung Diseases. N Engl J Med. 2019;381:1718-27.

7. Kolb M, Raghu G, Wells AU, Behr J, Richeldi L, Schinzel B, et al. Nintedanib plus Sildenafil in Patients with Idiopathic Pulmonary Fibrosis. N Engl J Med. 2018;379:1722-31.

8. Distler O, Highland KB, Gahlemann M, Azuma A, Fischer A, Mayes MD, et al. Nintedanib for Systemic Sclerosis–Associated Interstitial Lung Disease. 2019;380:2518-28.

9. Misra DP, Negi VS. Interferon targeted therapies in systemic lupus erythematosus. Mediterr J Rheumatol. 2017;28:13-9.

10. Furie RA, Morand EF, Bruce IN, Manzi S, Kalunian KC, Vital EM, et al. Type I interferon inhibitor anifrolumab in active systemic lupus erythematosus (TULIP-1): a randomised, controlled, phase 3 trial. The Lancet Rheumatol. 2019;1:e208-19.

11. Morand EF, Furie R, Tanaka Y, Bruce IN, Askanase AD, Richez C, et al. Trial of Anifrolumab in Active Systemic Lupus Erythematosus. N Eng J Med. 2020;382:211-21.

12. Evans S. When and how can endpoints be changed after initiation of a randomized clinical trial? PLoS Clin Trials. 2007;2:e18.

13. Morand EF, Mosca M. Treat to target, remission and low disease activity in SLE. Best Pract Res Clin Rheumatol. 2017;31:342-50.

14. Tselios K, Gladman DD, Urowitz MB. How can we define low disease activity in systemic lupus erythematosus? Semin Arthritis Rheum. 2019;48:1035-40.

15. Golder V, Kandane-Rathnayake R, Huq M, Louthrenoo W, Luo SF, Jan YJ, et al. Evaluation of remission definitions for systemic lupus erythematosus: a prospective cohort study. The Lancet Rheumatol. 2019;1:e103-10.

16. Sammaritano LR. Contraception and preconception counseling in women with autoimmune disease. Best Pract Res Clin Obstet Gynaecol. 2020.64:11-23.

17. Marder W. Update on pregnancy complications in systemic lupus erythematosus. Curr Opin Rheumatol. 2019;31:650-8.

18. Mendel A, Bernatsky S, Pineau CA, St-Pierre Y, Hanly JG, Urowitz MB, et al. Use of combined hormonal contraceptives among women with systemic lupus erythematosus with and without medical contraindications to oestrogen. Rheumatology (Oxford). 2019;58:1259-67.

19. Schett G, Emery P, Tanaka Y, Burmester G, Pisetsky DS, Naredo E, et al. Tapering biologic and conventional DMARD therapy in rheumatoid arthritis: current evidence and future directions. Ann Rheum Dis. 2016;75:1428-37.

20. Brahe CH, Krabbe S, Østergaard M, Ørnbjerg L, Glinatsi D, Røgind H, et al. Dose tapering and discontinuation of biological therapy in rheumatoid arthritis patients in routine care – 2-year outcomes and predictors. Rheumatology (Oxford). 2018;58:110-9.

21. van Mulligen E, de Jong PHP, Kuijper TM, van der Ven M, Appels C, Bijkerk C, et al. Gradual tapering TNF inhibitors versus conventional synthetic DMARDs after achieving controlled disease in patients with rheumatoid arthritis: first-year results of the randomised controlled TARA study. Ann Rheum Dis. 2019;78:746.

22. Parida JR, Misra DP, Wakhlu A, Agarwal V. Is non-biological treatment of rheumatoid arthritis as good as biologics? World J Orthop. 2015;6:278-83.

23. Stouten V, Westhovens R, Pazmino S, De Cock D, Van der Elst K, Joly J, et al. Effectiveness of different combinations of DMARDs and glucocorticoid bridging in early rheumatoid arthritis: two-year results of CareRA. Rheumatology (Oxford). 2019;58:2284-94.

24. Choy EH. Clinical significance of Janus Kinase inhibitor selectivity. Rheumatology. 2018;58:953-62.

25. Fleischmann RM, Genovese MC, Enejosa JV, Mysler E, Bessette L, Peterfy C, et al. Safety and effectiveness of upadacitinib or adalimumab plus methotrexate in patients with rheumatoid arthritis over 48 weeks with switch to alternate therapy in patients with insufficient response. Anna Rheum Dis. 2019;78:1454-62.

26. van Vollenhoven RF, Fleischmann R, Cohen S, Lee EB, Meijide JAG, Wagner S, et al. Tofacitinib or adalimumab versus placebo in rheumatoid arthritis. N Engl J Med. 2012;367:508-19.

27. Kingsley GH, Kowalczyk A, Taylor H, Ibrahim F, Packham JC, McHugh NJ, et al. A randomized placebo-controlled trial of methotrexate in psoriatic arthritis. Rheumatology (Oxford). 2012;51:1368-77.

28. Appani SK, Devarasetti PK, Irlapati RVP, Rajasekhar L. Methotrexate achieves major cDAPSA response, and improvement in dactylitis and functional status in psoriatic arthritis. Rheumatology (Oxford). 2018;58:869-73.

29. Nurmohamed MT, Kitas G. Cardiovascular risk in rheumatoid arthritis and diabetes: how does it compare and when does it start? Ann Rheum Dis. 2011;70:881-3.

30. Kitas GD, Nightingale P, Armitage J, Sattar N, Belch JJF, Symmons DPM, et al. A Multicenter, Randomized, Placebo-Controlled Trial of Atorvastatin for the Primary Prevention of Cardiovascular Events in Patients With Rheumatoid Arthritis. Arthritis Rheumatol. 2019;71:1437-49.

31. Nurmohamed MT, Heslinga M, Kitas GD. Cardiovascular comorbidity in rheumatic diseases. Nat Rev Rheumatol. 2015;11:693-704.

32. Malgutte D, Waghmare I, Bhute V, Joshi A, Gokhale Y. Non-ischemic Cardiomyopathy: Role of Immunologic Work-up and Cardiac MRI in Etiologic Diagnosis and Outcomes. J Assoc Physicians India. 2019;67:30-4.

33. Mavrogeni SI, Kitas GD, Dimitroulas T, Sfikakis PP, Seo P, Gabriel S, et al. Cardiovascular magnetic resonance in rheumatology: Current status and recommendations for use. Int J Cardiol. 2016;217:135-48.

34. Markousis-Mavrogenis G, Bournia VK, Panopoulos S, Koutsogeorgopoulou L, Kanoupakis G, Apostolou D, et al. Cardiovascular Magnetic Resonance Identifies High-Risk Systemic Sclerosis Patients with Normal Echocardiograms and Provides Incremental Prognostic Value. Diagnostics (Basel). 2019;9:220.

35. Saminathan M, Sharma R, Gogna A, Rani A, Kapoor R. Correlation of Inflammatory Markers and Disease Severity with Cardiovascular Autonomic Dysfunction in Indian Patients with Rheumatoid Arthritis. Indian J Rheumatol. 2019;14:123-6.

36. Amigues I, Tugcu A, Russo C, Giles JT, Morgenstein R, Zartoshti A, et al. Myocardial Inflammation, Measured Using 18-Fluorodeoxyglucose Positron Emission Tomography With Computed Tomography, Is Associated With Disease Activity in Rheumatoid Arthritis. Arthritis Rheumatol. 2019;71:496-506.

37. White WB, Saag KG, Becker MA, Borer JS, Gorelick PB, Whelton A, et al. Cardiovascular Safety of Febuxostat or Allopurinol in Patients with Gout. N Engl J Med. 2018;378:1200-10.

38. Kang EH, Choi HK, Shin A, Lee YJ, Lee EB, Song YW, et al. Comparative cardiovascular risk of allopurinol versus febuxostat in patients with gout: a nation-wide cohort study. Rheumatology (Oxford). 2019;58:2122-9.

39. Ju C, Lai RWC, Li KHC, Hung JKF, Lai JCL, Ho J, et al. Comparative cardiovascular risk in users versus non-users of xanthine oxidase inhibitors and febuxostat versus allopurinol users. Rheumatology (Oxford). 2019; Online ahead of print.

40. Su CY, Shen LJ, Hsieh SC, Lin LY, Lin FJ. Comparing Cardiovascular Safety of Febuxostat and Allopurinol in the Real World: A Population-Based Cohort Study. Mayo Clin Proc. 2019;94:1147-57.

41. Barrientos-Regala M, Macabeo RA, Ramirez-Ragasa R, Pestaño NS, Punzalan FER, Tumanan-Mendoza B, et al. The Association of Febuxostat Compared to Allopurinol on Blood Pressure and Major Adverse Cardiac Events (MACE) Among Adult Patients with Hyperuricemia: A Meta-Analysis. J Cardiovasc Pharmacol. 2020; Online ahead of print.

42. Leutner M, Matzhold C, Bellach L, Deischinger C, Harreiter J, Thurner S, et al. Diagnosis of osteoporosis in statin-treated patients is dose-dependent. Ann Rheum Dis. 2019;78:1706.

43. Ozen G, Pedro S, Wolfe F, Michaud K. Medications associated with fracture risk in patients with rheumatoid arthritis. Ann Rheum Dis. 2019;78:1041-7.

44. Li GH, Cheung CL, Au PC, Tan KC, Wong IC, Sham PC. Positive effects of low LDL-C and statins on bone mineral density: an integrated epidemiological observation analysis and Mendelian randomization study. Int J Epidemiol. 2019; Online ahead of print.

45. Zheng J, Brion MJ, Kemp JP, Warrington NM, Borges MC, Hemani G, et al. The Effect of Plasma Lipids and Lipid-Lowering Interventions on Bone Mineral Density: A Mendelian Randomization Study. J Bone Miner Res. 2020;35:1224-35.

46. Khadilkar PV, Khopkar US, Nadkar MY, Rajadhyaksha AG, Chougule DA, Deshpande SD, et al. Fibrotic Cytokine Interplay in Evaluation of Disease Activity in Treatment Naive Systemic Sclerosis Patients from Western India. J Assoc Physicians India. 2019;67:26-30.

47. Wakhlu A, Sahoo RR, Parida JR, Rai MK, Misra DP, Agarwal V, et al. Serum Interleukin-6, Interleukin-17A, and Transforming Growth Factor Beta Are Raised in Systemic Sclerosis with Interstitial Lung Disease. Indian J Rheumatol. 2018;13:107-12.

48. Chan EKL, Damoiseaux J, Carballo OG, Conrad K, de Melo Cruvinel W, Francescantonio PLC, et al. Report of the First International Consensus on Standardized Nomenclature of Antinuclear Antibody HEp-2 Cell Patterns 2014–2015. Front Immunol. 2015;6:412.

49. Misra DP, Pani KC, Shenoy SN, Wakhlu A, Ghosh P, Hissaria P, et al. Enhancement of Knowledge and Skills in Laboratory Techniques for Autoantibody Evaluation: Utility of a Single-day Hands-on Workshop. Indian J Rheumatol. 2018;13:178-81.

50. Ghosh P, Dwivedi S, Naik S, Verma A, Aggarwal A, Misra R. Antinuclear antibodies by indirect immunofluorescence: optimum screening dilution for diagnosis of systemic lupus erythematosus. Indian J Med Res. 2007;126:34-8.

51. Rao J, Shobha V, Thomas T, Kini U. Standardizing initial dilution titers of antinuclear antibodies for the screening of systemic lupus erythematosus. Indian J Rheumatol. 2019;14:211-7.

52. Conrad K, Röber N, Andrade LE, Mahler M. The Clinical Relevance of Anti-DFS70 Autoantibodies. Clin Rev Allergy Immunol. 2017;52:202-16.

53. Kang SY, Lee WI, Kim MH, La Jeon Y. Clinical use of anti-DFS70 autoantibodies. Rheumatol Int. 2019;39:1423-9.

54. Handa R. Biosimilars in Rheumatology- Name Changers or Game Changers? J Assoc Physicians India. 2017;65:6-8.

55. Shobha V, Rao V, Desai A, Jois R, Srikantiah C, Dharmanand BG, et al. Prescribing patterns and safety of biologics in immune-mediated rheumatic diseases: Karnataka biologics cohort study group experience. Indian J Rheumatol. 2019;14:17-20.

56. Chandrashekara S, Shobha V, Rao V, Desai A, Jois R, Dharmanand BG, et al. Incidence of infection other than tuberculosis in patients with autoimmune rheumatic diseases treated with bDMARDs: a real-time clinical experience from India. Rheumatol Int. 2019;39:497-507.

57. Misra DP, Sharma A, Agarwal V. Rheumatology science and practice in India. Rheumatol Int. 2018;38:1587-600.

58. Chopra A. Disease burden of rheumatic diseases in India: COPCORD perspective. Indian J Rheumatol. 2015;10:70-7.

59. Misra DP, Ravindran V, Sharma A, Wakhlu A, Negi VS, Chaturvedi V, et al. Physicians Perception of Rheumatology Practice and Training in India. J Assoc Physicians India. 2019;67:38-43.

60. Handa R. Rheumatology in India—quo vadis? Nat Rev Rheumatol. 2015;11:183-8.

61. Jennette JC, Falk RJ, Bacon PA, Basu N, Cid MC, Ferrario F, et al. 2012 revised International Chapel Hill Consensus Conference Nomenclature of Vasculitides. Arthritis Rheum. 2013;65:1-11.

62. Jones RB, Hiemstra TF, Ballarin J, Blockmans DE, Brogan P, Bruchfeld A, et al. Mycophenolate mofetil versus cyclophosphamide for remission induction in ANCA-associated vasculitis: a randomised, non-inferiority trial. Ann Rheum Dis. 2019;78:399-405.

63. Misra DP, Naidu GSRSNK, Sharma A. Recent advances in the management of antineutrophil cytoplasmic antibody-associated vasculitis. Indian J Rheumatol. 2019;14:218-28.

INDEX

Page numbers followed by *f* refer to figure, and *t* refer to table.